Guruji

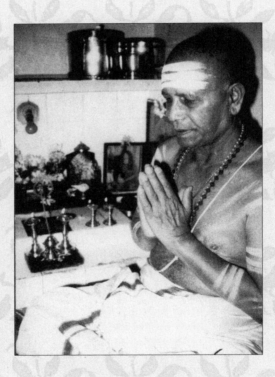

Guruji

◆ ◆ ◆

A Portrait of

Sri K. Pattabhi Jois

Through the Eyes of His Students

◆ ◆ ◆

Guy Donahaye and Eddie Stern

North Point Press
A division of Farrar, Straus and Giroux
New York
◆

NORTH POINT PRESS
A division of Farrar, Straus and Giroux
18 West 18th Street, New York 10011

Distributed in Canada by D&M Publishers, Inc.
Printed in the United States of America
First edition, 2010

Library of Congress Cataloging-in-Publication Data
Donahaye, Guy, 1962–
    Guruji : a portrait of Sri K. Pattabhi Jois through the eyes of his students /
Guy Donahaye and Eddie Stern.— 1st ed.
        p.   cm.
    ISBN: 978-0-86547-749-0 (alk. paper)
    1. Jois, K. Pattabhi.   2. Yogis—Biography.   I. Stern, Eddie, 1967–   II. Title.

RA781.7.D66 2010
613.7'046—dc22

                                                                    2010017755

Designed by Abby Kagan

www.fsgbooks.com

1   3   5   7   9   10   8   6   4   2

In loving memory of

Sri K. Pattabhi Jois

(1915–2009)

Yoga is showing where to look for the soul—that is all. Man is taking a human body—this is a very rare opportunity. Don't waste it. We are given a hundred years to live; one day you have the possibility to see god. If you think in this way, it is giving you good body, good nature, and health.

—Sri K. Pattabhi Jois, 2001

Contents

A Global Community ◆ 337

Preface

by Eddie Stern

My friend Harini, an Indian woman who lives in Mysore, shared a story with me that was told to her by a former neighbor, Doreswamy Iyengar, who had been an adviser to the maharaja of Mysore in the 1930s. One day Doreswamy came by with his sons. The sons, who had previously been stout, had slimmed down quite a bit, and Harini took note of it. "You have become so fit!" she said. They replied, "Oh yes, we have been doing yoga." Doreswamy said to Harini, "In the 1940s and '50s during Ram Navami [the nine-day worship of Lord Ram], there used to be stages set up all around Mysore for the musicians, poets, singers, and actors to perform. Pattabhi Jois and I lived on the same street. During the Ram Navami, he would get up on the stage and start doing all of the *asanas*. He would walk on his hands, jumping here and there, twisting, rolling, and turning circles. My friends and I used to say, 'What is this Pattabhi up to? He is jumping around like a monkey, what use is all this?' We did not take him seriously then. But now we look at him and think, 'Look how great he has become, what knowledge and fame he has, what a great thing he has done to spread yoga all around the world.' Yoga was here for us as part of our culture, but we did not even know its greatness until now. But Pattabhi never stopped holding on to its greatness."

Such inspiring stories remind us of the absolute dedication that Pattabhi Jois maintained toward *ashtanga* yoga beginning in 1927. Here in the West, we sometimes forget that yoga was not always a respected endeavor in India. In fact, yoga was looked upon by the general population as being a practice for either monks and renunciants or charlatans and sorcerers. When I went to India for the first time in 1988 with the intent to learn yoga, I was completely ignorant of the culture, geography, and basic ideas that gave birth to the Indian philosophies. My knowledge of yoga was scant. I assumed that all Indians knew yoga and was surprised to discover that most did not. Though there were many people of deep wisdom and devotion who embodied an overall gentleness, there were not many practicing yoga. By 1991, when Guy Donahaye and I began our studies with Pattabhi Jois in Mysore, yoga still had not achieved the cultural regard that it holds now both in India and in the West. When asked by Indians why I was in India, I would reply that I had come to learn yoga. Most would remark, "Oh, yoga; very good for health." Of course, having good health is indeed a worthwhile, if not imperative undertaking for those in search of some type of spiritual understanding. But it was the spiritual quest, and usually not health, that was the driving impulse that led many of us Westerners to India.

In 1991, India had only just begun to allow Western exports into the country. Pepsi, Coke, and many other name brands and fast foods had not yet begun to pollute the countryside. Bottled water was not always easy to find, and a trip to the post office seemed to be a daylong affair, as was booking a long-distance telephone call or going to the bank to change money. Everything demanded time and patience, qualities we were unfortunately short on. Though I did not have the hardships of those who came in the 1970s, there were still a lot of adjustments. A hot-water bath was a complete luxury, e-mail did not yet exist, and Mysore still required several days of travel to reach from my home in New York City. The day-to-day challenges, however, were offset by the Indian people, who had a sweetness that was palpable. Not a day would go by without complete strangers inviting us to their homes for tea, a meal, or a three-day wedding.

The daily difficulties made the experience of being in India and studying yoga all the more valuable, as did the simplicity of the lifestyle and the recognition of how little we need materially to be happy. I relished the time I could spend there, with no idea that the near future would bring large crowds of yoga students to Mysore in 2002, after Guruji's new school opened in Gokulam. In the years before that, there were few students in Mysore; when the number reached twenty or twenty-four, we would think it unbearable; and when it would shrink to four or eight, we would feel that all was normal again.

One thing that set Pattabhi Jois's teachings apart from other yoga communities that had made their way westward, and which made the quest for information all the more challenging, was a lack of literature. B. K. S. Iyengar had written *Light on Yoga*, Paramahansa Yogananda penned *Autobiography of a Yogi*, and Swami Vishnu-devananda had *The Complete Illustrated Book of Yoga*. We only had the firsthand experience of Pattabhi Jois's few English words, and his fearsome hands that put us into positions we would otherwise have chosen not to attempt. Due to his limited English, everything was broken down to its simplest equation—and perhaps that's what we, as largely overintellectualized Westerners, needed; *mula bandha* was simply "Tighten your anus!" Instructions on breathing were, "Breathe freely!" Queries on almost any subject could be answered with, "Take practice, all is coming!" In Kannada, his mother tongue, Pattabhi Jois could passionately relate the yoga texts, philosophy, mythology, and stories of the sages and *rishis* in such a way as to bring tears to his eyes. But in English, there was a large language barrier.

Pattabhi Jois's instructions, therefore, became something of a treasure hunt. If I put the effort in and researched what he was talking about, I could discover what he was trying to convey. If he mentioned a quotation from a particular book, I would take it as a cue to look for that book and read it. Finding the verse, of course, was another story. The attempts made, though, were always rewarded in one way or another. In fact, it is in the nature of the Indian tradition that the student should strive to understand the teacher, for in striving, and not from being spoon-fed, is knowledge revealed. The yoga texts note that the teacher can show you what to do and how to do it, but the student must fill in his or her own experience by constant, dedicated practice.

Before the advent of writing, all ancient cultures—including India's—passed down history as oral tradition. Today, India still relies on oral tradition to pass on knowledge. A subtle practice such as *ashtanga* yoga could not be learned just from a book; a teacher is necessary, one who has practical experience, one who is a valuable link in the oral chain. The Naga Baba Rampuri, a Westerner who has been living in India since the end of the 1960s, has said that when you wander for years around the subcontinent, you meet many saints and *sadhus*, each carrying a different piece of the oral tradition. Little by little, the various stories and knowledge come together to form a fuller picture. Knowledge is not entrusted to any one single person; it is spread around so that each one of us carries a piece. By searching for and listening to our fellow seekers, especially the more experienced, we can expand the limits of our knowledge.

As students of Pattabhi Jois, we too are part of an oral tradition. Through his instructions and teachings we form a link in the chain in which he is a part. In the 1990s, when working on the translation of *Yoga Mala*, Pattabhi Jois's book on *ashtanga* yoga, I noticed that he never tired of telling the story, sometimes several days in a row, about which students came to India to study during what years. I later realized that he was telling this story again and again to keep it alive—alive in himself and alive in the world.

Since the publication of *Yoga Mala*, the importance of archiving and collecting the teachings of Pattabhi Jois has been readily apparent. The knowledge he has, no one else seems to have. Therefore, the talks and instructions he has given are infinitely valuable, and will soon be lost if not recorded. When I came across the interviews that Guy Donahaye was amassing during the work on his documentary, I heard Pattabhi Jois's wisdom being conveyed through the voices of his students—a unique and refreshing take that should be made available to the ever growing legion of *ashtanga* yoga students. Though the interviews were not originally intended as a book, a book indeed has taken form, forged by Guruji's enthusiasm (before his death, in May 2009) and the loving and engaged support from his daughter, Saraswathi; his son, Manju; his grandson, Sharath; and his granddaughter, Sharmila, as well as all of those interviewed.

There are two notable students of Guruji's who have not been included in this book. The first is André van Lysebeth, who is no longer alive. He can duly be credited as the first Westerner to study with Guruji. In 1964, during his travels in India, he spent two months with Guruji, and later went on to write several books on yoga. In his book *Pranayama*, he included two photographs of Guruji, and in one of the captions said that Guruji lived in Lakshmipuram, in Mysore. That clue led many aspiring yoga students to seek Guruji out. The second student not interviewed here is Maria Helena Bastidos, who runs the yoga organization Yogocen in Brazil. Maria Helena met Guruji in 1973 and was the first person to invite him to come out from India and begin his teachings abroad as a delegate to one of the many yoga conferences that she held in São Paulo. Maria Helena continues to hold conferences in Brazil and

India, and is an earnest investigator of Indian thought and practices. She was not interviewed for this book simply as a matter of logistics.

Like the words of the wandering *sadhus* in India, I believe the interviews collected here each contribute a piece of the expanding story of Pattabhi Jois and his teachings of *ashtanga* yoga. Each interview holds small gems of wisdom, new ways of looking at the yoga practice, an unknown perspective on Pattabhi Jois that expands our appreciation of his genius.

In a recent conversation, Manju Jois noted how important it is for us, as yoga practitioners, to acknowledge with gratitude the contributions of those who have opened doors for us, for it is by their efforts and path-clearing that we have achieved and learned as much as we have so far. This book is an opportunity to acknowledge such "door-openers." In fact, Manju was instrumental in making sure that we did not neglect any of the early practitioners, as well as in helping to arrange interviews with Guruji's oldest Indian students. But first and foremost, it is an opportunity to extend our unending gratitude to the incomparable contributions of Pattabhi Jois, without whose enduring patience and devoted teachings we would not have learned anything of *ashtanga* yoga at all.

EDDIE STERN
New York City, November 2009

Preface

by Guy Donahaye

Sri K. Pattabhi Jois, who became affectionately known as Guruji by his students, was born on July 26, 1915, in the south Indian village of Kowshika, a tiny hamlet of Brahmin farmers about one hundred miles north of Mysore. He was the fifth of nine children. His father was an astrologer and priest who educated him in traditional Smarta Brahmin ways,* in the language of Sanskrit, and in the art of chanting the Vedas. Each day he would walk five miles to school in the neighboring town of Hassan. He was a spirited boy with lots of energy who loved to play soccer, act, and sing, and who had a somewhat mischievous nature.

One day in November 1927 he came across a yoga demonstration at the local Jubilee Hall given by a master of the name T. Krishnamacharya. He was very impressed by what he saw and went to Krishnamacharya's house the next day to ask if he could become his student. He was accepted and the following day commenced yoga practice. At that time, yoga was not held in high regard. There was a commonly held fear that it would withdraw one from participation in society. For that reason, Guruji did not want to tell his family and went secretly to practice every day before school. His practice developed well and his guru was pleased with his progress. In 1929, at the age of fourteen, he decided on his own to move to Mysore to further his study of Sanskrit. He ran away from home

---

*The Smarta Brahmins are especially concerned with the preservation of certain sections of the Vedic literature and ritual practices, and are devoted to the teachings of Sri Shankaracharya, an eighth-century saint whose Advaita Vedanta philosophy is still very popular in India today.

with two rupees in his pocket and enrolled at the Maharaja Sanskrit College in Mysore. Krishnamacharya settled in Mysore in 1931, so Guruji, to his delight, was able to continue his yoga studies with him until 1953, when Krishnamacharya moved to Chennai, or Madras as it was then called.

Mysore, City of Palaces, was known for its sandalwood, silk, and ivory, and its universities and other institutions of higher learning. It was the capital of a large kingdom and Maharaja Krishnaraja Wodeyar, who was a wealthy and enlightened ruler, put enormous efforts into improving the lives of his subjects. At that time, he was suffering from diabetes and infertility as well as a number of other ailments that no doctor had been able to cure. He had heard of Krishnamacharya, who had a reputation as a healer, and when he moved to Mysore the maharaja asked him to come and cure him, which he did through a combination of yoga, diet, and herbal medicine. His successful efforts earned the king's highest respect and appreciation. Wodeyar became a fervent advocate of yoga. He gave a wing of one of his palaces to Krishnamacharya to run a yoga *shala*, and he funded lecture tours and demonstrations throughout the state at public halls, schools, hospitals, and military installations, and even made a law that yoga be taught in schools.

On occasion, the king would call upon students from Krishnamacharya's school to give demonstrations for his guests at the palace. Guruji, one of Krishnamacharya's senior students and one of the maharaja's favorites, was awarded prizes and money and was also called on from time to time to teach the maharaja yoga. In 1937, Wodeyar established a yoga department at the Sanskrit College and installed Guruji as its head even though he had not finished his course of study. The maharaja gave him a scholarship and free food in the dining hall, as well as a salary. Guruji continued to teach there until his retirement in 1973.

Guruji was known as an erudite scholar, keen to research both the textual sources of yoga practice and how yoga was being taught around the country. In 1948, he established the Ashtanga Yoga Research Institute in his home in Lakshmipuram, a suburb of Mysore, to research the therapeutic effects of yoga. He would habitually elaborate his teaching with extensive reference to the scriptures, but claimed that from what he was able to see, Krishnamacharya was the only one who had understood the correct method of practice. "I have only one guru," he used to say with a broad smile.

Guruji was very devoted to his teacher, who was a brilliant man possessed of an encyclopedic knowledge and was also very strict. If a student was one minute late to class, they were made to stand outside the door in the full sunlight for an hour. During lectures, when traveling throughout the kingdom, Krishnamacharya would often use one of his young students as a platform: the student would assume a posture of Krishnamacharya's choice and he would then stand on the student and deliver his talk for half an hour or more. This would both demonstrate to his audience the power of yoga (mind over body) and test his students to the extreme. He was an intense personality and although only five feet tall, people would scatter in fear as he walked down the street.

Krishnamacharya had studied yoga in the Himalayas for seven years with his teacher, Rama Mohan Brahmachari, whom he described as a tall, bearded saint living in a cave at the foot of Mt. Kailash with his wife and eight children. Part of Krishnamacharya's studies with his teacher concerned an ancient text, the *Yoga Korunta*, which is the source for the method Pattabhi Jois went on to teach. There are several unique features to the system presented in the *Yoga Korunta*, especially insofar as it integrates philosophy and practice with detailed explanations of how the practice of *asanas* and *pranayamas* should be performed.

Although Guruji became known throughout the world primarily for teaching a specific sequence of *asanas*, this was probably the result of having to manage the large volume of students who came to study with him in later years. In earlier days, he adapted his teaching more to the individual's needs. He spent time teaching at the Ayurvedic hospital in Mysore, and used to work therapeutically with individuals with all kinds of conditions such as diabetes, elephantiasis, and leprosy. (In fact, Krishnamacharya had given him a sick man to heal for his teaching examination.) When at one point students stayed away from his yoga *shala* because he was treating someone with leprosy, he did not care. Helping a student in need was more important to him.

Guruji had boundless energy and enthusiasm for teaching. He usually arose at 2 or 3 a.m. and began class around 4:30 a.m. He would often teach until midday and then again for several hours in the evening. He would teach every day except on the full and new moons until his family begged him to spend more time with them. Then he began to take Saturdays off as well. He so loved teaching that even when he was in severe pain when having his teeth removed, or immediately following a cataract operation, or after having been in a motorcycle accident, he was immediately back in the classroom. While assisting students who were struggling to find balance on their hands, he would frequently be struck in the face by flailing feet. He lost several teeth this way, but he did not care.

Guruji was married in 1937 to Savitramma, the daughter of Narayana Shastri, a renowned Sanskrit scholar. She was fourteen years old and he was twenty-two. They had three children, Manju, Ramesh, and Saraswathi. Ramesh died tragically in 1973, and Amma passed away in 1997. Saraswathi and Manju both went on to be come great yoga teachers in their own right. Saraswathi has two children, Sharmila and Sharath, who are also teachers. Sharath assisted Guruji from 1990 until 2007, when he became the effective director of the institute. The whole family learned yoga from Guruji and continue to pass on his teaching after his death.

In 1973, at the age of fifty-eight, Guruji traveled abroad for the first time. That was also the year when Nancy Gilgoff, David Williams, and Norman Allen first came to Mysore. From this moment, Guruji's connection with the West grew steadily. In the first few years, there were just a handful of Western students in Mysore. By the time Eddie Stern and I arrived in 1991, there were perhaps twenty-five students for the month or two around Christmas, and then the rest of the year was much quieter. In the old *shala* in Lakshmipuram there was space for only eight students to practice at the same time. By the end of the '90s, twelve students were squashed in the room, with classes starting at 4 a.m. and finishing after noon. Guruji was in his eighties and still working an eight- or nine-hour day of intensive labor. The *shala* was bursting at the seams. The line of students waiting to enter class trailed up onto the roof. To handle the increasing numbers, he built a new yoga *shala* in Gokulam, another suburb of Mysore; he completed it in 2002.

The new *shala* could accommodate five times as many students at the same time. The shift to the new *shala* coincided with another phenomenon: many students now arrived in Mysore already having some familiarity with *ashtanga* practice. By now, Guruji had traveled widely and there were growing numbers of experienced teachers spreading *ashtanga* yoga around the world.

Sri K. Pattabhi Jois taught yoga uninterruptedly for seventy years, until the age of ninety-one. He was a powerhouse of energy, a yoga master, a husband, a father, a scholar. He had a great sense of humor and a brilliant mind. He enjoyed robust good health into his nineties. It was only after a severe infection in 2007 that he withdrew from teaching. He was stoic and unchanging to the last, bearing accolades and difficulties with equanimity. By the time he died, on May 18, 2009, his teaching had become a global phenomenon.

In 1991, I was living in England in a community of spiritual seekers in the middle of the Sussex countryside. Since my teens I had been on a path of spiritual exploration that encompassed the full spectrum of esoteric philosophies and had been trying to meditate for years. I struggled to find regularity in meditation practice and the ability to keep my mind concentrated as acutely as I desired. I was searching for a new modality, something that would help me concentrate better, put my body at ease, and perhaps give me a glimpse of ultimate reality.

Was it karma or just good fortune that led me to my first yoga class, given by one of Sri K. Pattabhi Jois's students? Raphael Dabora lived on a nearby farm and was teaching yoga at a local Montessori school. I had never taken a yoga class but I had read about Patanjali yoga ten years earlier in P. D. Ouspensky's *New Model of the Universe*, and been fascinated by the various "magical" powers yogis were said to possess. I had no idea what to expect. We started the class with the Sanskrit mantra and continued with sun salutations, the prototype for the breathing/movement system known as *vinyasa*, which strings the postures of the *ashtanga* yoga system together into a sequence.

From the start, I found that stretching combined with mindful breathing evoked blissful sensations in my body. My mind, too, was guided through an interesting trajectory of awareness. Instead of randomly flitting from one experience and thought to another, now it was channeled in a narrower stream. I immediately recognized that this might be what I had been looking for: a method for bringing the mind under control.

The breathing-and-movement synchronization generated intense sweating and a sense of lightness, and soon I felt like I was flying. By the end of class, as I lay resting on the yoga mat, my mind and body were pulsating with energy. I felt as if I had been through a purification from the inside out, as though my whole body and mind had opened up and I was transparent.

Raphael recognized my interest and gave me a "cheat sheet" of the *ashtanga* primary series; suggested I read B. K. S. Iyengar's *Light on Yoga*, *The Yoga Sutras*, and the *Bhagavad Gita*; invited me to his home; and showed me how to cook for a yogic diet.

A few days later I departed for the Bay Area. After struggling for three months alone in my apartment, often injuring myself horribly in my ignorance, I became convinced that I should go to India to meet Raphael's guru—Sri K. Pattabhi Jois, or "Guruji" as he called him.

I arrived in Mysore in September 1991. Each morning as I walked or cycled to the yoga *shala* in the dark for the early-morning class, which started at four or four thirty, depending on the volume of students present, I heard chanting and the ringing of bells, smelled burning incense or the coconut-husk fires used for warming water, saw the housewives sprinkling water on their doorsteps, sweeping, and decorating them with intricate chalk *rangolis* (sacred patterns) and flowers. Arriving at the *shala*, I could hear Guruji chanting to himself as he came down the steps to unlock the door or, if I was a little late, the pneumatic *ujjayi* breathing of the students who had already started their practice echoing through the windows.

Sharath would just be finishing his practice in the front row. Eddie and I were side by side in the back row. At five the side door creaked open and Guruji slipped into the room. Suddenly the atmosphere changed. Everyone came up to standing position with Guruji's commanding "*Samasthiti!*" for the opening mantra. I still remember feeling the hair stand up on the back of my neck, nearly moved to tears by the intensity of the moment.

Apart from this opening invocation, Guruji hardly said a word, except an occasional "Yes, you do!" He sat on his stool, watching us closely (even when we didn't think he was), or assisted us with deep adjustments, and occasionally taught a new posture. There was no avoiding anything in that room. Guruji's eyes were always on us.

Pattabhi Jois's yoga is radical. It is difficult to describe in words the kinds of experiences one goes through, but suffice it to say there are times when one encounters one's deepest fears and is pushed to the limits of endurance, both mentally and physically. Guruji inherited this intensity of teaching from his guru, Krishnamacharya, who according to Guruji was a "very dangerous man"—this always said with a laugh.

Many people would walk away from this kind of intensity. In the end of Krishnamacharya's time in Mysore, he had only three students left. His approach at that time was too radical for most people. But for those of an intense nature who desire radical transformation, they find it here.

If you walk away when the going gets tough, then you do not evolve. Guruji understood the healing and transformation process from many decades of teaching, and no doubt his own personal experience. He stayed with me throughout and helped me to heal and transform.

When being adjusted in a challenging *asana* by Guruji, I sometimes felt on a precipice staring down into the abyss at the prospect of death or debilitating pain, but also feeling that maybe salvation somehow was at hand. Then I was met in the present moment, because nothing will distract you from the moment when you face imminent death, by Guruji's smile: *"Why fearing?"* (*What are you attached to? What do you cling to?*)

"Just trust and relax!"

But I'm going to die!

"Just breathe!"

And then suddenly, before you know it, he has put you in the posture! The state of heightened awareness may persist for the duration of the adjustment, and during this time nothing else whatsoever troubles the mind. Afterward, there is a moment of suspension of belief, bliss, euphoria, openheartedness, ecstasy.

Oh! I didn't know that was possible! Put my troubles on one side for a moment, put aside all my preconceptions about what I am capable of doing.

If one can do that for a moment, it affords one the ability to put these troubles aside at will later on, to look at these troubles and let them go. With letting go one arrives at the state of calm and confidence, which is often seen in the demeanor of long-term practitioners.

The many wonderful benefits of *ashtanga* practice—such as good health, energy, and strength—keep us interested in the practice, but the ultimate spiritual benefits seem elusive. Thankfully, through practice, practice, practice eventually the inner nature of yoga also begins to manifest. For me, the most important lesson Guruji gave was to engrave a deep *samskara* for practice in my mind. From practice, everything follows. This is not an empty mantra but a reality. The teacher is there to give you reassurance that you are on the right path, but the real inner teacher is in the practice itself.

For deeper understanding to arise, the mind must be transformed. But to get a feeling for what yoga is, you have to practice. How can you convey the flavor of honey to someone who has never tested its sweetness? It is the same with yoga: you have to experience it to understand. Initially this experience is impossible to articulate verbally. It is more like a flavor that we enjoy. But as the mind is transformed through yoga practice, we become better able to perceive the reality underlying our existence, and consequently to understand the philosophical basis of yoga and the direction it suggests we move in order to widen and deepen our experience of this reality.

In the beginning I did not understand. But after many years, I began to. Yoga practice transforms the mind and body; it purifies, strengthens, and heals. A troubled mind has a reduced capacity for understanding and a diseased body will always cause distraction and trouble to the mind. Through *asana* practice, the body is healed and the mind is progressively purified and refined, and becomes more capable of grasping subtle truth. In addition, one begins to see the effect yoga has in one's own biography as the years pass, and to understand its essence in an experiential way.

Guruji always used to say that he taught "real" or "original" *ashtanga* yoga, the *ashtanga* yoga of Patanjali as described in *The Yoga Sutras*. He told us this was the most important text to read, though, he said, it was difficult to understand and required much interpretation. Although *The Yoga Sutras* give the most complete description of and context for *ashtanga* yoga, the same system of yoga is described and referenced in many other ancient texts, and this was something Guruji was fond of demonstrating.

Ashtanga yoga describes eight steps for attaining the goal of yoga. The first four are "external" and the others are "internal."* The first two steps are *yama* and *niyama*: nonviolence, truthfulness, not stealing, sexual restraint, non-greed, cleanliness, contentment, purification, self-study, surrender to the divine. These first two stages are challenging and take a

---

*In fact Patanjali talks about five external and three internal limbs, but Guruji always spoke of four and four just as is described in the *Yogayajnavalkya Samhita* (which he loved to quote).

long time to master. They are hindered by an unsteady mind and a weak or diseased body. The third stage, *asana*, or posture, is the starting point for Guruji's method. *Asanas* help to bring health and mental clarity, making performance of *yama* and *niyama* easier. *Pranayama*, or breath control, takes the purification a step further. *Pratyahara*, or sense introversion, results from perfection in *pranayama*—the senses turn inward and look for the Self. *Dharana*, the fixing of concentration; *dhyana*, or meditation, where the mind flows exclusively in one direction; and *samadhi*, union with the divine, proceed in this sequential order.

According to *The Yoga Sutras*, yoga is mind control. When the mind is under control, you experience yourself as its master. If you are performing an action and your mind is elsewhere, then it is not under your control, you cannot concentrate, and the mind is *your* master. Once the mind is perfectly controlled then we cease to identify with it and the inner Self is allowed to manifest without hindrance or obscuration. *Ashtanga* yoga describes the practical method for attaining this control, first by purification through *asana* practice and then by bringing the mind under control through a combination of *yama*, *niyama*, and *pranayama*.

Guruji emphasized intense *asana* practice. The *vinyasa* (breathing/movement system) combined with the *asana* sequencing "boils the blood" and eliminates toxins through the skin as sweat. Daily practice is emphasized, with certain days for rest, over a long period of time—"ten years, twenty years, your whole life long you practice." It was always hot and sweaty in the room, not from artificial heating but from the bodies of the practicing students. Guruji used to say, "With heat, even iron will bend," referring to the way in which even tough, hard bodies could be bent into shape.

Under the guidance of Krishnamacharya, Guruji arranged three sequences of *asanas*—primary, intermediate, and advanced—which were subdivided into four further sequences. The primary series, yoga *chikitsa*, was designed to purify the muscles and organs of the body, while the intermediate series, *nadi shodhana*, was designed to purify the nervous system and mind. Once a certain mastery had been attained in these first two series, Guruji would teach an intense *pranayama* practice which would take the process of purification deeper.* Students with lots of energy and flexibility would also proceed through the advanced series.

*In later years he taught *pranayama* less and less.

According to Guruji, the groupings of *asanas* and their *vinyasas* were described in an ancient text called the *Yoga Korunta* that Krishnamacharya had studied with his teacher, Rama Mohan Brahmachari, in the Himalayas. In addition to the instructions for performing *asana* and *vinyasa*, an entire system of integrated practice was described, which incorporated the Patanajali *Yoga Sutras* with commentary and instructions on *pranayama*, *bandhas* (core muscular and energetic locks), and *drishti* (points where the eyes should focus). According to Guruji, Krishnamacharya had once found a copy of the *Yoga Korunta* in a Calcutta library, but it was badly damaged by ants and incomplete. No other copy has ever been recorded to our knowledge.

One element of the practice that was not in the *Yoga Korunta* or part of the early teachings of Krishnamacharya was the *surya namaskara*. This sun prayer, which initiates the *asana* practice, was devised by Guruji based on references to ancient texts. The result of Guruji's research can now be found all over the globe in nearly every yoga class.

Guruji used to say it takes at least ten years of daily practice before a new understanding can arise. This understanding would result from the purification of mind and body. *Ashtanga* yoga is a step-by-step process. Guruji emphasized the third limb of *ashtanga* (*asana*) as the starting point because perfection of the moral codes of *yama* and *niyama* require some degree of mental control to begin with, and he believed *asana* practice to be the most effective starting point for that. Perfecting *yama* and *niyama* at the stage when *pranayama* and *pratyahara* begin to be engaged is mentioned in the *shastra*, the ancient body of literature on yoga, among other things, and is not a new idea. Everything Guruji did was based on the *shastra*. Once, when questioned about a particular style of yoga, he responded, "They have no [reference to] *shastra*!" That was his only comment, and all he needed to say.

Guruji encouraged his students to marry and have families. He saw this as a way of helping students to become more settled and engage with the *yama* and *niyama* in a practical way. He used to joke that family life was seventh series—the really difficult one.

The four external limbs of yoga are very challenging. When students would ask Guruji about "meditation," one of the internal limbs, he would say, "What? Mad attention?" He contended that if you can't keep your mind still for even a moment, what could you possibly achieve in terms of deep absorption and the rest? He held that once the four external limbs had been perfected, the internal steps would be easy. But perfecting the external limbs takes a great deal of time and effort and requires patience, faith, devotion, and much more. Guruji modified Krishnamacharya's dictum, that everybody who could breathe could do yoga, to "Everybody can do yoga, except lazy people."

Prayer is another pillar of Guruji's teaching. Devotion to God, family, and guru brings one closer to the goal. The external limbs relate to our experience of the world, to our bodies and our minds. The internal limbs are the doorway to the soul. Guruji was steeped in his own family tradition, which followed the guru Sri Shankaracharya* and the Advaita Vedanta philosophy. Shankara taught that our experience of ourselves as separate, discrete beings is an illusion. In fact, we are all part of one continuum. Separation has been caused by *maya*—delusion. In reality, everything is just part of one ocean of existence called brahman. Advaita Vedanta is a philosophy of non-dualism—there is only one unitary existence. By contrast, Patanjali's philosophy is generally seen as a dualistic system that acknowledges the existence of the soul, called *purusha*, and the body/mind, or *prakriti*. Shankaracharya's philosophy acknowledges only brahman, a universal being upholding the entire universe which, although it appears real (that is, permanent) to us, is actually in continuous flux and therefore transitory and devoid of permanent form. So according to Advaita, if there is no permanent form, there is no basis for attributing real qualities to that form.

How does a dualistic philosophy such as the one articulated in *The Yoga Sutras* merge with a non-dualistic system of thought such as Advaita? Both were obviously deeply influential in shaping Guruji's approach to practice. Guruji's explanation was that the external limbs of practice—*yama, niyama, asana, pranayama*—deal with the external world and our relation to it and are therefore by necessity of a dualistic nature since they involve a relationship between ourselves and the world. Guruji maintained that the internal limbs—*pratyahara, dharana, dhyana, samadhi*—are Advaita insofar as they concern the non-dualistic state, the experience of the Self, which is none other than God.

———

*Shankaracharya was also a fervent advocate of yoga and spoke a great deal about the importance of the *bandhas* and *pranayama*.

In 1998, I began work on a documentary about Guruji's life and teachings with Lori Brungard. It was my intention to paint a portrait of the man through the eyes of his students while at the same time revealing both what the interviewees believed to be the essence of his teaching and the results of their own inner work on the path of yoga. In the course of shooting we collected about twenty-five interviews with some of Guruji's closest students and family members.

In 2007, I published transcriptions of some of these interviews on the Internet. I received many enthusiastic e-mails. One such e-mail came from my dear friend Eddie Stern, who suggested making this book and motivated me to gather more interviews in order to complete this collection. He contributed several interviews, raised funds, and provided the text for Nick Evans's interview with Saraswathi, which originally appeared in the pages of *Namarupa* magazine.

Putting this book together has been a wonderful process. It has taken me to many far-flung parts of the globe, introduced me to wonderful people, and reunited me with very dear old friends. In some ways this collection of stories represents a sum total of contemporary experience on the path of *ashtanga* yoga, for here you will find represented the words and perceptions of many of Guruji's most senior teachers. If you add together the number of years of practice represented in this book, you have the results of six hundred years of practice.

Originally, many of the interviews were recorded on video. I wanted to make my subjects as comfortable as possible, so I asked them to tell stories first and then led the conversation toward the more intimate and profound. I specifically wanted them to speak on certain subjects that are often subtle, so the process was sometimes a bit roundabout, and the questions might sound naïve at times. I also wanted the material to be accessible to all readers, so often I've left in my own comments in the hope that they may help elucidate the matters under discussion.

In the tradition of Advaita Vedanta there is a technique called *vichara*, which means questioning. It was a method by which Ramana Maharshi taught his students to sink deeper and deeper into their inner experience until they could experience the true Self. With each question the aspirant asks, the response comes: "Who is asking the question?" At first, when looking for this "who," the aspirant experiences a void. But with repeated asking, the layers of accumulated dross which have attached to the soul fall away, and the Self begins to be experienced in its luminescence. In a similar way, questions posed to another may sometimes offer the opportunity for deeper reflection and plumb their being for answers they may not otherwise have articulated. I feel honored that I have been given this opportunity to be witness and recorder of such a process. Gathering, editing, and meditating on these interviews has significantly broadened and deepened my understanding of yoga. It is my hope that this valuable collection of wisdom will do the same for you, dear reader.

GUY DONAHAYE
New York City, November 2009

Guruji

Manju Jois

Manju Jois is Guruji's eldest child. He started practicing yoga with his father at the age of seven and began assisting him when he was thirteen. His demonstration in 1972 at the Ananda Ashram in Pondicherry was witnessed by David Williams and Norman Allen and fueled their desire to meet and study with Guruji, which led to the international spreading of *ashtanga* yoga. Manju travels and teaches all over the world and eventually settled in Southern California.

How old were you when you started to practice?
Oh, let's see, I was seven years old. It was just like a game for me, just to watch and then you try to do it because it's fun. It was not done seriously, he was not making me do things. We just went voluntarily and started playing with the postures, that's all.

When did Guruji start teaching you formally?
Formally when I was twelve years old. Then we had to practice every day—in the morning and evening. He started teaching me and my sister individually, giving us a private lesson. That's how it all started.

You started with private lessons?
Yes.

Then you joined his regular classes?
No, we were always private, never with any of the other students because he wanted to make us into good teachers, he wanted to make sure we were going to learn right.

He was training you to be a teacher?
Yes, absolutely.

When did you start learning to be a teacher?
I was just twelve or thirteen years old when I was starting to jump on people's backs and stuff like that. That's how I started. And he never stopped me from doing that and he was always guiding me what to do . . . where to push, when to push. He started training me when I was very young. So that was really helpful for me because it was so natural, the way I learned it.

Was he teaching at the Sanskrit College?
Yes, at the Maharaja Sanskrit College. He was conducting the classes for the Sanskrit students and others to take. And that's where I used to do yoga, and that's where I used to help all these people who were coming there.

Was the school at the Jaganmohan Palace already closed at that time?
Yes.

Was Krishnamacharya around in those days?
I met Krishnamacharya when I was seven or eight years old. He came to Mysore to give a demonstration with his son, and that's the first time I met him.

Do you remember seeing your father practicing yoga?
Yes, yes.

Could you describe what it was like seeing your father practicing?
Well, for us it was fun to see my father doing yoga, putting himself in all these postures. It was really amazing. He used to pick a posture sometimes and he would like to stay in that posture for a long time. That's how he used to practice. And that's how he started teaching us. There's no need to do millions of postures, just try to master one at a time. Then you can go to the next one. I really enjoyed watching my father doing yoga. Sometimes we all used to do it together, too: me and my sister and my father.

That's interesting. He teaches lots of postures to people, but to you he was advising the way he was practicing.
Well, yeah. He liked to master the thing, you see. So he was always telling us: "Master that, master that." Then you can go to the next one. But we are like little kids, we want to learn more, you know what I mean? "Oh, can I do this? If I can do this one, can I skip this one? Or can I go to that one?" Sometimes he let us do that, but at the same time he always had an eye on us to go back to finish that one. That's what he did.

So basically you started teaching with your dad when you were twelve or thirteen years old. How long did that continue before you left India?
I left India in 1975. But before that, I traveled to a lot of places. I would take my friend and we would go to universities in different parts of India and give demonstrations and talks on yoga. It was very fun, actually.

When did Guruji open the school in Lakshmipuram?
Mmm, that was about . . . a long time ago, maybe '61, '62. I don't know.

He was teaching in both places at the same time?
Yeah, he was teaching at the Sanskrit College at the time. Then he was about to retire and wanted to have his own place. So he started to build that small yoga studio there.

How many students did Guruji have in that studio?
We had, like, fifty students.

What kind of reputation did Guruji have among his students?
They respected him a lot. We used to get people with sickness in the body like asthma and diabetes and all sorts of problems. And those are the ones who used to come to yoga because they tried everything and finally the doctors used to send these people to my father to do yoga. That's the kind of group we had, people with problems.

So doctors would send their patients to Guruji after they could not cure them?
In those days they did not have modern medicine. And the doctor would

say, "Look, the best thing for you to do is yoga." Because we used get a lot of doctors, too, at the time. And they don't want to believe it, but they want to believe it—that is the kind of attitude they had.

Anyhow, when they started seeing the results with these people, who were getting healthier and healthier, then they would send patients to my father. "The best thing to do is just go to Pattabhi Jois, and do yoga, and then he would cure this." We got a lot of good results from doing that, yeah.

So he had a reputation for that.
Yeah, the Indian students who used to come, most of them were sick. All kinds of problems. That's why they started studying yoga. But we want to get a good yogic exercise. They used to come for the therapy. That's how it started.

Did Guruji adapt the practice at all for the therapy for the different students?
Yes, yes he did. He did mostly for the diabetic students. He'd make them sit in *janu shirshasana* A, B, C for a long time; *baddha konasana*, all the *upavishta konasanas* work here mostly [points to abdomen], you know. So that's how he started.

How did he figure that out?
If you read the *Hatha Yoga Pradipika* it will explain which posture helps in what kind of disease. That's why you had to study not only yoga *asanas*, you got to study the books, too. It's like a medical book.

Can you describe a specific instance of a cure? Guruji once told me that he cured elephantiasis.
And leprosy. We did have a student who just started leprosy in his ears. At that time there was not medication for that. He came from Tamil Nadu. His father brought him because he was the only son he had.

So my father started teaching yoga to this guy who was a leper. Then some of his students left because they didn't want to be there, because "Oh my God!" You know, they don't want to be in the same place.

They told my father, "If this guy is doing yoga here, we're not coming." And my father said, "Okay, that's fine. This is important for me."

So he started working with the guy. And then slowly the guy started to heal. His ears start getting better. Then after that, he decided to go back to his hometown and start practicing every day.

If you can cure leprosy, you can cure anything. So then people started getting attracted to cure through yoga.

What do you think was your father's main interest in teaching yoga?
I think mostly he concentrated on healing. Healing is much more important for him. Once you start healing yourself, his philosophy is that yoga would take you automatically to the meditative state, you see.

If you are not well inside, you can't do anything—no meditation, no nothing. So that's how it will draw you into the spiritual path.

See, that's why he says the yoga *asanas* are important—you just do. Don't talk about the philosophy—99 percent practice and 1 percent philosophy, that's what he taught. You just keep doing it, keep doing it, keep doing it, then slowly it will start opening up inside of you, then you are able to see it. So that's why he likes to concentrate on that aspect—the healing process.

Does the student take responsibility for their healing process, or does Guruji make any kind of diagnosis of the student?
Ah, well, a lot of people will say, "Oh, Guruji has the answer for everything!" My father sees that, that's why he gives them work: "All right, do it! Do it! You'll find out." That's what he does: he diagnoses, but he doesn't say, "Okay, you have this problem . . ." He figures out how to cure it.

I've noticed that he has a different attitude to different students. Do you think that's one of his techniques?
I think so, yeah. He studies the students. He doesn't like impatient students. A lot of people go to my father and say, "Okay, I'll be here for two months." And they expect they are going to learn a lot of stuff in two months. And then, when my father says, "No, no, you've got to stay here more, you got to come here more often and continue this" and people get impatient, he cannot stand that. That's why he gets mean.

Because for him to learn this practice, he put in a lot of energy and time, and he's been punished by his guru. His guru did not teach him very easily, he tried to see how much patience he had to learn this.

He would say things like, "Come at eight o'clock or twelve o'clock to my home to do yoga." They had to be there exactly at twelve o'clock at his guru's place. If they were late, then he would make them stand in the sun for an hour and see, you know, what happens. So my father went through all those things. Then when he sees these impatient students, then he would say, "Hey!" [*Laughter*]

What is your impression about where the asanas come from? Did Krishnamacharya make it up? Did Rama Mohan Brahmachari teach it to Krishnamacharya?
You mean the *asanas*?

The specific asana sequence.
Well, actually, it's all taken from books. If you take the *Hatha Yoga Pradipika*, it teaches a few postures. Then *Yoga Korunta* it teaches, and *Shiva Samhita*. All these books, you see, have it. So what they did was pick all the postures and then they sat down and kind of researched how to put it in a sequence. That's how they created the whole thing.

When you say "they," who do you mean?
Krishnamacharya in his *Yoga Makaranda*. That is the way my father teaches. When B. K. S. Iyengar took it, he just picked here and there. This is more like therapy. But everybody has their own ideas of what to do. Strict *ashtanga* yoga is how my father teaches: *vinyasas*, breathing—that's the real *ashtanga* yoga.

But this was created, you think, by Krishnamacharya? Did he put the sequences together?
I think so, yes, yes.

It's interesting that this lineage of ashtanga yoga comes through a series of householder teachers. We usually think of a yogi as someone sitting in a cave, renouncing the world. At least that's the Western impression.
Well, actually, that's a very good question, because in India it is like you're learning music or something like that. The family knows the music and they become the teachers. So for us, it is just like that. We do not have to be like a guru or go hide in a cave or something like that. It's just one of those professions we learn.

The priest teaches how to chant to their children, then their children become the next priests. And then every day they chant in their home, everybody learns that just by hearing it. The wife can chant. She doesn't have to sit and read a book or anything because every day she hears the same thing and naturally the kids will learn it in the same way—they know how to teach and how to do it.

Guruji says he only has one guru. But there's also another lineage of gurus through Shankaracharya, the family guru.
Right.

Can you explain a little bit the difference between those two, how Shankaracharya belongs to the family lineage and how Krishnamacharya is his yoga guru?
There's no relation between Krishnamacharya and Shankaracharya. Shankaracharya is the guru for the Smarta Brahmin. Krishnamacharya's guru was Ramanujacharya. You see he's an Iyengar. That's a different, what do you call it? A sect. Shankaracharya is the guru for Smarta Brahmins, as we are called. We follow the Shankaracharya philosophy.

So Krishnamacharya is Guruji's yoga guru, for asanas *and so on, but not so much for philosophy?*
I think Krishnamacharya follows the philosophy of Shankaracharya. You see, Ramanujacharya [Krishnamacharya's lineage guru] is a religious leader. There are three categories: Ramanujacharya, Shankaracharya, Madhvacharya. There are three gurus.

Shankaracharya represents Advaita, that's what we study. And Ramanujacharya is Vaishnava, that's a different study, that's what they follow. And Madhvacharya preaches Madhva *sampradaya*, it's called. They have different categories, different ways to teach, because Ramanujacharya and Madhvacharya, they don't talk about yoga or anything—it's more spiritual. Only Shankaracharya is more into yoga. See that's how we started. It came from Kerala.

How does Guruji communicate the spiritual aspect of the practice to Western people?
Well, actually he just does not put in a spiritual aspect when he teaches the Western students because he knows this is very new for them. Philosophy is too confusing. So he slowly wants them to practice their yoga.

Slowly, you know . . . because, actually, Hinduism is very, very hard to understand. You got to go deeper and deeper, deeper and deeper. It's an old religion. It consists of yoga and philosophy and all sorts of spiritual things. A lot of things I did not know until my mom passed away. Then, when I had to do all those rituals, I said, "Oh my God, so many things to learn here." There's no ending.

So Westerners, we had to take them very easy. That's what my father does. Just do yoga, don't talk. Don't ask any questions about spiritual things and this and that. No, you're here, you're doing karma yoga now, that's what you are doing. Just start working on that! That's how he teaches.

He regards it as karma yoga?
Karma is action, you know that's the actual meaning. Karma is action, so you're acting when you're practicing yoga—*hatha* yoga, *raja* yoga, *ash-tanga* yoga. But actually yoga is one. It has all these different names.

You are doing what I call karma yoga—you're working on your kar-mas. That's why you feel pain. And you're going through it slowly—that means you're slowly burning your karma up. So once you come out of that you feel great. Then you can concentrate on other things, and the next step.

Why do you think Guruji is not teaching much pranayama *anymore?*
Well, Guruji wants people to learn yoga first, *asanas*, master that. I think he used to teach *pranayama* only to people who had problems like asthma or something like that. Even in the *Hatha Yoga Pradipika* it says you should not do all the *kriyas* and *pranayamas* if it is not necessary. These are things you only do when it is really necessary. You have a health problem or something, then you do that.

If you have a problem with your breathing, you do the *neti kriya*. When you have an intestinal problem, you do the *dhauti kriya* but you don't practice that every day. If you are doing fine, no problem. If you start doing that without reason, you are going to get sick from it.

The first thing is to keep up with the *asana*, that's what my father says. Just keep doing the *asanas*, postures, master them. It takes a whole lifetime to do that.

He used to say that there was no limited life span in old times be-cause the rishis controlled the whole situation. When they decided to leave [the body] then they used to leave and that's it. But that's the whole thing, you see. When you start having control over yourself, then the next step you go to is *pranayama*. Your body's under control, your breathing's under control. So when you start controlling, you are going to be in the driver's seat!

How are the other angas *[limbs] of* ashtanga *yoga included in the practice we know?*
Everything is included in *ashtanga*. My father always used to say, "Don't say I'm doing meditation." It is not apart from your practice, the whole practice is the meditation. With your breathing, with your practice, you become one with yourself. That's "union." Yoga is called uniting, you know.

You go through the cycle, you start getting hotter and hotter and then you start sweating, you're feeling really good, then you totally become one with it. That's the whole thing. You can't just say, "This part I did, this part I did, this part I did." So that's why it's 99 percent *asana* and 1 percent theory. That's the whole thing.

Can you tell us how you met David Williams?
Long time ago, I was traveling all around India and I went through Madras. This guru who used to have an ashram in Pondicherry called Gitananda, he's a very good friend of my father and used to come visit my father in Mysore. He always wanted me to give a demonstration, he enjoyed my doing that.

So he asked me to come to his ashram and stay there as long as I wanted. When we were on the road, my friend and I decided, "Oh, maybe we should visit Gitananda." So we went to Pondicherry.

Then immediately he wanted me to stay and told me, "You can stay as long as you want, all you have to do is just give a demonstration in the morning like a led class." I would do the yoga and people would follow it. I said, "No problem," because I practice my yoga in the morning anyway, so instead of doing it in my room, I can go and do outside.

That day he announced, "Yogi Pattabhi Jois's son is here and he's going to teach you, he's going to show you *ashtanga* yoga." All these people were there who came to study yoga and philosophy. Gitananda said, "Okay, Manju is going to do this, so you can all follow."

Then I said, "Before I teach you anything, I would like to give a little demonstration, then you will know what you're going to do." So I start giving a little demonstration and all these people in the audience were really impressed because that's why they came to India, to study this kind of thing, but they did not know where to go. Gitananda gives a lot of philosophy but no *asanas*.

After my demonstration, this guy with long hair came to me and introduced himself. His name was David Williams, he's from the States, and he asked me, "By the way, where did you learn this? It's what I'm looking for. I want to learn this." And I said, "Well, I learned it from my father." "Oh, where does your father live?" "He lives in Mysore." And then he said, "Oh, I gotta go there to see your father."

Same day he left and I gave him the address. He went to Mysore to see my father. Then he started studying with my father.

Could you talk about your mother's influence on your father?
Oh yeah, my mother totally used to be the backbone of my father. She supported him in every way, whatever he did. That's how she was. She actually chose my father. My mother, she fell in love when she was watching him doing yoga at the Sanskrit College when she was a kid. She used to come there every day. They used to do yoga and then she was in love with him and that's how they got together.

Then she went and told her father that she already found a husband for herself. Her father started laughing and he said, "Who is that?" She said, "Oh, this guy I know. He does all these yoga postures." So then my grandfather told her, "Well, why don't you just bring him to be introduced to us." Then she asked my father to come to her home so he can meet my grandparents.

So he goes there, and she introduced them. My grandfather looked at him and said, "Oh yeah, he can take care of my daughter, no problem. He's pretty strong." [*Laughter*]

So that's how they started. Then they got married. She put up with everything with my father. He's not a very easy guy to deal with, but she was there for him all the time. She supported him every which way possible and played a main role in my father's life. We dearly miss her.

Did he teach her ashtanga *yoga?*
Yes. They both used to do yoga together. She used to give demonstrations

at Krishnamacharya's place at Jaganmohan Palace and she was very good, very good.

What kind of atmosphere did she create in your home?
Fantastic atmosphere, always at peace, you know. Funny. She got a great sense of humor and usually never made anything a big deal, she was always easygoing. My father misses her a lot. He gets intense sometimes and she was always there to soften him. She had a great quality, great sense of humor, and she was wonderful. Very loving and caring.

Sharath and Sharmila say that Guruji was really a father to them, too, because their own father was away so much. It sounds like he really took care of them.
Oh yeah, my father's a great father, you know. He looked after us really well. Sometimes my mother got sick and he would cook for us. He took good care of my mother at the same time. He used to do everything: washing the dishes and washing up clothes and bringing her food to the bed. They were very dedicated to each other, you know.

Can you think of any funny or interesting stories that illustrate the character of your father?
Actually, my mother used to correct him all the time. Sometimes my father wasn't thinking. He'd just be there teaching yoga in his shorts, and then once in a while he'd come out of his yoga school and he'd look out on the street and not realize he's just wearing his underwear. And Mom would be sitting right there, and she used to say, "Now, get back! Get back! Where do you think you're going?"

She never let him out. And he said, "Ah, I just came to look around." You know. "What are you going to look around at? You came out here to show yourself, how great you are. Get in! Get in!" And my father looked at her and he would go, "Grrr." He just grunts and walks away. And that was really funny for us to watch. [*Laughter*]

I remember you telling the story of how you went out to the cinema and came back at ten o'clock at night or something and he expected you to give a demonstration.
Right, right. One time I went with my friend to a movie. We used to

catch a night show. When I came back, I was exhausted. It's ten o'clock or ten thirty. I come home and there are all these people from Pondicherry. Gitananda brought all his group. They were all waiting, and my father is telling, "Yeah, my son will be here. He's going to give you a demonstration."

So everybody is sitting and waiting, and I come home. My father says, "Where did you go? Now get in here." And I said, "What's wrong?" I did not know. And he said, "No, you are going to give a demonstration now." I had some food at the restaurant, movies, eating out . . . then came home. I said, "What? You want me to give a demonstration now?" And he said, "Yeah, they're all waiting."

Then I have to take off my clothes and put on my yoga clothes and start giving the whole demonstration. The next day I talked to my father. "You should never agree to those kinds of things." [*Laughter*]

Do you think he's become less strict?
No, no. My father? He never changes. [*Laughter*]

New York City, 2000

The Seventies

·

How Ashtanga Came to the West

David Williams

David Williams commenced his studies with Guruji in 1973, and in 1975 brought Guruji to the United States for his first visit. After establishing the first *ashtanga* school in the United States, in Encinitas, David settled in Maui, where he has lived ever since. He continues to practice and to teach internationally.

I've been practicing yoga since my senior year in college at the University of North Carolina, in 1971. I've had uninterrupted yoga practice for thirty-one years. People say I'm disciplined. I tell them it's not really discipline, I'm just fascinated to see what will happen with me if I do yoga practice in my life.

When I was in college, I heard about yogis in India who got older and wiser. I looked around North Carolina and I didn't see anybody getting older and wiser. I was fascinated by this.

At a farm I saw a friend standing on his head and putting his legs in lotus, and I asked what he was doing. He said he was doing yoga. I thought I was in pretty good shape, but I knew I couldn't do any of this and I asked him if he would teach me. He said yes, and that was the beginning. The more I got into it, the more fascinated I got and I decided I should go to India and find a yoga master.

Looking back now, I realize I went like a detective looking for the greatest yogi. Wherever I went, I asked people and took yoga classes. My search took me all over India. In the spring of 1972, I was in Pondicherry at Swami Gitananda's Ananda Ashram. That's where I met Manju, the son of Pattabhi Jois. Norman Allen and I were friends, and we met Manju and his friend Basaraju, who were traveling around India giving yoga demonstrations at different ashrams.

We saw them do first series and I knew this is what I was looking for. I intuitively knew this was the next thing for me to learn. I asked Manju how he knew this and he said his father was a yoga master who lived in Mysore and this was what he taught.

My visa was about to expire, so I left India and saved enough money to return. Norman had just arrived in India, so he immediately went to Mysore and started learning the yoga from Guruji—Pattabhi Jois. Just as he was finishing up his first session, I came up to Mysore and started learning. I was with Nancy Gilgoff, and we stayed in Mysore for four months. I learned first series, second series, and half of third series, plus the *pranayama*. I felt very fortunate because Guruji had never taught any foreigners since Indra Devi in 1930s, and so he gave us a lot of attention. We were practicing twice a day plus doing the *pranayama*, and I was trying to learn it all as fast as I could.

At the time Guruji spoke very little English. I would learn by coming early and watching somebody else practice and memorizing the postures that were ahead of me. I set a discipline of trying to learn eight postures a day and this is how I managed to learn the first two and half of the third series at this time.

When my visa expired I came back to America and went to Encinitas, California, where I began to teach yoga. After I had been there for a little while I got a letter from Guruji saying that he would like to come to America. I decided that I would help him get here and would save $10 a week until I could bring him. I was excited about the letter and I went and told my yoga class that he had notified me. They said, "Don't wait on that, let's get the money together right now and send for him." By the next day, lo and behold, they had gathered $3,000, and we sent for Guruji to come to California.

Initially, we thought he was going to bring his wife, Amma. As it turned out, Manju came with him and helped him teach. His visa got delayed, as it has over the years at different times, and it was seven months before he finally arrived. By that time we had become a group of thirty-five people and were working on the series every day and preparing for his arrival.

Guruji and Manju came and stayed with Nancy and me and Terry Jenkins for four months, and we had daily yoga practice in Encinitas. After that ended, I wanted to leave California and go to Hawaii and discover paradise. Manju wanted to stay in America, so it was perfect timing. He took over my classes and I came to Hawaii. I thought I was coming for two weeks to check it out. I've been here ever since, twenty-six years, and taught yoga at many different locations and met thousands of people who I've been able to share this yoga with.

Can you describe your first meeting with Guruji?
In 1973, I arrived in Mysore by train and found a hotel room. I was with Nancy. The next morning I got a rickshaw driver who told me he knew where to go. We got in and he took us to the home of an astrologer who lived in the neighborhood where Guruji lived. It was the wrong address, but the astrologer knew who Pattabhi Jois was, and he sent the rickshaw driver to the right place.

When we got to Guruji's house he wasn't at home; he was at the Ayurvedic College, but was expected back in a while. Fortunately that day a fellow named Coconut Raju was there for yoga class. He spoke good English and decided to stick around and be our translator. We made friends with him and have been friends ever since.

Guruji came in a few hours later and said, "How did you find me?" I said, "Well, I met Manju and saw his demonstration of the first series and I'm a friend of Norman Allen's who has been here and I want to learn the yoga as well. I practice every day; I'm really fascinated by it. As a matter of fact, I've even taught a few people." So, this was my idea to get accepted. I said, "I think you should teach me, so that I don't return to America and teach people wrong." Guruji thought about it a little and he said, "Okay, stay in your hotel for three days and in that amount of time I'll be able to find you a place to stay nearby and you can start daily practice." So, indeed, that's what happened. He found us a little apartment right around the corner from his house and we moved in there and stayed for the next four months.

What was your first impression of Guruji?
He had a really nice smile. He was very intense with his focus and concentration, but I liked his smile. He was a very healthy-looking guy. At the time he was fifty-nine years old. He had great skin. He was a really radiant person and I knew whatever he was doing, I wanted to do it.

How would you describe Guruji's teaching in those days?
One would come to class and there were eight places for people to prac-

tice. Each person would come in and start their practice. I came at 6 a.m. and 6 p.m. I worked up to where I was doing about two and a half hours each time. We were doing half *vinyasas* and then after the practice in the morning, we would rest a little and then come back at ten thirty for *pranayama*. I was totally fascinated. I wanted to learn and put all of my energy and attention into that. For the next six years, until I had completed learning the entire system that he teaches, I put all of my energy into that. After that, I continued to be able to have mastery of it, and it's been my fascination now for thirty-one years.

I've often heard Guruji say he teaches real or original ashtanga *yoga. What is your experience with Guruji as a teacher—a true teacher of yoga?*
As I understood it, this series can be chanted move by move, breath by breath in Sanskrit. It's an exact formula that goes back thousands of years and has been time-tested to be the most efficient way that one can get themselves fit.

After practicing more and more years, I realize the perfection of the ordering of the postures. I say now that it's like a combination lock. If you do the numbers in order, the lock will open. If you just do any numbers, nothing happens. I feel this is the way with yoga practice. If you do the yoga practice in a certain order, your body and your mind open up. If you just do random yoga like is taught in so many places, it's much less efficient. So the greater amount of times I practice, the more I appreciate the order of the series. When I teach people, I try to teach them exactly the way I was taught and try not to modernize it in any way.

The other thing I found is that, after ten years, one starts to get a bit of a grip with the *mula bandha*. After twenty years, I realized this was the real strength of yoga. Now that it has been more than thirty years, more than ever I realize the real strength of the yoga is in what's invisible. I tell people, "What's invisible is what's important." The breathing and *mula bandha*; the name and the form, *namarupa*, is *maya*; it's an illusion. And the people who give too much emphasis to the name and form miss the real importance, which is the *mula bandha* and the breathing, the invisible internal practice.

Yes, I would say that there is a real obsession with the asanas, *the number of* asanas, *the series, and so on, progressing through it. How would you say*

Guruji focuses in on the invisible aspect—how does he teach the invisible aspect—even beyond the mula bandha *and breathing?*
From the beginning he told us that the yoga was 95 percent practice, 5 percent theory. If you do the practice, all will be revealed. To me, that's the spiritual part of having the revelations: by first getting the body fit enough so it won't interrupt you, so you can get into a state of meditation. The words "yoga" and "meditation" are synonyms. More and more over the years, I work to make my yoga practice a moving meditation, and then at the end of my practice, when I get up and walk away, I continue that meditation into my life, all day long. So I consider the practice to be the foundation of a twenty-four-hour-a-day meditation.

Were there many Indian students in the yoga shala *when you started practicing?*
Other than Nancy and myself, all the students were Indian. At that time, about ninety to a hundred people were coming each day. They would start at 4 a.m. and go until about 10 a.m., then in the afternoon from about four to nine or nine thirty. After several weeks, a fellow from En-gland, John McGeoch, came. He became the third non-Indian, and that was it.

Did you ever see Guruji practicing?
No. I'd always hoped to, but it never happened. My greatest wish at one time, maybe, was that I could have practiced with him. I asked Saraswathi why he didn't practice, and she told me he'd had a bicycle wreck and discontinued his practice and never resumed it. When I asked him myself, he told me he was putting all of his energy into teaching us and working on his legacy that way and not into his own practice. As I was the student and he was the guru, it was not for me to question. For my first twelve years with Guruji, I tried to put all questions aside and just surrender to the guru and do as I was told.

Were Manju and Ramesh teaching with Guruji at that time?
No, only Ramesh was helping. Manju was traveling around India with Basaraju.

Can you say something about Ramesh?
Other than Nancy, Ramesh was my best friend in Mysore. He taught me

quite a bit. He spoke very good English and could explain things to me, answer my questions, lead me around the market, and introduce me to Mysore. We spent a lot of time together. He was fascinated with us, I think, because he had not met any Americans other than Norman and his family. I liked Ramesh very much.

We described this practice as being an ancient practice which precedes Guruji and which will live beyond his lifetime. What do you see as Guruji's role in this?
Nancy and myself plus Norman, when he was in America, introduced Guruji to America, which began the spread of *ashtanga* to all of the world. In Mysore, Guruji just taught a limited number of Brahmins. After he started teaching us, *ashtanga* went worldwide, which was Guruji's wish. I think it made him very happy to see that happening. I believe more people outside of India are practicing yoga now than inside of India.

Why do you think that is?
A lot of people in India didn't have the leisure time to do it, for one thing. A huge amount of the population works for enough food to feed themselves and their family that day, and they are working from dawn to dark. Also, at least with this system of yoga, it was only taught to Brahmins up until we sort of released it to the rest of the world, and prior to, say, the 1960s, yoga in general was kept pretty much a secret. The guru taught the disciple and there was a lineage. Before mass communication, one person would learn one yoga system in their life if they got introduced to yoga. Now all of that has been blown wide open with mass communication and videos and all of that.

What kind of role did Amma play?
Amma played a very strong role in Guruji's life. She always had a smile. She was really friendly to all of us; it was a joy to see her. I always loved eating her cooking! Sometimes we went on picnics, and those were the best meals that I remember in India. She was really a fine, nice person. She wanted to relate to us, and as quickly as possible, once the foreigners started coming, she began to study English. She ended up learning to communicate pretty well. But from the beginning, even before she knew

English, she was very intelligent and figured out how to communicate. Everybody loved Amma.

Would you care to share some final thoughts?
Everything that I was looking for at that time in my life I received from Guruji. I went to India searching for the best possible yoga practice and I found his system and started learning it with diligence. Since then, I have still continued my search for the greatest fitness program. I ask everybody that I meet, "Have you found a better yoga system than this?" I still haven't found anything better than Guruji's *ashtanga* yoga practice. If somebody said to me, "Okay, you have fifteen minutes or one hour. Do something good for yourself. You can have all the equipment, no equipment, barbells, bicycles, whatever . . ." I would get down on the floor and start doing my salutations to the sun and going through the first series. I am entirely indebted to Guruji for every one of the hundreds of hours that he put into teaching me *ashtanga* yoga.

Maui, 2001

Nancy Gilgoff

Nancy Gilgoff became Guruji's student in 1973. She credits him with curing her of crippling headaches and other debilitating symptoms. Nancy taught with David Williams in Encinitas and moved to Maui where she lives and teaches. She travels widely teaching all over the world.

When did you first meet Guruji?
About thirty years ago, I was traveling in India with David Williams. We went to an ashram in Pondicherry and were looking for David's friend Norman Allen. Norman had gone and found Pattabhi Jois, so we followed along in the footsteps of Norman and went to Mysore. I was twenty-four years old and had no expectations at all about anything except world travel and went to Mysore. We were quickly brought into this man's family. I became enthralled with the whole practice and with who he was.

What was your first impression of Guruji?
I found Guruji to be openhearted and friendly. I enjoyed just being around him. I trusted who he was and enjoyed him as a person. I didn't know anything about yoga then. I surrendered to this friendly man who really seemed to want to do things with me. Guruji helped me in my practice and with who I was later to become.

So you started studying with him right away when you first met him?
Oh yes. We met him and then he told us to come back the next day and we came in the morning and he started to teach us *surya namaskara* A.

I've often heard Guruji say that he teaches real or original ashtanga *yoga. What is your experience of Guruji as a teacher of true yoga?*
What is true yoga? [*Laughter*] Ah, my experience of Pattabhi Jois as a yoga teacher is really my experience of it. When I met him I was quite ill, quite weak with migraine headaches, and within four months I felt better. I had no idea what yoga was. I never expected any health benefits.

So in terms of the practice of yoga over the years of studying with him, I have done some investigating and would say his knowledge of *asana* is genuine. I consider him to be the best *asana* teacher in the world . . . for me. He's certainly taken me through my own fire and has shown me a great deal of compassion. He helped my body to heal enough so that I could do the more advanced yoga practices.

When I first met him he told me my nervous system was very weak and that was why I had these headaches. He also told me right away where the headaches were coming from in my lower back, which I had no pain in, so that was kind of interesting. I didn't know if that was correct or not, I just thought it was interesting. And then as years went by I started to understand why he said that, and indeed I did have a scoliosis there, but all the pain manifested in my upper body.

Why does Guruji emphasize, in particular, the third limb of ashtanga *yoga as a starting point?*
The fiery practice of *ashtanga* that Pattabhi Jois teaches people is to heal the body—again this is how I understand it through myself—so that we can be strong enough to do the more advanced practices. Most people in the world come into *asana* practice with a body that isn't able to stand up to some of the intense *pranayama* and the fire that you need to do these advanced practices. I think that's why he also doesn't talk about the other practices. He's told me that a person needs ten years of this *asana* series before he really can talk about meditation or *pranayama* for some people—but definitely meditation.

Does he talk about the other limbs in his teaching or does it come at a later point?
He doesn't talk much about the others. He taught me *pranayama* within the third month I was with him. Now he doesn't teach that until much later. He doesn't really talk about those things too much with anybody.

It's left for self-inquiry, for people to go and find their own way with those. I've thought about it a lot over the years and came to see that his expertise is the *asanas*, and he's so wonderful at that. I think he was probably very wise to stay with what he does so well and let the rest of it unfold naturally. He will speak on any subject, but you have to ask him. Otherwise, in being around him and following the practice correctly, the other limbs will be realized.

Would you say that Guruji teaches a standardized form of asana *practice, or is it an individualized practice that he teaches?*
I would say there is a standardized form but within that form there's a lot of room for individual practice. So we have a set way of doing it, a specific order of practice, the set number of breaths. But within that there is certainly an individual practice. You see that with the way different people practice. Everyone has their style. I can see who taught whom as soon as they start their practice. I know if Richard Freeman was their teacher, Tim Miller, Pattabhi Jois. You pick up nuances from your primary teacher.

Does Guruji teach different students in different ways? Does he teach people individually?
A lot of his teaching seems to be based on their personalities. I've noticed with people who are very strong, he'll be more concerned with their strength and helping them build their strength in a positive way. People who are very flexible, he'll work with them in a different way. So yeah, there is a difference. For people like me, who were extremely flexible but very weak, he worked very much on the *bandhas* to build my strength, and build my energy internally.

We hear a lot about bandhas. *As somebody who's been exploring and experimenting with them over the years, can you say something about your experience?*
When I first began *ashtanga* yoga, of course I'd never heard of the *bandhas*, and when I met Pattabhi Jois, his English was pretty negligible, he spoke hardly any words of English. And so it was basically hands-on. I couldn't even jump back, I couldn't lift my weight up at all, and he would do that for me. And he also used his hands to do *mula bandha* for me. I found it to be energizing, and over the years I've investigated with as

much understanding as I can. It keeps unfolding. It seems to move my energy up more in my body. But at the beginning, I really didn't even have an understanding at all of the energy in the body, much less the *bandhas* themselves.

He just says controlling them, when he talks about it, if he talks about it at all. Is there any more subtle aspect to it as far as you are concerned?
As one becomes more used to the feeling of it, the energy moves up into the body more. You just start to become more aware of it in a subtle way as time passes. It's not such a large area of the body that one is taking in. You start to feel the perineum lifting and energy moving up in the body. At that point it has to join with the other *bandha—uddiyana bandha—*or it's not going to travel up in the body. I've been practicing almost thirty years now, and I'm just now, once again, thinking that I'm understanding a little bit more.

Guruji must have been one of the first teachers to take on female students.
There were not many female students even when I started with him. The men were downstairs and the women, the handful of women, were up-stairs. He had about a hundred Indian students a day come in those days, and David Williams, myself, and Norman. Then a woman named Sally Walker showed up, so he kept us in the room with the men. And generally, we spoke to no one in the room because they were all speaking Kannada, his language. We were just practicing off to one side, listening to their laughter and their jokes. The women were around but not very visible.

Do you think there is an intrinsic difference between the way men and women are taught yoga? Or is it appropriate to teach men and women differently?
I think they should be taught within the same framework but there should be a difference. A woman should be allowed to be a woman in the practice. And this particular practice is very much a male practice, as far as the general public has become aware of it. The men have predomi-nated in the field. As I travel more, that's one of the things that I hear people say: they are so glad that a woman is coming out and speaking about it and showing it can be done in a soft way and in a feminine way. I've just become comfortable with that myself, so it's kind of interesting.

There is a difference between men and women, and so we should honor that within our practices as well.

There seem to be more women practitioners but more male teachers.
Yes, I think so. I think that men are more motivated to be exposing themselves in that way.

I often find women's adjustments more sensitive—there's a softness—whereas men can sometimes be just too forceful.
Yeah, but there's some strong women out there doing that, too. [*Laughter*] But that is a subject in itself, that you know how to give the adjustments themselves. It's not about strength; it's about what are you trying to do with them. Are you trying to just take the external body and rotate it or put it in a place, or are you trying to get the energy moving in the body? And that's what I believe Guruji is doing. That's what I always felt with him, that he put my body in these postures and moved my energy. It wasn't about whether my foot went behind my head or not, although that was the external form. It was getting the energy moving in all parts of the body.

So he'd see a blockage or had a sense of you being stuck in some way and then would help to break that.
The energy does get blocked in the body and that can be from injuries and emotional things that keep coming up. There is a way to unblock it through heat and breath, and that's what the *ashtanga* series seems to do. It sets the body up to move the energy through it. If the *bandhas* are engaged, it helps move it more smoothly through the body.

You were just talking about how the energy can be blocked in the body. It's not only the body, it's the mind also very often, isn't it? I presume you've had experiences with Guruji taking you to where you think your limit is and beyond, you know, where you've experienced where your body somehow is blocked and he's helped to move you through that. Can you describe some incident where he's done that?
When I first met him, the posture that was my hardest was *baddha konasana*. My knees were very high and basically I couldn't bend over. He would take me down through the entire pose and my knees would go down on the floor, my chest would go down on the floor and my mind

would snap. The body was fine but my mind definitely snapped. I'd get up, I'd be fine. I saw it was my mind holding me back in that posture. As the years progressed I saw my mind being the stuck place most of the time. If I was able to take my mind out of it, the energy could move through my body more easily.

The other posture with him that I've had a lot of work on and am still looking forward to working with him more is *ganda bherundasana*, where you're on your throat and the feet come over. Generally when my feet touched my head I checked out, literally, and there I was. I even lost consciousness sometimes. When my mind was absent, my body did what he wanted it to do because I wasn't resisting and reacting at that moment. The mind definitely plays a big role in what's going on in the body and you learn that through the practice.

Richard Freeman described him as being a bit of a trickster, like a Zen master, speaking in riddles, making you sort of confused in a certain sense—you think you are going backward; instead, you are going forward or whatever. Have you had an experience with how he uses psychological methods to help you? Not just, "Yes, you go."
I feel a lot of times Guruji will be teasing in a way to make us move forward so that it takes us out of our mind-set and brings us into a place where it's both fun and where we're not so aware of what we're about to do. So in a sense, the fear goes. One of his lines is, "Why you fear?" And as he says it, you become aware of yes, it is about fear and why am I, what am I really afraid of? Am I afraid I'm going to fall on the floor? Am I afraid I'm going to break my shoulder? What am I afraid of? And as you examine it you realize that it's up here in the mind, not in the body, and you can let go of that. So yes, in terms of his way of teaching, he's a tease in that way. But again, it's very loving. I often tell people that he's the most compassionate person I've ever met because he'll take us into our fear and beyond it. When I'm teaching, if I read fear in someone, it's very hard to take them through it. So someone who can do that with you is the teacher for you because it's about fear, moving through it on all levels.

He says something similar about pain, doesn't he?
The pain element, there's good and there's bad pain. In terms of good pain, a lot of times you'll feel pain because you need to soften the mus-

cle. A lot of times you'll see that the mind is actually creating the pain. Again, because pain is contraction, when the mind shuts down so does the body. Once you can open the mind you can release a lot of the pain and contraction. He definitely takes you into that realm where you have to let go of the mind in order to do something. He generally is taking you quickly into the pose. There's a moment when the mind is not present and he will take you through that time. It's very quick, you go right into it, and that's the trick of teaching *asanas* well. If you are doing hands-on adjustments, it has to be fast before the mind can become involved in it.

Probably, first-time Baddha Konasana, *no problem.*
First time is much easier than the second because the mind is present, it expects it. So each time, as the mind shuts down and the body shuts down with it, you have to trick a little bit differently and go in there and work just a little bit quicker or wait until the person's mind steps out of the way again.

Guruji's been your teacher for thirty years. How does he teach you differently today than the way he taught you as a twenty-four-year-old?
I just saw Guruji in September, so that's a little less than a year, and normally whenever I've worked with him he's adjusted me almost in every posture. This time he was very busy—a lot of people in the room. Two times he did adjust me and they were the most direct, and I should say forceful in a way. But once again completely blew my mind at how amazing he was. He would come across the room and just get me right where I needed. I knew my energy in shoulder stand in my left hip had always sagged. Now most people wouldn't see that. And he came up the second day and kneed right in there, very sharp. But my energy went right through my body and I was really struck with how precise he is—I think he's become more precise and just goes right in. Now maybe it's because he knows my body and he can just go for a direct blow almost. It wasn't like an attack but it was just a real direct point of contact. Since that day I have never sagged again . . . at least not there. The other time he did it that day was in *yoga nidrasana*. I had woken up in the morning with my head stuck to the side and I couldn't straighten out my neck. I thought, "Oh, practice today is going to be really tough." And he came up and took me and just went boom, like this, pushed everything down, and I was ba-

sically in shock, surprise. When he let go everything in my neck cracked. It was totally fixed, it was a perfect adjustment. So I think he's gotten even more definite in his adjustments, which is really amazing because he was always great but it's like much more precise: this is it, boom!

That was really my second question. My first question is about age and does he adjust someone who's twenty-four differently than someone who's fifty-four?
As far as the difference in ages, I don't see there's much change. He doesn't read the body like anyone else I know. He reads the person. Someone who comes in who's in their fifties who's fit, he's going to adjust them as a fit human being not as a fifty-year-old fit human being. Age is really in the head; it's all in the mind. And it manifests through the body. A thirty-year-old can be walking around and really be in an eighty-year-old body. And so that's more how I think it's read, it's really the vitality of the person and it's very individual. With older people, he still expects them to work their hardest and to do their utmost. It can be that they're acting like a twenty-year-old as far as their practice goes or they can be in an older mind-set so they would act older.

Do you see ashtanga yoga as a spiritual practice?
I think at the beginning of my practice I didn't even have an understanding of what spiritual was. As the years have evolved, yes, I certainly would say that it's a spiritual practice. It's about transformation; it's about changing the mind-set. And that is what spirituality to me is about.

What is the purpose of daily practice and what are the nonphysical aspects of the practice?
A daily practice brings about a gauge in your life. For me, it's been a way to know who I am in the moment. And it's the only thing in my life that is something I do every day; it's the same practice. So no matter what else I'm doing—I'm traveling, if I eat differently—every day the practice being the same repetitive practice gives me a way to judge myself in a nonjudgmental way, a way of seeing. "How am I doing? How am I holding up to the stresses of daily life?" It's also the only time for me that I can take my mind out of my daily life and become free in a spiritual sense to investigate myself, my true Self.

Can you say what you think Guruji's definition of yoga is and how he imparts this knowledge to his students? Where does it come from and what is he teaching?

It's 99 percent practice, 1 percent theory. And to me, this is beautiful. The more I have been on the road teaching, I see more and more how beautiful that is. It's individual. He's teaching us to go within, to look inside, to investigate ourselves, not always to look to the external or someone else for the answer. The answer is in all of us and he's just given us a framework to work within that. I find that to be the greatest gift of all.

Could you say a little bit about Guruji's cultural origins and how that affects him as a person, and if he has moved from that by virtue of his connection with Westerners. As you said, initially he had one hundred Indian students and three Western students. Now he has maybe three Indian students and one hundred Western students. It's totally changed around. I'm sure his way of being has changed as a result of this cultural exchange that's been happening with Westerners.

In truth, he hasn't changed very much in terms of how he deals with the Westerners today and how he dealt with Indian students when I first met him. He's had a lot of Indian students. He was always a very loving, jovial kind of person, and very family oriented. He's very much into his Hindu life. He is a spiritual man coming from within the framework of Hinduism but he doesn't project that out to us too much. Those people who want to learn the cultural parts of his life have taken that on, but it's not something he presents or forces on anyone. I find his being involved in the West a lot has increased his understanding of the world. He's becoming more worldly in a way, but he very much has stayed the same man he was. The Westerners he hangs out with give him a limited perspective of what the West is. When we first met him and his family, I wore no jewelry and I was the first woman he had met from the West. And so he and his family would say, "Oh, American women don't wear any makeup, they don't wear any jewelry." I said, you know, "This is not the norm. I'm a little bit off the beaten track here." So they had that perspective. As they moved into the Western culture more, I'm sure that they've seen other aspects of the world but they, the whole family, very much have the same energy. It's very interesting really to see that.

Do you think the system originates in the Yoga Korunta *or with Rama Mohan Brahmachari, Krishnamacharya's teacher, or do you think Krishnamacharya developed it himself? Where do you think is the origin?*

As I was told originally, the system was found in Sanskrit by Krishnamacharya and Guruji and they translated it together. Guruji was in the Sanskrit College. I don't know where they found the papers. Some people say they were found on leaves. Now Guruji said he's never seen that. I don't know. It seems to be an old system. I feel that it was started a lot before Krishnamacharya and it was taught to young boys. My understanding was that it was taught to the young boys who were going to be the priests. And it was taught to them to purify their bodies and get their bodies strong so that they can go on to do more advanced yoga practices.

I've often heard yoga teachers talk about this as a system that Krishnamacharya taught to children. Do you have an idea why it seems so appropriate for Western people?

I think it is because the Western personality is competitive and very mindful—their minds and bodies are strong—the Indian peoples' bodies were not as developed in terms of genetics and diet. It was also the reason why Guruji at the beginning told Norman that Westerners couldn't do this practice. He thought only Indians could do the practice partly because of the way the Western mind was always going into competition and trying to go after worldly pursuits. As the years progressed and Westerners would come to it, the practice has certainly changed in the sense that there are more strength aspects coming into it.

Do you see Guruji as a healer? And what qualities in him make you see him in that light?

Guruji is certainly a healer. He healed me. I can only speak from my experience about who he is. And in truth I don't know that I'd be alive today if it weren't for him. I've certainly added quality to my life that I had not even expected when I went to him. I was losing energy very quickly. Sleeping twelve hours a day, had not much will to fight it, but I was a strong person in my being, that's why I kept going. So in terms of who he is, yes I always have seen him as healing me. I feel that it was from his yoga practice, that whatever drove him to Krishnamacharya's door when he was a young boy is the reason he's a healer today. And that's what he loves about doing it. You see him expand with love every moment he's teaching. He loves the practice. Same way that I feel when I'm teaching, I'm sharing this great gift that he gave to me and it's a healing gift; healing on many levels but certainly the physical level has been extraordinary in what's happened to me.

How do you try to incorporate his teaching in the way you teach? And if there are one or two qualities you try to emulate when teaching, what would those be?

On our first trip, when we were getting ready to leave, Guruji told us, "Do your practice. Someday you teach it. All is coming." And I believed him; I had no questions in my mind, I took that to heart. And I did my practice every day. Eventually I found myself, without wanting it necessarily, teaching, sharing this with people. I teach the way he taught me, which is what he tells me to do. Whenever I've asked him questions about teaching, he says, "Teach it the way I taught you." So I have a road map and I feel that I'm teaching the way I experienced it. I don't change things. I teach through his method of using hands-on. Because he was so hands-on with me, I learned how to do hands-on adjustments. I'm mimicking him in a way, but translated through my body. I learned through his hands, not through words.

I use my hands more than I use my words because that is how I was taught. And I now understand that people learn differently. Some people learn through talking, some people learn through seeing, and some people learn through touch. So I've expanded that and I've learned that really through my special-education teaching, which I also have done. Each of us learns differently. I happen to be a person who learns through touch, so Guruji taught me the method that worked best for me. David was a person who learned through sight and through hearing, and so he worked with him that way. Very rarely did he adjust David. David didn't need the same kind of teaching. I'm learning more and more to work with different kinds of people. As I read their energy more, I work differently with them. Some people I can do more aggressive adjustments with and others, if I went up and did an aggressive adjustment, they would just freeze on me. Some people I can feather-touch, just lightly touch them, and their body will open up, whereas, if someone feather-touches me, nothing will probably happen. I need to have someone actually move my body. So it's reading each individual and remembering as we go from person to person that it's a different person instead of teaching everyone in the same way. In a large group we have to use more words, but it's really just to keep the form going. The fewer words, the better.

What was it like having Guruji as a guest in your home?
Guruji has blessed our houses with visits many times. The first time was for four months with his son Manju in California. And it was pure delight. Always fun to have him there. Very easy. Basically, his son or his daughter takes care of him in terms of cooking and all of that. It is not our responsibility to do anything except to be with him and take him around. He loves to tour and be a tourist in new environments, and it's fun to go shopping with him, although I don't usually like shopping. It's delightful to see him and watch him discover things.

Guruji comes from a lineage of householders. How important is family life in the system of yoga Guruji is teaching? And how does that affect the quality of this practice?
Guruji's family is extremely important to him. His immediate family is the core of his life, I feel. He also has an extended family with all of us who are his students. I think traditionally most human beings are going to be householders. There are very few people who are going to be renunciants, and that's as it should be. If we didn't have householders, we wouldn't have the human race anymore. So there's a way of being within the daily life of a householder that has integrity and compassion and love within it, and I think that's what he teaches by example because his family is a very loving family, and they extend that out to other people and allow other people to come in and be close to them.

Is that how he teaches the yamas *and the* niyamas?
Possibly, yes. His teaching is definitely very rarely through words. You are with him and you learn who he is and how he reacts and how he treats people by his doing it. He's not really going to give you much on the verbal plane. We used to think it's because he couldn't speak English, but now he speaks English very well although he still doesn't converse. If you ask him a direct question it's amazing how much knowledge he has on different subjects, but someone has to ask him the question.

That is intentional, obviously, in some way.
I don't know, you'd have to ask him that. I don't know. You know, I was
with him recently when a friend of mine, who's an incredible body-
worker, asked him a question about the body and the two of them got
into a discussion that left the rest of us in complete wonderment: What
were they talking about? But they had this exchange going that was so
deep and so beautiful to watch and they both were so excited and into it
but most of us hadn't an idea of what they were talking about. It was way
beyond our comprehension. And the same with his study of Sanskrit and
the *Sutras* and all of this. He's so schooled in them, but very few people,
really, could talk to him about those things. There are very few people
who understand it, and that's one of the things about the practice being
everything. You don't talk about things you don't know about or with people who can't understand it. You have to ask the right questions to receive
those kinds of answers.

*After Guruji passes on, what do you think would be his legacy? What would
continue on after him?*
All of it, all of the people practicing will continue on. I think that all of the
people in the past who've continued yoga practices are part of the same
legacy. Within the framework of each practice there are different people
who are going to continue the form. I once asked a teacher of mine, Baba
Hari Dass, "What do the students owe a teacher?" And the answer was,
"To do your practice." And I think that the legacy of yoga, the only reason
that I get to practice it now, is because many, many people went before
myself, went before Pattabhi Jois, went before Krishnamacharya, and created this lineage that we can all use as our lineage, and to evolve with it.

*One definition of guru is the remover of darkness or the one who sheds light.
Would you consider Guruji to be your guru in that sense?*
The word "guru" in our culture has such overtones and undertones and
all of this. To me, yes, I have no problem with calling Pattabhi Jois my
guru. I think of a guru as a teacher and someone who exhibits compassion and helps someone go beyond their normal frame of reference of
who they are, shows us the way out of our self-image. So yes, Guruji has
certainly been someone who has done that for me, way beyond my imagination. He took me way past who I thought I was, who I thought I could
be, and has helped me develop into the person I am today.

Can you tell us any interesting stories of the time you spent with Guruji in Mysore or when Guruji has come to visit you?

When we were first in Mysore with him, he took us once to Bangalore to the circus, and we were watching these girls go over backward. Their heads were touching their butts and they were so flexible and we kept saying, "Guruji, look at this, this is so amazing." And he kept saying, "Yes, but it's not yoga." And we were, "But Guruji, look at these people!" So for me, at that point I started to examine what he was really talking about. How could this not be yoga? I couldn't understand the difference. To me, at that point it was still about flexibility and about only the external form. And it took years of him working with me and kind of pushing me along to see that it isn't about the external form; it's more about the internal happenings. A gymnast is not a yogi although they may be very flexible.

When he first came to the United States, we took him into a grocery store. He would go into the spice racks with all the little jars and open them up, pour them in his hand, sniff them, and kind of look at us like, "There's no life, you know, in these spices!" and kind of "tsk, tsk, tsk." Nobody in the store ever stopped him. You can just see us with this little man in a dhoti, waiting for the man to come and tell us that you can't just open the jars and close them again and put them back on the shelf. But nobody ever stopped us. It was really wonderful to see.

On his first trip he wanted to tease his wife. She had not come with him, which he said he would never do again. We bought him a pair of pants. He had never worn regular pants before, and he wanted to get off the train in Mysore in pants to tease his wife. So the night before he left California he tried on these pants, and we were all laughing so hard we were crying because he looked so different in pants. And he got off— apparently he did this—he got off and Amma was beside herself in hysterics laughing to see this Western man.

Were they Calvin Klein?

Not in those days, they were probably cheap polyester we bought him. I don't know what we bought him actually, but they were not Calvin Klein. He's moved up in the world. This is how he's changed.

That brings up another subject, which is Amma. Could you talk a little about being the first Western woman that Guruji met and taught yoga to?

How did Amma influence or help that process, and what role did she play in your time in Mysore?

Amma would greet us after class with a nice beautiful strong cup of Mysore coffee and sit on her little stoop in front of the house and tell us a story. And I remember, I would not braid my hair then; I used to always wear my hair loose and she would sit and she always braided my hair for me, and stroked my head like, "It's good to braid your hair." And she put a little coconut oil in it and things like that. There were a lot of different things she would talk to me about. She was quite fun to be with herself. She also spoke very little English when we first met but seemed to develop a better grasp of it during that first trip. When I couldn't practice because I had my period I would spend time with her because I couldn't talk to Guruji. I would go over and sit with her on a bench and she would tell me that this was a good time for women. That it was a time to be quiet and not have to deal with the world so much, and not have to deal with men. And they could, you know, separate in a way, and it was to enjoy this time. Ah, she was quite the woman in her way. She took care of the house, fed us, made sure that everyone felt comfortable. Very open and welcoming all the time.

Is she the one who explained to you that you shouldn't practice when you had your period? And that you shouldn't be in Guruji's presence? Is that how that happened?

As far as not practicing during your period, I don't remember exactly how it was first presented to me but I was told not to come over. We were told to just stay away from the whole scene over there. We would go out to dinner, I remember, and we were questioned a couple times, "Why is Nancy going out?" And we would say, "But you know, she has to eat." They generally would stay home. So I believe it was probably Saraswathi who started to explain some of the tradition, because Saraswathi's English was very good. And we also spent a lot of time with their son Ramesh. And Ramesh's English was also perfect. And so Ramesh gave us a lot of the understanding of the culture. When we first got there both Saraswathi and Ramesh were not allowed out of the house too much because of the local culture. They were pretty open people, but society had said he was a single young man, he was not to go out without friends. And Saraswathi was living with the family with two children, so she wasn't to go out without friends or family. They let them go out with us, so we were quite popular with both Ramesh and Saraswathi. We could take them shopping, go to the movies. And they pretty much taught us how to be in the society.

Was Ramesh teaching with Guruji?
Ramesh was a teenager when I met him and was always in the yoga room. He was wiry and, as I told Sharath—I had not seen Sharath since he was five years old and I just saw him, and he's, what, maybe thirty now, and I called him Ramesh many times when he was there—he reminds me so much of his uncle. Ramesh was learning handstands in those days. And the yoga room was very small. He would be doing handstands and as I said, was very wiry, and he was just falling this way and that but never fell on anyone. The second time I was there he was already in college and going to school and teaching full-time and basically that was his life. So he was very much in that room all the time. There were several times when Guruji traveled and Ramesh was the person left in charge of the room.

Like when Guruji would come to California?
No, no, he would go off on a meeting for a day or two and Ramesh would be left in charge of the classes. But Ramesh was very much present in those rooms the first two trips that I was in Mysore.

Did you live in Guruji's house?
No, when we went to Mysore for the first time we were in a hotel and then he got us what was affectionately called "the dungeon" and it was two doors up from him. And it was just a big long room that had a cement floor and we laid little mats on it. And there was no kitchen; the kitchen was filled with straw. So we always went out and ate. We wouldn't have known how to cook on their stove anyway. And we had a little toilet and a little spigot out of it. He could call us from his house. A British man named John had shown up, and John was staying on the other side of Guruji. If Guruji knew that John hadn't walked home because we would play cards or something until late in the evening, we'd hear Guruji, "John, go to bed. John." And so John would leave. We were always being observed.

Was Guruji teaching at the Sanskrit College at that time?
I think he may have just retired from the Sanskrit school when we met
him but maybe he was actually still teaching there. He was probably just
coming up to retirement when we met him. Basically he was in the room
all day. It's interesting to me now because people tell me, you know, he's
in there until two o'clock in the afternoon—as if this is a lot. Well, he
used to be in there from five in the morning until two o'clock in the afternoon then he'd take a two-hour break, and then he would go back in
the room until ten at night. He was always in that room teaching. And
Manju had told us that it used to be that the practice was every day except the full moon and new moon, and the family finally said, "We need
you home one day," and that's why people started taking Saturdays off,
because Guruji's family wanted him home some. So he started taking
Saturdays. But his life has been revolving around that room.

Burlington, 2001

Brad Ramsey

Brad Ramsey began his practice with David Williams in Encinitas in 1973, and with Guruji and Manju when they made their first trip to America in 1975. He started assisting Manju, eventually renting a church where he taught along with Gary Lopedota. Brad moved to Hawaii in 1980, where he lives in retirement from teaching.

Tell us how you got into yoga and how you met Guruji.
It started when David Williams and Nancy Gilgoff moved to Encinitas. Cher Bonelle and I were already doing the *28 Day Exercise Plan*, that Richard Hittleman book. Cher's son was taking a Pilates class, and after the class David was using the studio for his little *hatha* yoga class. We started doing that with him and it was really enjoyable. Later he said, "There's this other yoga. It's not for everybody but you are welcome to come over to my house and try it." So I started working with him through primary and part of intermediate. Then he organized for Guruji to come over, and rented a church in Cardiff. That was where I met Guruji and Manju. And that was a real experience. That was the beginning of *pranayama* and more serious practice. Manju stayed, and at one point his class was large enough that he needed some help, so he asked me if I cared to apprentice with him. I worked with him for at least a year, maybe closer to two years. Then a group of us rented a church closer to my home in Carlsbad, right on the border between Leucadia and Encinitas, and I taught class there until I moved to Maui in 1980.

In about '76, '77, I had a chance to go to India and get the full experience of studying with Guruji there. That was a real eye-opener. Then I taught. Taught here with David Williams, and on the Big Island. Then we moved to Kauai and I stopped teaching. That's the story in a nutshell.

Can you remember your first impression of the practice, when David showed it to you, in comparison to what you were doing before?

It was really hard. Even salutation A was very difficult. I was one of the stiffest people that I've ever seen in my teaching experience. Just to get through three and three salutations, to get comfortable with that, was months of work. All the little *hatha* yoga things I had done before were no preparation whatsoever for that kind of physical effort. But I was really attracted to the synchronization between the breathing and the motion, and the idea of the locks, that was new to me also. The whole system just made sense to me. I still think it's the most perfect system ever devised, the most efficient method of physical transformation that I've ever seen.

Do you remember your first meeting with Guruji?

I was working at La Costa Country Club at the time, and when his agenda was definite, when we knew he was going to be there, I asked them to lay me off so that I could collect unemployment and study exclusively with him and not have to shuffle. My work schedule would have interfered with the time when he was here. So after that, I was pretty much exclusively doing yoga and working with Manju. And with my own classes, a little income started coming in and I was able to eke out a small living. So that worked well for many years.

You continued to teach hatha *yoga, or you taught the series?*

After working with Manju, I never taught anything but the series.

So there were a few years of teaching with Manju before you went to Mysore.

Yes. I finished my apprenticeship by then and we were already in our own little deconsecrated church. I had a pretty good-size class in Leucadia. Some of my friends helped me finance the trip and it was wonderful. It was really wonderful to see him at home. He'd returned to California, and he and Amma stayed with Manju and taught at Manju's place. I would do yoga there, then they would come over to the other church, my church, and teach there. It was a busy schedule: started early with Manju and then at nine o'clock at our church, little St. Andrews.

Do you remember your first impression of Guruji?
I thought he was amazing. He radiated quiet brilliance. His English was not good at the time. But still, if you listened, you could get the gist of what he was saying, and the more you listened to him the easier it got. Having Manju there was a great help. You could start to pick up some of the nuance of the Kannada. But Sanskrit has always been easier for me because you can study it and it's in all the literature.

We had theory class every night. You'd get it after a while in spite of his English. And his English picked up; every trip, he would get a little better. I think he was getting more foreign students then, so it improved fairly rapidly. He never had the facility with it that a lot of Indian men do, but his Sanskrit was impeccable, so it was a trade-off. I didn't have trouble understanding. When you meet your guru, you just know. It's there or it's not. I don't think it's something you grow into. It's automatic.

Can you describe how it was studying in Mysore with him?
It was intense. It was painful. He would take care of his Indian classes in the morning. His Western class was in the afternoon, so meals were kind of a problem because you could take a little something for break-fast, something easily digested, but then you had to wait until six or seven o'clock at night to eat again. But in a way it was good, because we had time to do *pranayama* in the morning, maybe some light stretching, walk around Mysore a little, and then head to class in the afternoon. And it wasn't crowded. The yoga *shala* was very small at that time. So we'd do our practice, and then *pranayama* again, and then go find a place for dinner.

You said it was intense. Can you say a little more about that?
It was extremely painful. I don't think there's one part of me that wasn't sore. He wasn't as restrained on his home turf as he was in the U.S., so it was transformative. That's where I really got my leg to stay behind my head, and that took a lot of torque, a whole lot. I felt like I was being dis-membered. My body was changed.

Why do you think we allow ourselves to go through so much pain?
The benefits, I guess. You can feel it working, you can feel the quietness after. And I don't think it's the endorphins; it's because the system really works. You can almost hear your mind shutting down. Even the pain, if

you give that up to God, I think that's part of the practice, really. I don't know. Manju always says, no pain, no gain. And there is a great amount of truth there, I think. The pain is almost necessary. The pain is a teacher also.

Usually you take that as a message to stop what you are doing because you are about to do some damage.
Yes, that's the American way, probably the rest of the world, too, but Americans especially. In a lot of schools of yoga, if it hurts you are doing something wrong. And if you were a perfect physical and mental specimen already, then I can see how that might be true. If you are altering the status quo in an unpleasant way, you might want to stop if you were already perfect. But if you feel growth coming from it, and see things changing that need to be changed . . . the series is just a mold toward a body that meets the requirements for spiritual advancement, I believe. I don't think you can get there without pain. I never met anybody who did. For me, it hurt from the first day to the last, at least something. There's always something.

I think for everyone there comes a point where the pain gets moderated, you learn how to practice in an intelligent way and sustain yourself, rather than trying to break through.
That's true, it does get better.

It's a hard lesson to learn, and a difficult one.
Sometimes even to make the effort is painful.

Why do you think that is?
It's the nature of the beast. It's a birth process really.

I guess it's one stage more awake than total dullness and total ignorance. The pain is the beginning, a sign that the body and the mind are waking up, things are moving.
Evolution. And an important part is giving it up to God and making that part of the practice.

Guruji says that a lot, doesn't he? He tells us, "Pray to God."
Yes. When it hurts, put your mind on God instead of your pain, whatever

your concept of god is—whether he is the great architect or the basic element of the universe, which everything is made out of.

So I guess the purpose is to take your attention away from your personal experience and be with the universal, to get away from your personal suffering. Yeah, that's what practice is. Getting outside the little voices in your head.

Clearly you felt that he was your teacher, but he also represented something unique as a yoga practice.
Energy. *That* you feel; the rightness in things, when things are right—it's a goal. You can use images. For the *puja*, the mantra recitation that we learned, Ganesh was the one that we address. But that's just one manifestation. You know the Hindus have their whole pantheon, with different ways of visualizing the attributes of God. There are so many, and you can pick any one. For yogis, Ganesh works good. The remover of obstacles. His pop, Lord Shiva, is a great one, too, and Krishna . . . all these help. *Bhajans* are a great way to practice, too. God songs. They get you very close very quickly. That's an important part of *sadhana* also.

Did Guruji instruct you or tell you about doing pujas?
He gave me the mantra that I use and the instructions for its use. I wake up at night, three o'clock's a good time, it depends on your sleep schedule, but it's supposed to be kind of unnatural, you know, not a time you would choose to get up. So that's part of the sacrifice, too: take a little bath, do *pranayama* completely, and then do your rounds [of *japa*]. Start out with 108, work up to 1,008. As long as you can stay awake and sit in lotus, that's good. And after a while you lose yourself completely. It's not sleeping because you're in lotus. It's a little difficult to fall asleep in lotus; it can be done but . . . At night it's easier to lose yourself, things are shut down more, so there is no nervous little chatter and then the mantra takes away the rest. It's a completely empty slate.

Did you explore Guruji's family background, his connection with the Smarta Brahmin and Shankaracharya lineage?
It didn't seem important to me. At that time, the prayer we used started with God: *Narayanam padma bhuvam vashishtham* . . . the whole lineage of gurus from God on down to *vande gurunam.*

He had you doing that as part of the opening mantra for the asana *practice?*
Yes.

More recently he used it just for the pranayama.
But he still starts with *vande gurunam.* That's just one little piece, about
one quarter of the whole prayer. It's time-consuming to do the whole
thing before you start, but it's beautiful. Before *pranayama* we would do
it again. That was one of the hardest parts. When I started, lotus posture
was very painful. Even to sit there for a few minutes and say the prayer
was difficult. By the time the prayer was over, I was already dying, and
then we'd have to do the *pranayama.* And learning *pranayama* from Guruji was a pretty wild experience, because when he holds his breath, a lot
of times he just goes out, you know, he's not there anymore, he forgets
to count. So everybody's dying, and finally you hear him go on to the
next one. But he's a classic, that's a mark of success in practices: *kevala
kumbhaka*—you don't need to breathe, there is no urgency about it. It's
like sleep apnea, but if it's ingrained in your practice there's no panic
when you come out of it. You don't gasp for air or anything like that, you
just realize you stopped breathing and you just continue where you left
off. Or if you forgot where you left off, then you go back to the last place
you remember and start there. It was a hard way to learn but it was worth
it. It's an important adjunct. The practice can be nerve-irritating, over-
stimulating.

You mean the asana *practice?*
Yes, and the *pranayama* is partially an antidote to that, like the cooling-
down period for an athlete.

Normally, he wants to see padmasana *perfect before teaching* pranayama,
but obviously in your case he felt that you were advanced in some other way.
It wasn't perfect, but close enough I guess.

*He says you should be able to sit in it for three hours. I heard you had a high
level of concentration. When people saw you practicing, they said they had
never seen someone with such incredible focus.*
I got lost in it. I would lose myself in it. I got everything I wanted to get
out of it.

You felt that in the moment, or after practice?
I feel it right now.

When you say you got everything you wanted out of it, I presume you don't mean just the physical practice.
No, I mean the place where it put my mind. It may not appear perfect to anybody else, but inside I'm very comfortable and I feel that I have achieved the goals that I have for myself. Really it's all preparation for your death moment, that's the whole idea behind it. Because if you can put your mind on God while you are hopping around on the floor doing mildly painful things, that's practicing for the last moment of greatest extremity. And if in your death moment you can put your mind on God, the theory is, you save yourself a whole lot of births, you save yourself many travails.

Did you come to India with an idea or feeling for divinity, or did Guruji help you, or did your practice deepen that understanding or experience?
It was immersion in the practice with Guruji, because of the *shlokas* he would quote, the verses he would recite, the little poems, and the stories—immersion into the spiritual side of life. I wasn't particularly spiritually oriented before, and I don't even consider myself so spiritually oriented now. But I feel that that immersion is like what baptism would be to a Christian, you're saved. Now I'm saved forever. I can't get lost. Krishna tells Arjuna, "Arjuna, it doesn't matter how far you go or what you do. You do yoga, you do it as much as you can. If you can't do it anymore, fine, next life you get to take up from there again. You can't lose ground." That was Krishna's promise. Some people believe it, some probably don't.

Did you feel it became real through practice?
Yes. I truly believe that that is real. Underlying all the little stories—you know, those are the Hindu bible stories really—the universal truth is there, and that order of things makes perfect sense to me now. Before yoga, it would have seemed a little hocus-pocusy, kind of mythological, but now there's an underlying reality that becomes apparent through the practice. The practice changes your life, and the whole point of changing your life, I believe, is to become spiritually comfortable.

That's an interesting way of putting it. It really means just "comfortable with the Self" or "knowing the Self."
Yes, you can't be lost.

It takes a while to come to that . . .
It varies for everyone. Some people say that if the parents were yogis, then the child born into a family of yogis has one of the greatest blessings a child can have, and the mark of a soul who has done the work in the past. They get that bonus, that little head start, so they can make further progress.

How do you characterize what Pattabhi Jois actually teaches?
He's a great technician. Manju is even better at the physical adjustments. Guruji has the transmittable power through his lineage. If you recognize him as guru, then the benefit is in his touch as much as what he is touching. It doesn't matter where he is putting your leg at the time, just being in contact with him, there's a flow. It goes back and forth, too: the guru also gets nourished by a good student. So the circle gets flowing, that energy circuit, and that really can only happen with your guru. Teachers can help you physically, but the transmission of power is usually exclusively the province of the guru. You have to accept that person as your own guru for the circuit to be complete and he has to accept you as his student. That's the natural order of things.

You mentioned the fact that he is empowered by the lineage. Perhaps it's possible just by mutual acceptance of those roles—student and teacher— that the same transmission could happen.
He would have had it from Krishnamacharya. He would have had his batteries charged, so to speak, so that he could impart that to the students who chose him and that he chose. And when it happens, neither the guru nor the student has a choice: that's like the pull of a magnet. If they are meant for each other, they attract. If they are not, there is some repulsion there.

I asked Guruji about karma and the fact that he is my teacher. The way I came to him wasn't a conscious process. I was drawn toward him. I asked him, Is this karma? And he said no, that's a complete misunderstanding— implying that the choice of guru is a free choice rather than something that is programmed. I don't know if I misunderstood him.

That's not the way it seemed to me. What's the other solution? Where does the free choice come from? I don't know if there is such a thing as free choice. That's a debatable point and it might be just semantics, you know: What is choice? What makes you choose this or that? To find a teacher is very rare. Most people never do. So to recognize one when you find him, that also is rare. And for him to recognize you? Everything has to work out. So I would say there is at least an element of karma involved, some past-life conjunction, not necessarily between those two souls but within the whole gestalt, the whole dynamic of spiritual progress in the world, that at this time these two people will have the guru/*shishya* relationship. Extremely rare.

They also say that when the student is ready, the teacher will appear. It's interesting to me that Guruji seems to have students across the range of preparedness. When I was there, there were people with no real interest in spirituality at all and those deeply connected to that already, and he seems to have had the ability to speak to a broad spectrum of people.
That demonstrates the powerful energy reservoir, doesn't it? To be able to open himself to that broad spectrum of people, it's very hard to do. I always like to keep things as small as possible. I never saw the advantage of a huge class, it just doesn't make much sense to me. I can understand, logistically, after achieving a certain level of being known, having students spread around the world, that large classes become necessary. I don't know how he does it, I don't know how a lot of these people do it. It seems to me that the level of transmission would be affected. But for Guruji, people keep coming back, so he's doing it right.

Do you feel it's mainly energetic, the transmission?
I don't know what else it would be, but it's physically perceptible. When you get the direct transmission it's like tunnel vision. It's definitely an energetic phenomenon, I don't know what kind. Maybe that's what spiritual energy or *shakti* is. It's very difficult to explain.

Presumably, you were able to understand Guruji better than many. He does teach philosophy and the theory part, the 1 percent, as he likes to call it. And it occurs to me that some of the transmission has to also come through that channel.
It really does help to study. I studied enough Kannada to be able to read

street signs. That's a hard language to learn to write, isn't it? Sanskrit makes a lot more sense to me. I' had my Sanskrit dictionary and a few books on beginning Sanskrit, and I studied enough to get the basic terminology, all the important terms that he would use that there are no literal translations for in many cases. I think that's part of it, too: to receive a clear transmission you need some kind of common language, some kind of pidgin that you can operate in.

So Guruji encouraged you to study or directed you in certain directions.
He'd recommend the books, but he didn't care at all. He thought it was kind of funny, actually, that a white guy would even attempt to learn Sanskrit because it took him twenty-six years to get his full *vidwan* degree. So he thought someone dabbling in Sanskrit was pretty funny. He would teach us these little poems and then throw in some tongue twisters and I'd say them back and he would just crack up at my accent. It's like us listening to a hillbilly—there was just something slightly amusing about hearing your language mangled like that. Amma was a sweetheart. She was very helpful with the language part, the Sanskrit accent. She was always singing—a beautiful contralto voice—and she knew so many God songs. In a way, she was partly my teacher. I think that was part of his energy, too. I learned a great deal from her.

How was Guruji influenced by her? How was his teaching supported by her?
She was his student. She went through advanced B. She learned all the postures and she took great care of him; she ran the house like a commanding officer. Outside the house, he was definitely the boss. He would do a lot of the shopping, boss her around a little bit, but in the house he was truly respectful. She was in charge, it was quite clear. She was a beauty. She used to say that when she started [practicing yoga], she was a baby elephant. I guess she lost a lot of weight.

Family life was pretty important for Guruji, and as this yoga has unfolded in the West, Guruji was always telling people to get married.
One way of *sadhana* is the householder way. Traditionally, you take care of that first. You set up your household, raise children, produce your heir, accumulate wealth, and then retire to the forest. That was the old style: husband and wife go to the forest together after their children were

raised and their householder duties were finished. Now, I don't know if it's because we are still descending into *Kali Yuga*, the old patterns are broken. All the greatest gurus were renunciants, but we don't always hear about their early life, whether they had experience as householders. Vashishta, Vishvamitra—these are guys that would hold poses for a thousand years to curry favor with their gods. They may have been householders in their early stages. We don't know. Sri Shankaracharya. At one point there was a female preacher talking in town and he went to hear her and she said, "You don't know anything about life, you are still a virgin. What could you possibly know about the human condition?" So Shankaracharya sat down in meditation and he told his students to look after his body for a while and he traveled into the body of a great king in the north of India and enjoyed his harem and his wealth, raised children, and did the whole experience in the most fulfilling way possible. He could have anything he wanted as a king. So he experienced the world that way, then went back to his body and continued his life as renunciant. So both systems are valid I guess.

And then he beat her in the debate, right?
Yes. There's another part to it which I left out.

Shankaracharya was very important to Guruji. The Yoga Sutras present a dualistic model—the purusha/prakriti *duality—whereas Guruji comes from the Advaita, non-dualist perspective. How do you think these different perspectives merge?*
I think it's all one. Theology is just another way of fixing your mind on the issues. I don't think it really matters because there really is only one way and in the end it's all one thing. These different ways of looking are more suitable for the individual—each individual chooses a way. It doesn't really matter a whole lot which way that is. There's no right or wrong. It all resolves into one. It's interesting to ponder, though.

Guruji recently said the external angas *of ashtanga* yoga *were dualistic in nature, and the internal ones were Advaita (non-dual)—the internal experience of God or self-realization.*
That's true. *Yama* and *niyama* are external, and with *asana* and *pranayama* it begins to be internalized, and the rest [of the *angas*] are all putting your mind on God, concentrating on God. That's where duality ends. Even in

asana there is right side, left side, right way or wrong way—these things can be dualistic. But after *pranayama*, there isn't a right or a wrong, a this or a that, there's just one.

In mastering the asanas, too, there's that overcoming of the sense of duality. That's true. You lose yourself, and there are no extremes as long as breath, movement, and *bandhas* are locked up. Theoretically, if you practice, that stillness is available to you, and that's the essence of nonduality, that stillness. There is no this or that.

It seems that from an early stage what you were looking for was not out there but something internal. It was not a search but just becoming comfortable with the existing reality.
That has to be true. You can't find happiness out there. It's just not out there to find.

It takes a while for people to realize that. Perhaps forever.
It does.

Had you been studying philosophy and yoga before you went to India?
Not at all. Before David, I read exactly one book about yoga, that Richard Hittleman book. It was baby stuff, you know, a little cobra, a little locust, no breathing. You just lie on the floor, maybe do it a couple of times, no counting breaths or anything like that. You'd just hold for ten seconds. It didn't say anything on how to breathe except blow your stomach out when you inhale, you know, balloon breathing: a lot of mistakes. But even that was enough of a teaser. By making my body feel better afterward, it opened me up to more complex stuff. Everybody has to start someplace.

You started with the purely physical as your interest.
Yeah, until after the first time I did the series and I felt that silence ringing in my head and that was *way* different. That was a new thing.

Did that inspire you to study more?
It's addictive and that's the way it works. Nobody would go through that unless it was addictive.

Say something about Guruji, the way he teaches and how he motivates people.
I don't know how he does that, I guess his power precedes him. Any good teacher can motivate his students. Any good teacher can make the student want to please the teacher, because they know that is pleasing themselves. He was exceptionally good at it because of the power he had inherited and accumulated. He was special. He'll be back.

Some people think he had a physical mastery, the ability to understand the body and move it. As far as you are concerned, it seems to be more energetic.
It was energy, I think. He was a good technician. But Manju is a better technician, smoother, fewer injuries, deliberate or unintended, whether it's good for you or not. If you want somebody to make steady progress, you don't have to rip them apart the first time you see them, you can kind of tease them into it. That's each one's dynamic. Manju's just smoother. Guruji was a little rougher but I think, too, he was looking at energy fields instead of the body. What he was seeing wasn't, "If I step on this guy's knee, he's going to scream and he's going to be out of action for a couple of weeks." He was seeing energy circuits—"Oh this needs to go there"—and I believe that sometimes he was not conscious of the physical dynamic at all. That wasn't what he was looking at and that's the way it's supposed to be with a guru. A teacher has to be more aware, because unless you have the psychic cachet to see a person past whatever infirmities they are going to suffer because of your ministrations, unless you have enough voltage to get them through that, you should not be messing with them. Unless you have the power to do that, you can't hurt people. It's against human nature.

You think Guruji acquired that shakti through his asana practice or his connection with Krishnamacharya, or you think he was born with some amazing energy?
It had to be a high birth for him to get where he was going, even to meet up with Krishnamacharya. I think he got the transmission from Krishnamacharya and that upped his voltage. His practice certainly did—that's part of it, too. But any single element—birth, transmission from guru, or practice—any one of those by themselves wouldn't explain the power. It has to be a combination of them all.

How do you understand the transmission of shakti?
You can feel it. You know when it happens. When he gave a mantra, it's a direct conduit, it's accompanied by physical sensation, a coolness. Part of working with the guru in the *asanas* is you can feel heat coming off his hands and electricity, so that's part of it, the direct transmission. When he is telling you something special, some part of this power is being passed to you and that's a special feeling, too, and it can't be mistaken for anything else.

That would be a cumulative thing over a period of time.
I think so. You couldn't handle any amount of direct voltage until you have had a lot of little jolts to purify the conduits. A lot of *nadis* need to be cleaned before they can even carry voltage. One thing that was interesting in our practice in India was that every Saturday would be *neti* day. When I got there he was using his old *neti* string, a really old one, a piece of bicycle valve tube, what we call surgical tubing, but black like bicycle inner tubes are made out of, and one of his old Brahmin threads. He'd double it and roll it on his leg and spiral it real tight, and it felt just like sandpaper—it was, of course, linen. So every Saturday we lined up at his little sink in the yoga *shala* and he would make some of the Indian people come, too. If they were snorting in class or blowing their nose or something, they'd have to come and they were the first in line. We always got there as early as we could because the sink was just cold water. The first time I went there this little Indian kid, I think his dad made him come because he had a kind of asthmatic sound to his breathing, really clogged up, and the kid was practically crying, "No, no," and they were rattling back and forth in Kannada and Guruji was like, "Hey, you get up here!" and the kid is crying and screaming and Guruji says, "Open!" So he puts the tube up the kid's nose and reaches into his mouth to grab it, and "Aargh!" throws up all over Guruji, who jumps back and starts yelling at him. So he does the other side on the kid, and I'm next. "Oh, no, don't worry," [says Guruji] and runs his hand over it like that [to clean off the *neti* string].

Did you ever contract any infections?
A little bit, because they were still burning a lot of dung at that time. A little bit of respiratory congestion.

But not from the string.
No, I never did. That's another sign of great energy. I thought I'd be as
sick as a dog.

Did he teach you any other kriyas?
Nauli. We always did that. Manju was big on *nauli* also.

What was his suggestion about practicing nauli?
He liked it between salutation A and B every day.

Did he say specifically why he was teaching it or how often you should do it?
Manju said every day. Guruji wasn't concerned. It was part of your private function—to make sure that your bowels were moving correctly and
so on. He figured that was not his business, and if you couldn't take care
of that, then what are you doing here, clown? But Manju was pretty specific because it demonstrated that you came prepared, not loaded up
with breakfast at Denny's. That makes sense. It's also good to know you
are as clean as you are going to get before you start delving into your series for the day.

In Yoga Mala, *Guruji says to do* nauli *in* kukkutasana, *which is fairly challenging.*
That sounds interesting. What amazes me is all the *vinyasa* numbers
were there in his first book, the exact method was right there. The Indian
men didn't want to spend hours going through the full *vinyasa* numbers.
It's very time-consuming, takes twice as long as flipping from side to side
with the occasional jump-back. But it's really worth the energy, cuts
down on injuries drastically. The physical benefits are hugely acceler-
ated, the body comes to neutral between every posture at *samasthiti.* If
your back was bent forward before, now it's straightened up again. If it
was bending back before, now you are back in neutral and ready for the
next thing. So the *vinyasa* part is essential to the series and I think that's
why it works so well. Breath with movement. There is no movement
without a breath. There's not one thing you do that doesn't have a number and an inhale or an exhale attached to it. That being the case, there
is no place to chat, stop and scratch yourself, drink from your water
bottle—there's no place to do that. It's one uninterrupted flow. And I

think that's where you really achieve the quiet, where you lose your monkey mind.

Did he teach you the full vinyasa *back to standing?*
Yes. When they first came, David and Nancy learned in class with the Indian people, so they were doing sometimes just side to side with the jump-back between postures. I don't know if they observed the full *vinyasa*. But when David Swenson and Paul Dunaway came back from India—that was just before I left to go there—they had a white people's class, and he taught them that. So when I went I asked to learn that way; in the white people's class, that's the way he taught. I understand they have now abandoned that to some degree, but again, that's probably time constraints. With vast numbers it would be really hard to control. Takes a lot more space, too.

It has struck me more and more over the last few years that what is really being transmitted is energy, heart, or whatever you want to call it. People are able to practice in all these different ways and still receive from Guruji the same essence.
I hope that's true, that it doesn't matter which way you practice. I can only speak from my experience, and I've seen people make their optimum progress with full *vinyasa* in the shortest time.

He seems to have changed and to have taught people in different ways.
Then I feel very fortunate that I got what I got.

Do you have a sense of the origin of the practice?
He would tell the story of the *Yoga Korunta*, written on palm leaves or something like that. Now that's possibly apocryphal, but there are other mentions of the *Yoga Korunta*. I don't know if he saw it or not. I'm sure Krishnamacharya saw it.

The academics tend to believe that the asanas *are a modern invention. There are no pictures—*
Yes, I've heard those skeptics.

Can you say something about the importance of food for the yoga practice?
That's one of the first things that has to change, unless you are already

vegetarian, like David Swenson or Paul Dunaway. Their whole lives. Somehow they were raised in an environment that was vegetarian; that's a sign of a higher birth. That's one of the signs: that you start out with a good diet. If you don't start out that way, it's the teacher's job to give you a little guidance on what's acceptable and what's not, just to get you started. Then you have to do your own research and explore the different methods. One of the seminal pieces of literature that helped me change my diet was Arnold Ehret's *Mucusless Diet Healing System*. It's a really radical thing, and you go through some transitions that are similar to the ones you experience in *asana*. It doesn't always feel good. When you start eliminating some of the residue of past indulgences, it's quite unpleasant. That correlates to the pain you experience as you progress through the different *asanas* and work on clearing different parts of the body. But food is basic, for the beginner at least. The regular practitioner, they should know exactly what they can and can't eat instinctively. They will be able to tell by their practice, so they are guided in that way. For the beginner, it's the teacher's job to give a few clues. If you were having a stiff day, Manju would say, "Oh you had cheese last night." Probably true, too, but after a while, a little cheese won't kill you. You grow into your diet like you grow into your practice. And the same is true with the devotional aspect, the *bhakti*. You need to experience that through a teacher also, to feel the power inherent in worshipping God in song. And that, too, is addictive. It's like we were saying, you feel that upwelling, that's an emotional cleansing, I think. And the tears that come are proof that something is moving. It's not because you are sad or unhappy, it's because it's beautiful.

Do you think bhakti *is important for everybody?*
Everybody is devoted to something. Devotion to money doesn't work very well for most people, as far as bringing happiness. I would say devotion is an important tenet. Guruji was scrupulous about his prayers. He was a big believer. Even when he'd be reciting some *shlokas* and he'd have no book in front of him, he'd recite for a while and you could see his eyes go like he's turning the page in his mind because he'd gone over his little book so many times. It's ingrained, it's part of their Brahmin training. But for him I think it was part of his life. Every day. I don't know how many times a day.

I wonder if it performs a different function or perhaps has an amplifying effect on the asana *practice. Can the* asanas *bring you to a similar place, or does one really need the addition to open the heart?*

I believe it does, because I have seen people who are so good with *asanas*, you know, circus people are great, they can do impossible physical things, but it's not yoga, because the *asana* is posture not just of the body but a mental posture, too. And I think that part, the mental posture, has to go someplace, and that for me is devotion. That leads back to putting your mind on God. It's going to go someplace until you learn to shut it down. So *bhakti* is like the temporary reservoir for that. And for some people that becomes more their practice than the *asana*. That is their meditation. Ramakrishna—there's a great story—his was pure devotion, there was no practice involved. He drank wine until he was silly, sang songs to the Mother—that was his practice.

The beginning of the sadhana pada *says:* tapas, svadhyaya, *and* ishvara-pranidhana. *Three elements are required: purification, study, and devotion. Perhaps the three essential elements of practice.*

Well put.

You mentioned that food brings you pain, but also the practice brings you pain. Is there a way of distinguishing between pain that is caused by incorrect diet and pain that is a by-product of transformation through asanas?

That requires scientific observation and exploration for each person. Once you know what foods are bad for you and you eliminate those from your diet and you do a little sweating and enough work so you are fairly confident that the pain you are feeling isn't all uric acid crystals or whatever, your excuse would be for whatever you ate in the past. In my case, I think that's what it was. In my family, it wasn't a meal unless meat was served. So that required a long period of elimination and the pain during *asanas* was worse. When I had corrected my diet to the point where I felt good with myself, then the pain in the *asanas* got less on the gross level. But it would change and get more severe on the nervous level. It shifts between the bodies [koshas]. First *yoga chikitsa, nadi shodhana,* and *sthira bhaga.* First you have to do the yoga therapy on yourself with the primary series. Then with the *nadi shodhana,* with the intermediate, you are reaming out your nervous system. Then finally with the advanced, *sthira bhaga,* you build strength—not just physical but emotional and spiritual.

I've been pondering how the pranic *body and the physical body are related, and it seems to me that* yoga chikitsa *is very much concerned with the muscles, organs, and circulatory systems, and* nadi shodhana *is concerned with cleaning the* nadis. *Are these* nadis *physical or are they in the* pranic *body?*
I don't think you can dissect a corpse and point to a nerve bundle and call it a *nadi*. It's not like that. It's more like the acupuncture model of the human body, that there are energy channels where the power flows. I'd say it's more the *pranic* body, and for that reason *pranayama* is really important. One thing about *asanas*: we were talking about circus people that are too good to be believed. In many cases like that, the ego grows out of proportion to the amount of spiritual development, so you end up with an egotist instead of a yogi. You should have a baby yogi developing but instead you have a blossoming power tripper. For many teachers, their image is important to them, and that to me demonstrates imbalance.

It's been one of my questions all along: Does advanced practice necessarily imply advanced spiritual development? And does that then imply that those who are only able to do a few surya namaskaras *have less opportunity to have that kind of insight?*
Yep, that's the big quandary. But from my experience your progress in *asana* has only a minor role in your spiritual progress. *Asanas* are the first step, *yama* and *niyama* are much harder than *asana*. But for some people *asana* isn't possible at all, like in Heather [Troud]'s case. That's not to say she couldn't be a spiritual giant. That's not the way it works. The body should be shined up to the best degree possible, as far as you can take it. If you can get to an advanced level, that's wonderful, but it's not vital at all. *Asana* is kindergarten. You are playing, jumping around.

It seems, though, to some extent that yama *and* niyama *naturally happen, they are integrated in the practice in the sense that if you are aggressive and ambitious, you hurt yourself and so you learn how to soften, and if you eat the wrong things, the body becomes impure, and you become aware of that. There's a feedback system that helps you evolve to some extent.*
That's why *ashtanga* yoga, when it's done correctly, is a self-teaching system. All the steps kind of sneak up on you at once. It's not like, I gotta work on this limb today, and next year I'm going to concentrate on that limb. You teach yourself what you need at the time.

What about the bandhas? *Can you say something about them and how Guruji teaches them?*
That was one of the major things about *ashtanga* that grabbed me immediately—how much sense it had. I was really fortunate. On Guruji's first trip to America, his English was pretty pitiful. He explained as best as he could in English, but if he could see you weren't holding *mula bandha* correctly, he had no qualms whatsoever about reaching behind you and just putting a little squeeze on the rectum. The reflex is to pull it tight immediately, to tighten up. When teaching *pranayama*, he was very strict about *uddiyana bandha*. He would have each person sit in front of him and he would press in very hard on that section you need to hold very tight to keep the air locked properly. People who don't do *pranayama* don't understand the importance of *uddiyana bandha* a lot of times. It's locking up the energy so it goes to the right places. That and the chin lock are very important, and using the three together is like playing the piano and using the pedals. To make the music come out properly, it's absolutely vital that some degree of mastery be attained. And it's hard during *asana* because you are moving and shifting position. It's much easier when you are sitting in lotus. Like you were saying, *kukkutasana* would be a great place to practice *nauli* because it's challenging. So after learning *pranayama*, control of the *bandhas* comes more easily during *asana* practice and as you shift position [*vinyasa*]. *Mula bandha* is vital. That's one thing that separates *ashtanga* from most other systems. If you are holding *mula bandha* properly and keep breathing, you can try to pick up a piano. Either you will be able to pick it up or you won't, but the likelihood of hurting yourself is very slim. It's a protective device; it prevents hernia and all manner of displacement of organs. It's vital. The system wouldn't work without it, and teachers who don't concentrate on it are not doing their students a favor. Their students will progress in spite of the lack of knowledge, but it will be nothing like the pace they could achieve if they had a little instruction. It's the cornerstone of the practice, really.

What is your understanding of Guruji's teaching with the mula bandha? *Is it just a contraction of the anal sphincter, or is it the perineum?*
It's a pulling up rather than a squeezing close. It's not exactly like fighting off a bowel movement. I think it's pulling up, yes, in the region of the perineum.

I asked him about ashwini mudra, *which is the action of pulling up on the anus, and he said absolutely not, so that would imply that it's farther forward.*
Yeah.

Everyone seems to have their own opinions. I found him giving instructions in uddiyana bandha *in primary series. For instance, in* utthita hasta padangushtasana, *he's emphasizing squeezing with the hand at the waist. Also in* prasarita padottanasana B, *again squeezing the belly with the hand. I've seen that a number of times, and repeatedly emphasized.*
He's big on that. That's an important part of that posture.

It must be the combination of the two, and generally he doesn't speak about it very much, does he? If he does, it's more about mula bandha *rather than* uddiyana bandha, *except, as you said, in* pranayama *class. A lot of people read Swami Satyananda Saraswati's book,* Moola Bandha: The Master Key.
That is a great book. He's a cool guy.

I also thought it interesting that Guruji would not say, "Contract your anus," he would say, "Control your anus," which to me has a much greater implication. What about Guruji as a healer? Do you see him as a healer?
I wasn't really there for some of the research he did with diabetes and various other aliments. I've seen the system work wonders with scoliosis. I don't know how much of that was in his healing powers or just in the efficacy of the series, but he was quite remarkable. He could have been a great doctor, too. Well, he was a doctor, just not of medicine but of yoga therapy. He didn't deal a lot with sick people. He could have, but that's very time-consuming and you have to be on that mission. He chose to bring it instead to people who were basically starting out in good health, they just needed a little tuning up. That's the way he was able to reach so many people. If he would have concentrated on the healing of diseases, his output would have been much more limited because it's more time-consuming, progress is slower.

He did work a lot therapeutically, particularly in the earlier years, in the Ayurvedic College.
He was an expert. I missed that part of his work. He never talked much about it. He spent so much time in so many schools.

It's easy to forget that he had a whole life before we even met him. You observed him working with Heather. Can you describe that?

Her mom would bring her to class and he would carry her up the stairs and lay her out on the floor. Then Guruji would just go through a whole range of motions. He would move every part of her body just like physical therapists do today, move her legs back and forth, work all the joints, work her feet, walk on her hands, because you know how they tend to curl up a little bit, all the limbs do with disuse. And he would do it for about an hour, go over every part of her body, probe really deeply at all the organs, work on her spine. I think that's where he was mainly using his energy instead of a physical application because there was nothing that could be corrected physically, it was more in the *pranic* body, and for that he used the more delicate energy. It was amazing to watch, like a very good physical therapist combined with a natural healer, almost a faith healer.

What about humor? Guruji's quite a funny man.

He was. He cracked me up. He was quite the joker; he loved to laugh. We would take walks and he would point out different plants. There was this really common weed. "That one very good for teeth." "Yeah? That's good for your teeth? What do you do with it?" "Rub on teeth, shining white!" So I was, okay I'll try it. Picked it up, rubbed it on my teeth. It was the worst thing I ever tasted, just sickening, like echinacea, the way it tingles in your mouth, but worse. It had little thorns or something like that that stuck in my gums. Guruji was, "Good? Good?" He thought it was funny. He was quite a character. He and Manju laughed a lot together. And Amma, she was just sparkly, she was very witty. Manju got a lot of her sense of humor, too.

What do you see as the role of humor in teaching yoga?

If you don't laugh, you'll end up crying. Even when dealing with people, if you don't keep a light touch about it, they can really get you down. So a little humor goes a long way.

Most people end up crying at some point in the yoga practice.

That's true. I did. Usually after, when I was trying to get into the bathtub. Crawling in.

As we used to leave the shala, *there was a lady who cooked for us, Na-garathna, perhaps after your time. These healthy Westerners used to come to the* shala *and then we used to just stagger out and limp over to her place for breakfast. A trail of us at dawn, the sun was rising and one was holding a hip, another a knee, the other a shoulder.*
March of the invalids.

Any special memories of Mysore?
David and I had the same experience; he used to talk to me about it. He'd be sleeping and then in the middle of the night he would wake up and say to Nancy as she was stirring, "What posture are you on?" *"Janu shirshasana* C." "Well I'm way ahead of you, I'm on *marichyasana* D." We were just dreaming of it, it went so deep. The intensity of it, that was special.

What would you say is the most important thing that you learned from Guruji and the practice?
Persistence. Just keep at it, just do it even when you don't feel the same eagerness that you felt the day before. Just get up and do it again, for as long as you want to.

Anything you want to add?
No messages to the universe from me, just keep on doing it. I don't know if this is really the descent into *Kali Yuga*. You've heard all the theories, like that there are another 428,000 years to go into *Kali Yuga*. I'm not sure. I pray for a hopeful outcome for the world. I see things getting minutely better, and Guruji is partly responsible for that. He certainly reached a significant percentage of the population. Before him, what was there? This turned into a big movement because of him. Bless his name.

Maui, 2009

Tim Miller

Tim Miller started practicing with Brad Ramsey and Gary Lopedota in 1978 in Encinitas and met Guruji soon after, on Guruji's second trip to the United States. Tim traveled to Mysore many times, and took over Brad and Gary's school when they moved to Hawaii. He continues to live and teach in Encinitas and also travels and teaches widely.

What first attracted you to ashtanga *yoga?*
I was fortunate when I moved to Encinitas in 1976 that it was the one place in America that *ashtanga* yoga was being taught. It took me a little over a year to discover it, but I lived half a block from an *ashtanga* yoga center when it opened up early in 1978.

I happened to be walking down the street one day and saw an old church that had been vacant since I'd moved into the neighborhood. It had been freshly painted and the yard had been cleaned up; there was a new sign out front that said ASHTANGA YOGA NILAYAM and a picture of a dancing hermaphrodite. I said, "Well, this looks interesting." And there was a gentleman standing in the yard doing something, I think he was eating blades of grass or something like that.

So I stopped and started chatting with him and he started telling me about the yoga, saying that it was a very rare and powerful form of yoga that was taught only in a couple of places in the world and that in two months he would make me as limber as a gymnast. So I asked him about the class times and came back, I believe it was the next day, to an early-evening class.

I was working at the time at a psychiatric hospital and had had a little exposure to yoga during my college years. Based on that limited experience, I was teaching a yoga class to the psychiatric patients. Realizing that I really knew very little about yoga I thought it would be a good idea to try a yoga class. Discovering this place seemed fortuitous.

It was a rather primitive setup. There was no electricity in the building so when I arrived it was dark inside and people were lighting candles. A gentleman walked over to me and asked if I was there to take some classes. I wasn't really dressed for it. I was wearing a pair of jeans and a flannel shirt and I thought I was just going to come in and watch, so to sound noncommittal, I said, "Well, I guess so." Not really meaning then, at that moment.

He said, "Okay, well come on over here." So I went over there and he started showing me *surya namaskara*, which I was doing in my flannel shirt and blue jeans and so I proceeded to become very hot and wet within in a few *namaskaras*. Anyway, he took me through roughly the first half of the primary series in that first day.

It was quite a mind-blowing experience. It took me to a place that felt very familiar, very deep, peaceful, like something that perhaps I'd done before or something that I definitely wanted to be doing again. I was hooked from day one on the practice and kept coming. That was early in 1978.

How did you become interested in studying with Pattabhi Jois?
I was working with a couple of American teachers who had been students of his son, Manju. I had been studying with them for seven or eight months. And they raised enough money to fly Pattabhi Jois and his wife, Amma, over. He taught right there at this little church for three or four months back in 1978. He was the big guru. I'd been reading books about Eastern philosophy and whatnot, masters of the Far East, and had heard stories about this man. I thought that when he arrived he would sort of materialize in the center of the room in a ball of light or something.

When he opened the door in black loafers and white shirt and glasses he looked quite ordinary, but then when he came into the room and started to teach, it was obvious that he wasn't ordinary at all. So again, it was just fortuitous that I was in the right place at the right time when he came there. That was his second trip to America and to Encinitas.

So how was studying with Guruji at that time?
When I first studied with Guruji in '78 his command of English was

fairly limited and these first couple of trips to the States he was teaching all Mysore style. This was a fairly good-size room and there were probably thirty to thirty-five people who were all practicing Mysore style at the same time. He was trying to cover such a large room with so many students, so his proximity to you would inspire 200 percent in the *asana* for fear of being adjusted.

He was quite a powerful man at that time. He was in his early sixties and his adjustments were quite strong. Although he had a good sense of humor and seemed quite light he still inspired a certain amount of terror when he came close by.

I was just learning the second series at the time and after classes, after *shavasana*, he would arrange those people who were doing second series or beyond in a big circle and teach us *pranayama*.

The first time he sat with us in a circle and took his shirt off, took that first deep breath and kept expanding his chest like a bullfrog, like Dizzy Gillespie's cheeks when he plays the trumpet, he gave us a rather radical introduction to *pranayama*: long retentions of the breath, lots of trembling and sweating. He was also teaching theory classes at Manju's house three times a week.

Because of his limited command of English, he was a little difficult to understand, but Manju acted as his interpreter. He would go on quoting scripture and laughing and crying and on and on for several minutes then he would turn to Manju for the translation and Manju would give us, you know, ten words. Obviously, we were missing a little bit in the translation!

On that first trip we didn't really get to know each other very well. There were a lot of students, old students who had worked with him on his first trip to the States a couple of years before. David Williams and his crew of people from Maui were all there.

I continued with the practice and then, in 1980, he spent a couple of months in Maui, and I went there and worked with him. It wasn't until early in 1982 that I was able to save enough money to make that first trip to Mysore. By that time I'd been doing the practice for four years and had already learned the first three series. It was when I went to India that we really got to know each other for the first time.

How was the yoga shala *in Mysore different then?*
Being there was just a much more intimate experience. There were very

few foreign students, maybe three or four at different times. Part of the time I was the only foreign student in the class. But I also met Norman Allen there at that time, who was Guruji's first American student.

It was obviously quite different from the situation now, when there are seventy to seventy-five students and a long queue to get into the room. His focus was on teaching his Indian students, many of whom had been referred by their physicians for various medical problems: heart problems, diabetes, asthma—conditions like that.

So they weren't the young strong athletic types like the Westerners who came to practice.
They were generally older and not necessarily that fit. Also, their approach to the yoga was—how can I say this kindly—maybe not as exacting as the Western students have come to practice it. They would move fairly quickly through the poses, and they were all busy, getting it in before they went to work, a different situation than us Westerners, who, basically, practiced and then had the rest of the day to recover before we came back and did it again.

I stayed three months. We had a nice rapport and I had an amazing experience in India just shedding layers, and I was convinced after that experience that I should teach yoga. I asked Guruji at the end of my time there if he would be willing to give me a teaching certificate. He kind of hemmed and hawed and finally agreed to do that. I was unaware at the time that he had never given a teaching certificate to a Westerner before, so I didn't quite realize the significance of that event until some time later.

Did he give you an examination?
The certificate actually states that I passed public examination, and the only thing that was something like an examination was a yoga exhibition at the Lion's Club in Mysore in '82. It was long and involved many lectures and a yoga demonstration consisting of Indian students, men and women separately.

Guruji's daughter, Saraswathi, did a little demonstration. Norman and his girlfriend, Purna, did a demonstration. I came out and did the whole third with Guruji talking me through the whole thing. He was pacing me through the *vinyasa* very quickly. He would say the name of the *asana*, count it out, and I would have to follow all the way through in front of three hundred or so Indian people. So I guess that may have constituted my public examination.

So you would say the atmosphere today, the energy in the room, is quite different than what it was before?
Yeah, the energy in the yoga *shala* today is decidedly different than it was then, just through the Western influence. It's the Western students who have brought out the best in Guruji as far as presenting the teachings and the way they were intended to be. The Western students, since they can devote all their energy to practicing the yoga, can be quite zealous in their practice. It's much different than the way I saw the Indians practicing when I first came.

I often hear Guruji say he teaches real, or original, ashtanga *yoga, Patanjali* yoga. *What's your impression of him or experience of him as a teacher of true yoga?*
He's probably the last of a vanishing breed of teachers of traditional yoga. He really seems to carry the energy of Shiva, that energy of both annihilation and creation. There's this mixture of love and fear that I've always connected to him. I know when I work with him that I'm going to be transformed and it'll bring stuff up. And yet the love that I have for him instills a certain amount of trust in the process, in his wisdom and in his ability to guide me through that process.

You talked about shedding layers during your first experience in India. To what extent is Guruji instrumental in that process?
Guruji makes it clear that it's the practice itself that's important and that he's just the channel through which the practice flows. He's not there to do it for you. Whatever transformation you work out is a result of your own practice and work and discovery.

How important is it to have a teacher? What is Guruji's role in the process of transformation?
It's very important to have someone who knows the authentic techniques of yoga and who can impart them accurately and systematically and intelligently, compassionately. Without that, you're just sort of scrambling in a mishmash of techniques that don't necessarily meld together to formulate some sort of integrated process.

On my first trip to India, in particular, oftentimes after practice, lying in *shavasana*, I would feel certain emotions surfacing. Sometimes I would just sit there and weep, not in a dramatic way, tears would just be running down my face and it was incredibly purifying and powerful. I would get up after and go out in the streets and feel almost as if I was transparent or something. Things were just moving through me, and somehow a great sense of spaciousness had been created inside me.

Do you feel that Guruji was just somebody who gave you the techniques and you did the work? Or was he a motivator in some way?
He's definitely a powerful motivator as well. He's a master at extracting as much from people as they're able to give. He has an incredible work ethic that he adheres to, which has always been very inspiring as a yoga teacher to look to as an example.

Could you describe his work ethic?
He's just an extremely hardworking man, motivated by his deep love for yoga.

What would his typical day be? When does he get up? When does he finish?
I had the opportunity to be a guest in his home that first time in India. I would get up about four thirty in the morning and would creep outside my room and see Guruji sitting in the living room on his deerskin doing *pranayama*, right about four thirty. He wouldn't ordinarily take a hot bath, a cold bath was fine for him, but knowing I was a Westerner and used to hot water, he would go down and build a little fire in the cistern so I could have hot water in the morning.

At that time he didn't have the same number of Western students that he does now. He had more Indian students. They would begin to arrive at four thirty in the morning, and he would just work straight through until whenever the last batch was finished, then oftentimes do his own laundry or whatever, all that stuff, like take a bath or do an elaborate *puja*, and maybe finally he'd get around to taking a meal at two or three o'clock in the afternoon.

I knew when mealtimes were because, when I was staying with him, I would sit there dying of hunger wondering when lunch was going to be and often it wouldn't be until very late. His willingness to give his own strength and energy to work with people in the poses has lessened somewhat over the years. In the old days, if one couldn't get oneself into a position, Guruji would get you in there himself. It's always amazing to watch him, especially working in a guided class. His incredible enthusiasm and energy in adjusting people coaxes them to extract more from themselves.

Would you see him as an example of a moral, ethical person in the way he lived his life?
There's the work ethic, which has always been very inspiring, his devotion to his family, his devotion to his spiritual practice, his *puja*, his teaching, his humility, his sincerity. There's a lot of misconceptions floating around out there that gurus are somehow not expected to be human in some way. But his humanity is a great example. He likes things that are very human, you know. He likes money, for one thing. He makes no bones about the fact that he enjoys being prosperous, although that prosperity has arrived rather late in his life. He enjoys reading the newspaper, he enjoys watching TV, he's very human, which is nice.

How significant is it that this lineage of teachers are householders?
Guruji's emphasis has always been to lead a balanced life, and that the life of the householder is the life best suited to most of us and that the life of the renunciant is suited to only a small fraction of people. Certainly, if yoga is to have some sort of impact in the world, we need to be *in* the world, not off in a cave somewhere. He's a shining example of that and the dharma of sharing the practice with people.

Every one of his children and grandchildren practice yoga, and they were taught by him. Was Amma also taught by Guruji?
Amma, Guruji's wife, was one of his first students. She was terrified of him. I think she was thirteen or fourteen when they got married, and apparently she barely spoke to him for the first year of their marriage. I think he was quite demanding as a yoga teacher. He was in his early twenties at the time and the only example of a yoga teacher he had was Krishnamacharya, who from all accounts was very stern and strict. It was probably the only way he knew how to teach at the time.

How important did Amma become in Guruji's teaching and in supporting him?

I think Amma was all-important as the support structure all during Guruji's life. She stayed in the background, cooked for him and took care of him and also advised him. She was an extremely intelligent woman whose advice he often sought. She was the real power behind the throne. She called the shots to some extent.

How would you describe the ashtanga vinyasa *system that Guruji teaches?*
The *vinyasa* system of *ashtanga* yoga has always been very attractive to me because, I think, of the element of breath and movement together. Breath initiates movement. Movement seems to deepen the breath, and the *ujjayi* breathing adds the audio quality to the breath; the *vinyasa* adds a kind of choreography to the breath. For myself, the breath has always been the main focus of the practice.

Of all the different styles of yoga I've been exposed to over the years, this one seems to be the most breath-oriented. Breath certainly seems to be the core of yoga. Other yoga classes I've taken that don't really focus on breath don't seem to work at nearly as deep a level. Breath is something that really opens up the internal space; it takes you to new places.

How is Guruji's teaching different in Mysore than abroad?
Guruji's teaching in Mysore is, of course, what we refer to as Mysore-style teaching, which means that each student is practicing independently at his own level whether it be first series, second series, or third series, and learning new poses one *asana* at a time as they begin to approximate the poses that come before. In the States, except for the two visits when he was teaching Mysore style, he'll do a conducted class, which I assume is the way he used to teach when he taught at the Sanskrit College when he was teaching large groups of students with the traditional counting, "*Ekam* inhale, *dve* exhale, *trini* inhale." It's a different experience where everyone is doing the same thing at the same time. There's a certain group energy that is cultivated out of that; it's quite powerful. Both ways are good and valuable. I've had the good fortune to spend a lot of time with him when he's teaching in the States, and to assist him in many of the conducted classes and to learn through assisting him to teach that way myself. It's been very valuable for me.

What was it like to be his assistant?
First of all, it's always been a great privilege and honor. There's a certain

art, when you're used to conducting the class yourself, to taking the background role, to being a support person, just to look and see where you're needed and go and adjust the people that need the help. In a sense it's easier to work that way because you're not concerned about pacing the class and counting the *vinyasas*. It's also been a great opportunity to learn about adjusting. Working with him in that setting, watching him adjust ten or fifteen people in a row in *marichyasana* D, you begin to pick up certain techniques and to appreciate the mechanics of why he adjusts the way he does.

Was he quite particular about how he wanted you to adjust people or did he give you free rein?
I was always quite observant of the way he worked with people and I think he would watch me. He never really criticized or corrected me, which I guess was an indication that he was satisfied with the way I was working with people.

What would you say is the essence of Guruji's teaching?
There are a few things that come to mind. One is the element of *tapas*—of purification through a fiery ordeal—that certainly we all have a lot of purification that is necessary, but to go through that process in an atmosphere of support and love and humor. Doing the practice intensely takes you to some interesting places, not all of them good but all of them educational. Even though he's a tough guy and he makes you work very hard, I've always gotten the feeling from him that he's right there with you. He's very generous in his support and very loving and very interested in each student.

You talked about techniques, but at the same time it's a spiritual practice. Can it be both a technique and a spiritual practice? What is the relationship between those two things?
Yoga is a scientifically based technology that gives us certain techniques by which we can awaken or uncover our inherent spirituality. The idea is that we are inherently spiritual but that there are perceptual blocks to our realization of that. I look at yoga as a way of removing the obstacles to a perception of our true essence.

It's what Patanjali talks about in *The Yoga Sutras: yogas chitta vritti nirodhah*—yoga is the cessation of the fluctuations of consciousness. When that happens then: *Tada drashthu svarupe avasthanam*—then the true nature of the seer, the inner being is revealed. So yoga is all about techniques for removing the blocks to our true perception of ourselves. It's a scientific method for the realization of the fact that we are spiritual beings. In that sense it's obviously a spiritual practice.

One of the principles that Guruji emphasizes again and again is the second sutra. Do you have any perception as to why or how it actually happens? And would you say that ashtanga *yoga, with* vinyasa, *works particularly well for controlling the mind?*
The technique of *ashtanga* yoga has worked well for me. I've dabbled with other schools of yoga just to get a sense of what they were about. Some styles emphasize the techniques, you know, the biomechanics of yoga. And it was interesting and I certainly learned some things.

But for actually working toward the state of yoga, that state of cessation of fluctuation of consciousness, *ashtanga* yoga has been the most effective path for me. I think the reason is the element of breath, how breath is emphasized in the practice, that breath is the real connection to consciousness. Breath, in a sense, is the vehicle of consciousness. Many of the techniques of *ashtanga* yoga are oriented around breath: how to make our breathing a more conscious process. We add the audio quality with the *ujjayi* breath, we add a kind of choreography to breath with *vinyasa*, we have the idea of an energetic root of the breath with the concept of *bandhas*. Using the breath as the main focus seems to be a very powerful technique for stilling the mind. I've found that practice influences my consciousness much more strongly than other things that I've done.

The other aspect that Guruji emphasizes is prayer, devotion to God. Personally, I've always found it very difficult, but I think a lot of people find it difficult because we don't have that connection with God in the West that is so immediate in India.
Guruji often says that *ashtanga* yoga is Patanjali yoga, and in the second chapter of *The Yoga Sutras*, the chapter on practice [*Sadhana Pada*], in the first sutra, Patanjali gives us three crucial ingredients for success in our yoga practice. The first thing he mentions is *tapas*, literally meaning

to burn, to burn away impurities. Through *tapas* one purifies the *indriyas*, the organs of perception, which lends itself to a greater capacity for discrimination and self-reflection.

The second aspect is *svadhyaya* [self-inquiry], and he says, through self-inquiry we come to recognize what he calls the *ishta devata*—our personal deity, our own individual connection to some aspect of the divine that we can come to know through self-inquiry. The predecessor to that is the process of purification. So it's a process of physical purification and then mental purification through self-inquiry which ultimately leads to the realization that you have help from unseen forces. There is an energy or entity referred to as Ishvara, that universal internal teacher, who exists and is there for us if we're receptive to the guidance coming in.

The last part of that equation is *ishvarapranidhana*—literally, bowing to God or recognizing in awe and humility that there is a timeless eternal teacher working on our behalf, and that a way of connecting to that teacher is through the lineage of yoga teachers. As we begin the practice we say, "*vande gurunam charanaravinde*"—I bow to the lotus feet of the gurus, the lineage of teachers who've passed down this knowledge as a way of embracing the living teaching to help connect us with this timeless universal teacher: *Ishvara*. This is what they called Shiva in Mysore.

They say that humility attracts the divine and egotism repels it. The problem we as Westerners have is we are reluctant to surrender the ego. I remember having a conversation with Joel Kramer about this. He wrote a whole book about the guru/disciple relationship, *The Guru Papers*. His point of view is that you should never surrender to another human being. I said, "Why not?" And he says, "Why surrender?" I said, "Just to see what's on the other side of surrender. If you never surrender, you never go there, you never find out what is on the other side of surrender."

My first experience with this was soon after I first met Guruji. After class I would watch some of the older students go and do the traditional gesture of touching his feet. Traditionally, touching the feet three times and applying the dust of the guru's feet to the eyelids was a way of taking the understanding of the guru and using that to further your own awakening. I was kind of put off by it initially, as most Westerners are.

Then one day I was feeling a bit more vulnerable, and perhaps more grateful, and I went and clumsily attempted to do what I saw other people doing. As I touched Guruji's feet, I just felt an overwhelming emotion of gratitude engulf me, and I looked up at Guruji and he was just beaming down at me and he patted me on the shoulder and said, "Oh, very good, very good." It was like, "Ah, you're starting to get it." That's when I began to figure out why surrender works.

What is the value of daily practice: day in, day out, twenty years, thirty years? What is the inner quality produced by long-term practice?
My experience of practicing yoga now for about twenty-three years is that it keeps me connected to a process that is life-giving, light-giving, and health-giving. The rewards of yoga are tangible and immediate, and especially in the beginning. Staying connected to the practice for me just ensures that this evolutionary process continues to unfold itself in some kind of organic way, creating greater health, greater wealth, greater possibility, greater opportunity, greater things.

It's one of Guruji's favorite sayings.
"Do your practice and all is coming." Yes, it's true. I think it's very important for people to develop patience in the process. Things may not come at quite the speed that people would like them to come and oftentimes people become attached to the physical progress in the poses, using that as sort of yardstick to measure how well they're doing in the practice. I suppose everyone goes through that phase at some point, and maybe some people never get out of that phase.

For me it's been a long process of recognizing the value of the *yamas* and the *niyamas*, the process of making yoga real in my life, how it affects my relationships with other people, my relationship with myself. You're only on the mat for, at best, a couple of hours a day. What are you doing the rest of the time? You can't practice yoga for two hours and then go out and act like a jerk the rest of the time. I mean, I suppose you could and people do, but I can't see the point in that. Ultimately, one needs to—especially if one's a teacher—one needs to set some sort of example.

I was going to ask you about the more subtle aspects of the practice and whether they're in some way integrated into the asana *practice. Does one naturally evolve from the* asana *practice to the more subtle aspects of yoga?*
Well, that's the way it's supposed to work, doing a physical practice lends itself to refining one's awareness of the rest of the limbs. I can't say it al-

ways works that way in people. Yoga is about cultivating awareness, and you begin with something very tangible—your own body, cultivating awareness with that. That's a way of doing self-inquiry. You know, you put yourself through a variety of *asanas*. The *asanas* could be seen as metaphors for the varying situations we encounter in life.

You put yourself in a challenging situation and you summon as much poise, as much steadiness and relaxation as you can under the circumstances, and that's incredibly good training for life, but there's got to be some carryover. The *asana* is not an end in itself. It's just a training ground as a way of training the body, training the mind so you can use those skills in other aspects of your life.

How are the other angas *related to* asana *practice?*
All the limbs of yoga are interrelated. They're all designed to lend themselves to the experience of unity or oneness. In *The Yoga Sutras*, Patanjali did not arbitrarily come up with certain injunctions for behavior. He says: try these things, try acting in a nonviolent way, try telling the truth, try not stealing, try being moderate in your actions, try being generous, and I think you'll find that it lends itself to a greater experience of unity in the world. Try the opposite behavior and see what happens. I think you'll find that [following the injunctions] lends itself to that experience of oneness. Be clean, be content, be self-disciplined, be self-observant, be reverent to the divine, and it all lends itself to a greater experience of oneness.

Guruji is fond of saying that the first four limbs of *ashtanga* yoga are extremely difficult and the last four limbs are very easy. If we provide ourselves with a strong foundation in *asana* and *pranayama* and in our own ethical behavior, then the rest of the limbs will gradually evolve out of that foundation. He seems to think that certain of the limbs of yoga can be taught, and some can only be caught. One of the criticisms I hear of *ashtanga* yoga is that there is so much emphasis on *asana*. Why only *asana*, only one limb? There are seven more limbs. Again, we're working with something tangible, something that has brought ramifications in other spheres of life.

How do you think Guruji would articulate the most important aspects of yoga practice?

Guruji would say the most important aspect of practice is to do it and to do it in a traditional manner. He's a traditionalist.

Can you explain what tradition means as far as yoga is concerned?
As far as the physical method of practice, that there's a certain beginning, middle, and end to practice. There's a certain way that things are sequenced and there are valid scientific reasons and energetic reasons behind that and it doesn't work as well to take just a little of this and a little of that and mix it all together.

One of the things we're attempting to do in the yoga practice is to soften the *samskaras*, the impressions which are a result of our prior experience that cause us to be who we are. Not that all of these are negative; some of these are quite positive, but the *samskaras* make us behave in certain prescribed ways, to think in certain prescribed ways, and for our bodies to be certain ways. If we start creating our own practice, I think the danger is that we come up with something that reinforces the existing structure of *samskaras* rather than something that tries to mollify that or soften it to create the possibility of change.

What is Guruji's essential teaching and on what authority does this practice rest?
The proof is in the pudding. With yoga practice, it's not like we're asked to accept something on faith or on belief: Try this and see what your experience is. It's experiential. You do the practice and you have an experience. It's designed to be self-reinforcing. The experience is greater awareness of something. And if we want greater awareness, then we keep going; if we don't, then we stop.

Guruji always says 99 percent practice, 1 percent theory. What is the theory?
Guruji is fond of saying that yoga is 99 percent practice and 1 percent theory, but he's often happy to expound on the theoretical part of yoga. I think it's a reaction to different schools of yoga he considered to be too much in the intellect, with no real focus on practice. People love to talk about yoga because it's an interesting subject, but talking about yoga doesn't really do much for you other than exercise the intellect. There are branches of yoga that have omitted *asana* or *pranayama* and they say,

well, these are crude aspects of yoga, let's just keep what's refined. Let's just meditate; this is the real yoga.

Have you had the experience of Guruji demonstrating this to you? There must have been times when you were questioning, but at the same time there are moments in one's practice where you're right up against a consciousness-changing reality.

I'm not the kind of person who questions things so much in life. From day one, I've always had an incredible faith in the practice because I felt the tangible results, and I think I realized fairly early on that yoga is really about self-reliance and maybe the best thing you can do to the guru is to make him obsolete at a certain point. The best thing you can do is take the tools that he's given you and use them. And you have to work out your own process of self-realization. I mean, it's fun to ask questions, but I'm the kind of person who always wanted to answer my own questions.

Has Guruji transmitted something to you in a nonverbal way? For instance, when you touched his feet and felt overwhelmed by the experience? Have you had moments with Guruji where he's made you aware of something in a very dramatic way?

Certainly I've had the experience of being adjusted in *asana*. [*Laughter*] I've experienced a considerable amount of pain and that created some sort of internal experience that led me to a different place. But you know, there's nothing that really stands out. For me, Guruji is just a very steady, shining example of the power of yoga. I'm like Guruji in a way; I'm a plodding sort of a person. I get into a routine and I just continue if it's working for me. They say if you want to find the water you dig one deep well. Don't dig many shallow holes. I've found something that works for me and I've kept at it and am certainly extremely grateful to have a presentation of this lineage to work with.

Would you say his teaching has changed over the years?

Small changes have occurred over the years in Guruji's teaching: some in regards to sequencing, some additions, and some rearrangements of the advanced sequences since I first learned them twenty years ago. Now in Mysore what I see most is that, since there are so many people, they get a little less in terms of the adjustments and also the intensity of adjustments seems to be less, which again might be related to the number of people there. Although he is still quite a strong man for eighty-four years, he's not as strong as he once was. He also has the capable help of his grandson, Sharath, now, which is great. Not too much change, a little bit.

How do you incorporate Guruji's teaching in the way that you teach?
When I teach a conducted class, the main thing I've learned from Guruji is pacing, that there's a certain rhythm that the practice needs to be done at. Without the proper rhythm there's not the necessary heat built up, not the necessary flow that keeps people involved in their own breath. In terms of the Mysore classes, I've learned a lot from him about adjusting—not that I adjust in exactly the same way in all the poses. I see where his emphasis is in his adjustments. Basically, he's very oriented in his adjustments to opening the joints and muscles. Tendons and things like that become secondary.

How is practicing different from teaching?
When I first started teaching, the biggest challenge was to try to present something that had been imparted to me in a nonverbal way in a verbal way. I've learned from Guruji over the years through the "you do" method. Sometimes he would demonstrate an *asana*. He rarely does that anymore. Most often, he would give the name of the *asana* and you would figure it out as best you could. If you didn't figure it out correctly, he would physically adjust you. So I guess the main challenge in teaching Western students, a lot of whom have been used to yoga classes with detailed explanations of what to do moment to moment, is to try to retain the right-brain essence of *ashtanga* yoga, breath-oriented and flow-oriented, yet at the same time give people verbal cues to follow if they are not kinesthetically oriented.

In your experience as a practitioner and teacher, can you say how ashtanga *affects people? Does it change people's lives?*
Ashtanga yoga definitely changes people's lives if they stick with it. Almost always in my experience for the better. There's a certain primeval quality to it. There's light and goodness in the practice and one associates with that over a period of time. It tends to manifest in your life—greater health and happiness and feelings of personal satisfaction and so on. It seems to affect different people differently. As Guruji says, "The effect of the yoga has much to do with the person's *samskaras*"—the ten-

dencies they've brought into this lifetime from their accumulated experience from other lifetimes. Some people will see it right away as a spiritual practice; for some perhaps it will always be a physical practice. Either way, it's still going to be a beneficial practice.

What is the difference between an injury and an opening?
With an injury, there's usually some feeling of being set back. That there's tissue—connective tissue, usually—that's been damaged in some way, overstretched or torn, and when such a thing happens the body responds usually by contracting as a protective response to allow healing to take place. An opening is something that will accelerate your practice. An injury is something that will slow it down—not that injuries can't be very educational. Normally injuries happen if the person gets inattentive in the practice, or perhaps too ambitious. Sometimes, unfortunately, it's the teacher who gets too ambitious or inattentive. Or sometimes one part of the body will try to compensate for another part of the body that is stiff by overstretching, and it's not sufficiently open in a particular posture, so that can teach you something.

Is ashtanga *a standardized form or an individualized practice?*
Ashtanga yoga is a standardized form, but I think there's also a lot of leeway for adaptation to specific individuals. If you work with people on an individual basis, either privately or in a Mysore-style format, you can give each person a certain amount of individual attention and take into account things like age or physical condition or existing injuries or whatnot. I think it's both—standardized and adaptable.

What is the relationship between ashtanga *yoga as taught by Pattabhi Jois and the* ashtanga *yoga of Patanjali in* The Yoga Sutras?
The *ashtanga* yoga taught by Pattabhi Jois he refers to often as Patanjali yoga. He says, "This is Patanjali yoga." What he has said in the past is that certain aspects of yoga can be taught, certain aspects of yoga can only be caught. *Ashtanga* yoga is self-teaching to a large degree, and you need to begin the practice with something very tangible, like your own body, and work from there. Learn to apply awareness to your body, to your breath, to your gaze, and whatnot. And then, hopefully, those techniques of observation and attention will carry over into other aspects of your life, in how you relate to the world around you, which is what the

yamas are all about, and in what kind of a relationship you have with yourself, which would be the *niyamas*. Certainly *asana* and *pranayama* will prepare you to enter meditative states of awareness.

Do you see this as a spiritual practice?
Absolutely. That was apparent to me from day one. In the first chapter of *The Yoga Sutras*, Patanjali first gives the definition of yoga: *"Yogas chitta vritti nirodhah"*—yoga is a cessation of the fluctuation of the mind. Then he goes on: *"Tada· drashthu svarupe avasthanam"*—then the seer is unveiled in its true form. I had something of that experience in the very first class that I took. Through the practice my mind really shut off, and underneath the mind there was just this presence that felt more like me than anything else. This was the seer, that grounded being that was my essential Self and I suppose it could be referred to as the spiritual Self.

Could you say something about Guruji's relationship with Sharath, and how they work together?
The first time I came to Mysore, Sharath was about nine years old. And Guruji would try to get him to do yoga, but Sharath was really not interested. He was much more interested in playing cricket in the streets with his buddies. It wasn't until quite a number of years later, when Sharath was maybe nineteen or twenty, that he seemed to be ready to devote himself to the yoga and began assisting in the classes with the Western students.

In the beginning, he was not very skilled. He was struggling to find his way. There were a lot of Western students who had been coming for a long time who had much more experience in the practice than he did, and he recognized that. And so he learned a lot from those people because he was open to feedback about his adjustments. We would help him with his adjustments. We'd say, "Try this." Over the years I've seen him gain experience, knowledge, and confidence in himself. That's really quite beautiful to see, and his relationship with his grandfather is really quite beautiful.

Manju, Guruji's eldest son, ended up moving to the U.S. He was the heir apparent in inheriting the yoga *shala*. That didn't happen. The younger son, Ramesh, tragically died. So it's wonderful that Sharath has stepped into place to continue the legacy. They seem to have a wonderful relationship. Sharath seems to grow in stature every time I see him. He's become quite a good teacher in his own right.

You seem quite close to Guruji and his family, since you've been coming to Mysore for so many years. Can you say something about Amma passing away and how you perceived Guruji through that period?

The first time I came to Mysore in 1982, I had the privilege of staying in their house for a month or so. My bedroom was Guruji's office, which was also the changing room, grain-storage room, multipurpose room. It was quite an honor to be invited to stay. Not being a Brahmin, I wasn't allowed to eat with the family, so they would bring my meals to my room. Sharath and his sister, Shammie, would sit with me while I ate. Also, they would eat at what I thought were odd times of the day. I would practice very early in the morning, be finished by nine o'clock, and they oftentimes would not have had their first meal of the day until three o'clock. That was a great experience, too, because it really allowed me to get to know the family on a personal level and see how they interacted.

Amma was always sweet and generous and kind, and would refer to me sometimes as her American son. Over the years oftentimes I'd be one of the last people to finish practicing, sometimes two full series in a day—something crazy like all of the A section and all of the B section— and by the end I was exhausted and sometimes the last one in the *asana* room.

Amma would sometimes peek her head in and see me in there and say, "Coffee, Teem [Tim]?" And I'd say, "Oh, yes." So I would come into the front room and have coffee and chat with them. Of course, Amma accompanied Guruji to the States on several of his trips—in '78, '80, '82, '85, '87, '89, '93—so it was another opportunity to get to know them. We would take them on outings. In a sense, she was my Indian mother.

It was sad when she passed away. Last year [1997] when I was here, the wound and grief from her passing was still very much apparent in Guruji. He was still quite sad a good part of the time. And last year, this whole conference thing hadn't grown to the proportions it has now, so sometimes there would be just two or three of us sitting with him in the afternoon. We'd talk about Amma and he would get very sad. He would cry, I would cry. But this year, with a little more distance on the event, he seems to be regaining his strength and moving on. It's great to see that. We were all concerned when Amma passed because it hit him hard.

They were together for sixty years and she was a great support to him throughout that time. I still feel her presence strongly there in the yoga *shala*.

Where do you think the legacy of this practice will go after Guruji stops teaching?
Years ago, those of us who were practicing *ashtanga* yoga and feeling great benefit from it would say to each other that it's only a matter of time before this stuff catches on. We said that for a good many years without a lot of evidence. But in the last few years the practice is spreading quickly and quite a few of what I call senior Western teachers have been teaching for a number of years, grounded in the practice at a cellular level. When Guruji passes on, they will all certainly continue to spread the practice.

Hopefully by the time he's ready to retire Sharath will be very capable of taking over the scene in Mysore and people will continue to come, the practice will continue to spread throughout the world. In America, there used to be fairly limited geographical areas that the practice was being done in—California, Hawaii, New York, and Boulder. Then it spread into the northwest, Northern California, more in the East Coast, now it's spreading a lot in the Midwest—all different parts of the country—and throughout the world. There are people here from Malaysia, Norway, Slovenia, all sorts of places. As the practice continues to grow, it'll have an enormous impact on life and on the planet. I think Guruji sees that and firmly believes that. He always said, "Slow growing is good. Quickly growing very dangerous." It's good that we had all those years to lay the foundation, to make the roots strong. Now that it is starting to grow quickly, there is that good root structure. So we won't just topple in a strong wind.

Is there anything else you'd like to add?
Ashtanga yoga has been very, very good to me. I'm very happy to have found the practice and Guruji, and to have him as my mentor.

Mysore, 1999

David Swenson

David Swenson began practicing yoga at the age of thirteen and discovered *ashtanga* yoga four years later when he met David Williams and
Nancy Gilgoff in Encinitas and became their student. He first met Guruji in 1975 and made many trips to Mysore to study with him. David
travels almost continuously, teaching yoga all over the world.

What is ashtanga *yoga?*
I bring it down to a simple question: What is its application in daily life?
How much does it have to do with what we are doing on the mat and
how much does it have to do with the rest of life? In my mind *ashtanga*
yoga is just a tool, but the fascinating thing about it is that it's a universal
tool. It seems to have applications across the board. If a student is having
a hard time focusing, it tends to help them; if it's an athlete, it can help
physically in so many areas. It's just an incredible tool, and I don't know
anything quite like it.

The word yoga means balance, so the big question is: *Balance of
what?* You can talk about God and the individual. The universe is com-
prised of opposing forces—everything has an opposite. *Ashtanga* yoga
deals with two things, an internal world and an external world, the subtle
and the gross, the energetic and the mechanical. The first thing people
see is the gross aspect of the practice, the visible practice. That's the first
and most attractive thing to people: "I want to jump through, I want to
get my leg behind my head, I want to be able to do this and that and
achieve these physical things." That's what we can see, that's what we relate to, but there's a whole other world.

If you only focus on the physicality, you've created an imbalance. The
other aspect of the practice is the internal world represented by the *band-*

has, prana, ujjayi breathing, and the meditative aspects. The gateway to this is *drishti*. *Drishti* allow us to remain present with a focus and concentration that enables us to bring our awareness internally. The balance we seek is between the internal and external. The physical aspect of *ashtanga* yoga is like a tether that ties us to the earth and keeps us grounded, but the other part is the ethereal aspect. If you think of a balloon on a string tied to the earth, you have a balance between floating and being grounded at the same time. If you just focus on the energetics you can just get spaced out, too spacey, too much breath without the grounding, and your mind is wandering and lost and too ethereal. Too much physicality, you are too grounded, out of touch, the senses become too dull to tap into the subtle areas. *Ashtanga* yoga seeks a balance between these things.

But at the end of the day the only thing that really matters is does someone feel better from the practice? It doesn't matter why we come to this practice. People come for all different reasons, but once you begin the practice the balance of it starts to unfold. The only way to do this yoga for the rest of our lives is to seek the internal, subtle aspects and not just the external and gross. In a nutshell, I'd say *ashtanga* yoga is a universal tool to enhance life.

Can you say something about Guruji and how he teaches?
The greatest duty of any teacher is to encourage, to inspire, and to facilitate practice for the student, because the ultimate guru is the practice itself. The teacher's duty is to introduce the student to the *sadhana*, then to help them carry on with that. Look at the power of Pattabhi Jois. He's never really demonstrated a posture, yet he's inspired people all over the world to practice every level of *ashtanga* yoga. Also he's an incredibly learned man, a Sanskrit scholar who taught Sanskrit at the Sanskrit College in Mysore. He has committed to memory all the great scriptural writings of the Vedanta, Vedic writings, *Bhagavad Gita, Srimad Bhagavatam, Brahma Sutra*. He can quote them at will, yet his English is very limited, so he has never been able to convey through a lot of words this philosophy. Yet in the simplicity of his words, in addition to his inspiring one to practice the *asanas*, there is a depth of understanding that goes beyond the physical because Pattabhi Jois has been able to distill the information into a very concise commentary.

The greatest teachers in the world have this ability: to convey complex ideas in simple terms. There are many learned scholars in the world.

You can go hear them talk and go home and tell your friends about it and say, "Wow they were so smart! I didn't understand a word they said." What is the benefit of all that knowledge if no one understands it? So one of the great powers of Pattabhi Jois is that he's conveyed the essence and beauty and strength and power and the dynamic nature of this system in such a way that people of all levels, whether they have never heard of Patanjali, if they're a scholar or if they are physically able or not, he's made this yoga accessible.

How did you get into ashtanga *yoga?*
I grew up in Houston, Texas, and began yoga in 1969 at the age of thirteen. This was a strange thing to do in Texas, particularly at that time. My older brother got me interested. He was out in Southern California, Encinitas, surfing and was introduced to yoga because the spot he was surfing every day was called Swamis. At the top of the cliff was Paramahansa Yogananda's ashram. So he saw people doing yoga stretches on the beach and he bought some yoga books and when he came back to Texas, that was what he was doing. And I thought, wow this is cool, I want to be like my big brother. I think if he had come home riding a Harley-Davidson motorcycle and fighting in biker bars, my life would be very different. But he was into healthy things—health food, yoga—and we practiced outdoors in a park. There were no yoga schools, no yoga clothes, and no yoga mats. We practiced on a beach towel or whatever we could find.

The first book we had was *Yoga, Youth, and Reincarnation* by Jess Stearn. We also came across a book from Swami Satchidananda, *Integral Yoga Hatha*, and eventually Iyengar's book. And we would just take these books, practice a routine, and flow. It was a way for us to connect with nature and also feel something inside.

We were practicing one day and the neighbors called the police. Police cars came zooming up the park, the policemen jumped out of the cars, guns in their hands. "What are you boys doing out here?" We raised our hands and said, "Officers, don't shoot. We are just breathing and stretching." And they said, "Well, son, the neighbors called and said you are doing some kind of devil worship." They could not understand why these long-haired guys in white pants were flowing and moving under the trees. So this is the sort of environment I was in.

In high school, I was doing my yoga, I was a vegetarian, I was growing my hair long, I was surfing—was a big oddball. This was not a posh private school, this was your standard, average high school. They said long hair on a boy is a distraction. So my father went to the school board and he gave this presentation. "To my knowledge Jesus had long hair, Einstein had long hair, Moses had long hair, and the founding fathers of this great country had long hair, so I am not going to force my sons to cut their hair. What's the alternative?" And what do you think the alternative was? Short-haired wigs. I had to wear a short-haired wig! After three years of this, I couldn't take it anymore and left home. I wasn't really leaving home—I love my parents; I love everything about them, they have always been supportive. I couldn't take one more year of this wig on my head. So I went to Southern California and finished my last year of high school out there. I was sixteen and had to get a legal guardian to sign to get me into school.

Meantime a friend of mine said, "Since you are into yoga, come check out this yoga—it's dynamic, it's different." I said, "Sure, I'd like to." So in the early-morning hours—it's cold even though it was Southern California—they take me up these rickety stairs in back of a strange building. It was a combination of karate school, church, and yoga school. The early-morning light was shining in the windows and as I open the door and look in, I was taken aback. I felt like the room itself, the walls were breathing and pulsating with energy.

And in this light I saw steam rising from the bodies of the practitioners and I thought, Wow! The room wasn't heated, but they were generating this heat in their bodies from moving and flowing, and there was this young man and a young woman with long hair walking around, obviously the teachers. One of them walks up to me and says, "Hi, who are you? I'm David." And it was David Williams. It was David Williams and Nancy Gilgoff teaching a Mysore-style class. The first day David talked me through *surya namaskara* A, B, and the final three seated postures. That's all I got, but it was all I could take. My arms were tired, I could hardly get through it, but when I got on my back and looked down my chest toward my stomach, I saw steam rising and I just said, "Wow, this is something!" The pulsing of energy I had seen in the room I now felt a taste of it in my body, and it made me want more. I started coming every day. David and Nancy thought it was great that this young kid was so fired up about the yoga, so David took me under his wing, shared the yoga with me, and that was my introduction to *ashtanga*.

How long did you stay with them as teachers?
I still consider them my teachers. Once someone is your teacher, they are always your teacher in some way. I stayed with David and Nancy for a couple of years. Then my brother and I decided to make a surfing/yoga film. I was making trips to Central America, but still practicing every day, trying also to make this movie. I ended up back in Encinitas, and David and Nancy brought Pattabhi Jois for his first trip to America in 1975. To prepare for his arrival we were all just pumping and practicing, pumping up our practice and our breath, and David was telling us how to respect the guru. Keep in mind that Pattabhi Jois had never been to the West, so no one had met him except for David and Nancy and a guy named Norman Allen, who was living in New York. So we didn't have a clue other than the stories David told us and the photo or two that he had.

Pattabhi Jois arrived with his son Manju. They stayed for four months and proceeded to take us through the paces. He decided to have theory classes in the evenings, and taught us the *asana* practice as well as *pranayama*. The senior teachers were David and Nancy. They would go to Guruji and say, "Guruji, we think so and so should come and do *pranayama*." [You had to be invited into the *pranayama* circle.] You'd come in and you had a little test. You had to sit in front of him and he would place his thumbs on your belly, turn on his X-ray vision, look right into your body—it felt like he was looking into your soul, into your energy body—and make an assessment if you were ready or not. He was trying to see if we had an understanding of the *bandhas*. If not, he said, "No, not yet," and you'd go away. Or maybe you'd stay and would be included in the *pranayama*. We had to sit in the *pranayama* circle for an hour because he would take time with each person to show them individually. We would sit in lotus and after the hour, Pattabhi Jois, David, and Nancy would just lean back, pop their legs out of lotus, stand up, and walk away. "Are you coming, David?" I'd be there for another half an hour. "I'll catch up with you later," taking my legs out, going "Ah, ah" as the blood was coming back in. It felt like needles in my legs but the energy from the *pranayama* was amazing.

How did you first go to Mysore?
I carried on with the surfing-film idea and ended up working in Texas. One day I got a phone call from David. "David, this is David. Nancy and I are going to Mysore and we want you to take over all our classes for us

while we are gone." And I'm thinking well, Houston, Texas, or Maui? Houston, Texas, or Maui? [David Williams and Nancy Gilgoff had moved to Maui by this point.] I was on the next plane to Maui.

And the yoga room there was basic, capital B. The floor was made from dirt, and on top of the dirt was carpet that we got from hotel rooms that were remodeled. We would just roll the carpet over the dirt floor. We built the room with eight walls like an octagon. Four walls had rough-hewn wood where you could practice handstands. The other four walls were screened for ventilation. It was built like a yurt. The center of the room was a pole from the ground straight up to the sky, and from the tip of that pole down to the top of the walls were other poles.

Because of our lack of funds—we were a bunch of hippies living in tree houses and nobody really had much money—people used to just give us papayas and things for class. We stapled clear plastic on the roof as covering. This was a little silly but it was all we could afford. Clear plastic in a place called Lahaina. Lahaina in Hawaiian means "relentless sun," so this was basically a greenhouse, good for growing tomatoes. To practice yoga, you had to get in there really early before the heat. With the carpet over the dirt, anytime anyone jumped back their feet would make a little dent in the ground, so after thirty, forty, fifty people practiced there, the floor was dented. So every day we'd roll up the carpet, rake the floor, fill in the holes, stomp it down, roll the carpet back, and do it again the next day.

I was lying totally asleep one night and I just sat bolt straight up with my heart pounding and almost the words in front of my face rolling in space: "I'm going to India!" This was frightening because I didn't even know I wanted to go to India. And yet I said, "Wow, when they return I'm going to India." And to go to India was not an easy thing to do. David and Nancy would travel overland on trucks and buses from Europe and so forth. But now I was fortunate, I was able to fly. So I decided I was going.

Before David left Maui he had taken me up to advanced A sequence. When I learned *ashtanga* yoga, there were four levels: primary, intermediate, advanced A, and advanced B. Today those four levels are taught as six levels: primary is called first; intermediate is called second; advanced A is third and fourth; and advanced B is fifth and sixth. So when they came back I went off to India. It took me days to get there through some circuitous route: from Hawaii I flew to San Francisco, San Francisco to New York, New York to Paris, Paris to Tehran, Tehran to Delhi, and it was just crazy. Anyway, I finally made it to Mysore.

Pattabhi Jois was around sixty years old. Pattabhi Jois at sixty is like a teenager, just full of energy, wow! And there are three students, a total of three foreigners there. So there are the total of three students and I'm twenty-one years old and so enthusiastic and hungry for this yoga and wanting more and so he just obliges. He would give us so many *asanas*, like he'd bring *asanas* in a wheelbarrow and just dump them on us. He would adjust us in every posture. If someone couldn't jump back he would just throw them back every time. He had so much energy he didn't know what to do with it all, so he decided once-a-day practice wasn't enough. We practiced twice a day and even that wasn't enough. We'd practice two series each time: first and second in the morning, advanced A in the afternoon, plus an hour of *pranayama*, plus he taught us how to do *nauli* and *neti*. In the old yoga *shala* there was a little sink at the bottom of the stairs and we'd stand over the sink with our mouth open and he would take a *neti* string and shove it up our nostril, wait until he saw it drop down the back of our throat, reach in with two fingers and pull it out of our mouth and nose, and we'd go "ah, ah, ah" and then he'd do it again. It was a full-on intensive immersion, like diving into the deep end of practice with him. So that's how I ended up in Mysore.

And what did you do for the rest of the day?
Well, the problem was there wasn't much left to the rest of the day for anything other than finding food and resting and preparing for the next class. We had a practice in the morning and in the afternoon and for the other things we were doing, and your body is just totally tired, wiped out. It was like you take a wet rag and wring it out and there's so little left, all you can do is go out, find something to refill your body, lie down, rest, get ready for the next class. I stayed for four months like that.

How was it practicing when you went back home?
Difficult. Actually, the practice wasn't difficult, but reentry to a more mainstream lifestyle was extremely difficult. I had been living in Hawaii in a tree house, living simply and not needing a lot of money, and then being in Mysore. When I got back to the States, I remember arriving at the airport and a couple of immigration officers were talking to each other in the Texas accent: "Can't wait to get home and have me a nice

thick steak and an ice-cold beer." And that statement just sent my mind into this tailspin: "Oh my God, how do I fit in?" and "I don't fit in. Not only am I an oddity here, I'm an alien, I'm from another planet! I can't relate to people around me, I can't figure out how to work or get a job. How does all this yoga somehow apply to daily life? It doesn't make sense. I either have to separate from daily life or . . ." So it was frustrating, but I needed to find some source of income.

I looked in the paper and I saw there was a horse farm. The couple who owned it needed a house sitter. They traveled extensively for long periods of time and needed someone to live in the house and take care of their animals. I thought this was great. I don't have to deal with humans, I can deal with the animals, I can live simply, think a bit, and try to sort all this stuff out. So this was good and bad. It was good because I didn't need a whole lot and it did give me time to reflect. What happened during this reflection was all that I came up with was just a whole stack of questions, one of which was: Wow, where are the eight limbs? I'm just doing *ashtanga*, it's all *ashtanga*, but I'm just doing *asanas* and *pranayama* and I want to know about the rest, and so I decided to write Pattabhi Jois a letter. So I sit down and compose this letter: "Dear Guruji, Some questions seemed to have arisen in my mind concerning this practice. Where are the eight limbs? All we are practicing is *asanas* and *pranayama*. What about the *yamas* and *niyamas*? What about *pratyahara, dharana, dhyana,* and *samadhi*? Like, where's the *samadhi*, man? I'm doing this, where's the bliss?"

So while I was at it, I thought, I'm going to ask him some other questions that seemed to percolate up, such as: What is the meaning of life? Why are we here? Who is God? I thought these were reasonable things, so I put all this from pen to paper, mailed it off, and waited for months and months and never got a reply. I became so frustrated that I decided to find the answers on my own. I love this practice, but I've got to find what this is about. So it energizes me and I enroll in courses of study anywhere I can find, exploring these ideas. I enroll in philosophy classes at this Esoteric Philosophy Center. I studied palmistry and astrology and past-life regression and sound-color vibrations. I ate nothing but grapes and grape juice for forty days one time. I read Saint Francis of Assisi's books and meditations, and I was questioning and hungry and asking anyone I could for the meaning of life.

Well lo and behold! I end up in a Hare Krishna temple asking the same questions. They'd go down the list and answer all these questions and they backed it up with scriptures and books and Vedic communities and ways of life. So I think, I don't want to be a hypocrite and I want to know the answers so I'm going to try it. So I shave my head and become a Hare Krishna. And as a Hare Krishna guy I followed their regular principles, which were really intense. It was the life of a monk, a life of celibacy, practicing on my *japa* beads, chanting two hours a day, getting up in the wee hours of the morning, taking cold showers, and studying the traditional texts like the *Bhagavad Gita*, the *Srimad Bhagavatam*, all these different books. And going out and working hard and renouncing the fruits of our labor, giving it to the temple and living simply like a monk.

I was told that this *asana* practice was some kind of an illusion, you know this body of yours is going to get old and die. Toying around with these *asanas* is just *maya*, give it up, the real yoga is devotion. And I did, I gave it up for a while, a couple of years. And I traveled around and I taught and I helped open temples all over the place, but even the Hare Krishna devotees' bodies started falling apart—not sleeping much, the food was difficult—so some of the devotees started doing a little *asana* practice.

After five years I leave the movement because I started looking around and, wow, within the confines of the walls of this religion I see some people seem very spiritual, and some people seem to be very mundane, some people are egotistical and self-centered and mean, and some people are humble and compassionate, and it seems to have no relationship to what they are doing. It seems like you have the same chance for spiritual growth out on the street as you do with this religion. My parents aren't wearing robes, they aren't chanting, they don't do yoga-like *asanas*, yet they are very spiritual people, they exhibit unconditional love. I'm out of here, and I leave. I had zero money when I left there because I had given every cent to them.

I'm trying to figure out how to work. Not only can I not figure out how to work, I can't figure out how to dress—all I was wearing was a dhoti and kurta for five years. So I'm wearing mismatched clothing and thinking, what kind of job can I do? And I realize I had just graduated from the Hare Krishna school of business. For four years I sold stuff. I said, David, if you can sell a *Bhagavad Gita* to a cowboy on the streets of Dallas, you can sell anything. So I opened an art gallery in Texas, I represented artists, I wore business suits, carried a briefcase, but I was secretly practicing yoga.

There really was no avenue to teach then, so it was a personal practice, and I separated that from my daily life. Then I moved back to Hawaii and got a job at an art gallery and started going to classes again because Nancy was teaching regularly. I was loving it, it felt good to be back in the fold of old friends and practitioners. And she brings Pattabhi Jois to Maui. It's now 1989, twelve years from when I had last seen him. She brings me to him and she says, "Guruji, here's David." He says, "Oh, so many students!" and doesn't remember me. Now at first I was a little crestfallen and thought, well, you know in twelve years he's probably had fifty thousand students. I used to have long blond hair down to my waist. I'd cut my hair and my hair's falling out and I look totally different, so fine, he doesn't remember me. The next day I do my practice, I'm standing there waiting for him to assist me in a backbend. With Pattabhi Jois's assist, you stand on your mat, your hands across your chest on opposite shoulders, and you wait and he comes and steps in front of you and places one of his feet between your feet, grabs onto your waist, and you lean back and down. So I wait for him and he steps in front of me and I lean back and he feels the weight of my body in his hands and he says, "Oh, David Swenson!" He just recognizes my body, he remembers me from the touch because I look so different and I come up from the last backbend and if you have ever done this you remember, he stands so closely, like belly to belly. And so I stand up and now I'm face-to-face with him and he looks me right in my eyes and he holds his hands up in front of him as though he's holding some cymbals in his hands clapping them together and he says, "Hare Krishna, Hare Rama! Hah hah hah" and he just laughs.

And to this day I don't know if he ever got the letter, but it didn't matter any longer because the questions I had sought, or the questions I had and the answers I sought, had come full circle right back to where I was standing before with this practice. I said, "Wow, David! What were you thinking? He would just go down your list and answer them one by one? That's the silliest thing!" All he's ever said was 99 percent practice and 1 percent theory. Who knew? I realized, or had some kind of personal epiphany, that the full spectrum and potential for growth existed within this system as within many systems, and that spirituality is not determined by the practice itself but rather by the focus and intent of the practitioner and the choices they make and the quality of their character.

Sometimes people say, "I do spiritual yoga now and I don't do physical yoga." And I say, "Really? What's that?" And they say, "Well, we do a lot of chanting." And then I say, "Everyone that chants is spiritual?" It's not always true. Some people chant and are spiritual, some can chant like a rock star. Somebody can do yoga *asanas* as a devotional practice and somebody can do it to pump up their ego and look how strong and beautiful and powerful they are. The thing we do, the *sadhana*, the personal practice, is nothing more than a gardener tilling the soil in a garden, bringing fertility into our being. The seeds we plant, the choices we make will determine our spirituality, and so the eight limbs of *ashtanga* yoga, the potential for their presence, is there. All I have to do is be aware of how I use each breath and each word and action in my life, to take the benefits and the *prana* and the energy from the practice and the fertility that is cultivated in my soul from the *sadhana*, from this daily practice, and try to be objective and realistic and honest and say, Is the world a better place for my presence here? Which is a definition of a yogi in my mind. So I've come full circle with this, and there was that gap of time when I didn't see Pattabhi Jois, but the insights I gained from that, for me, were invaluable. I wouldn't recommend it for anybody else, but it was helpful to me.

Why do you think Guruji emphasizes asana *practice, the third limb of* ashtanga *yoga, as a starting point?*
The whole tree is one thing. As linear thinkers, we tend to say, "Oh there are eight limbs. What limb am I at?" We want to know. Number eight, *samadhi*, that's the gold ring. That's the prize. You start running through the limbs. You want to get there but ultimately it's a tree. You can't rush it. *Asanas* are the first thing we can relate to. Our body. You can see it, you can feel it, it's the first thing. But ultimately it's a little bit of a trick. *Asanas* are like toys for a child, they are toys for learning. At first we think it's all about the *asanas*, and later you realize, oh that was just a trick to get me on my mat and focus my mind for this period of time. You'll say, "Well then, why do we do the *asanas*?" And you'll say, "We don't have to, they are central in this system and a tool." But ultimately there's a difference between doing yoga and just making an *asana* of ourselves. We can make shapes, we can make *asanas* and move our body, and they have some physical benefit and they help to strengthen our nervous system, and I think those are some of the reasons Pattabhi Jois introduces them right away: to create some strength in the body and the nervous system

so you can deal with *prana* for *pranayama* and so forth. But at the end of the day, it doesn't matter if you can do the *asana* or not. Just because someone is flexible and strong doesn't mean they are advanced yoga practitioners or advanced as a yogi. If it were true, if that were the case, who would be the greatest yogis in the world? Go to Cirque du Soleil, the circus people, they can do any of this yoga in a snap. So the yoga, the learning, is in the endeavor and not in the result of some flexibility in your body or something. But he starts with the *asanas* because we can relate to it—you have to start somewhere. That doesn't diminish other systems that don't start with that. We all have different ways of learning and different mentalities, and how you come to the yoga and even the *asanas* are tools that at one point in the beginning mean one thing and later mean something else.

Do you think Guruji uses them consciously to teach the other aspects of yoga?
I think the duty of a teacher is to facilitate, encourage, and inspire practice in the student, to present the tool, to give all knowledge about the use of the tool. It is the duty of the student to use the tool to build their destiny. And so yes, Pattabhi Jois presents the yoga and shows how to use the tool. Now I can take that tool and slam it onto my thumbs and say, "Look how bad this tool is, look how bad this hammer is, it hurt my thumb."

You are saying it's for the student to experiment and come to their own conclusions. Or would Guruji use those tools to enlighten you about specifics, such as yama *and* niyama?
I don't think it is the teacher who enlightens one. The definition of guru: darkness to light. Let's say I'm walking around in a cave and I have a candle in my hand but I have no matches or any way of lighting it. I see some glow over there in the corner and I see someone holding a candle. They hold their candle out to me, I touch my candle to theirs. Now I have a flame and now I have light: from darkness to light. The guru has this information, this knowledge that he got from his teacher. He shares that knowledge with us. So there are different ideas about it. That story I told you, that long convoluted story, my journey, and coming back around to the eight limbs.

Now this is just me talking, these are just my own ideas here, so don't think I'm quoting Pattabhi Jois. Even if you never heard Patanjali's name and you don't know what the eight limbs are, the yoga begins to do its work. You water the seed of the tree through practice. The *yamas* and *niyamas* start to bubble up even with our not being aware of it. *Yamas* and *niyamas* are not the ten commandments of yoga, they are choices, things we choose to participate in or not participate in when we begin to practice yoga. It doesn't matter why you came to it. You came to it because you heard a celebrity does it or you are looking for the meaning of life or whatever, it's almost secondary.

But what happens is that we begin the practice of yoga and it changes our life. Things change, our choices change, our values change. Our friends say, "Come on, man, let's go party," and we say, "Is there going to be smoking there? What time are you going to be back? I got a yoga class in the morning." You start making choices around the yoga because when you practice yoga, you feel better and all of a sudden the choices, the *yamas* and *niyamas*, start to come up. *Asanas* are the third limb, that's obvious. Then he teaches *pranayama*, so there are the first four limbs.

There are so many distractions in the practice of yoga. In any yoga room, there are people hopping around, people doing wild postures, or when you are out in nature, whenever there are distractions, you learn to bring the mind back to the task at hand. Concentration, the next limb, is developed by learning to withdraw the senses, by staying present, by mono-tasking. We live in a society of multitaskers. But yoga is about mono-tasking, staying present and fixed. Don't worry about the next *asana*. This is where we start. "But I want the next posture, it's in the next sequence, it's in the next series . . ." Later we realize, "Oh, I have to stay present." Leg behind the head is no more or less advanced than standing in *samasthiti* ready to begin your practice, it's about how present I am in that breath, no matter where that leg is. And meditation, what is meditation? It's simply fixing the mind. So if the mind wanders, you bring it back, you can't tell someone: "Think of nothing." You are going to be sitting here thinking about thinking of nothing. So rather than say, "Think of nothing," meditation means you have something to think about, something to focus upon. Breath, *ujjayi* breathing, is such a single point. If the mind wanders, you bring it back to that. The *asanas*, they keep us intrigued, but really we keep coming back to the breath. And *samadhi*, maybe we reach that stage of non-duality. By presenting the *asanas*, Pattabhi Jois is giving us the tool to water the seed. I like to ask this question: If I eat an orange, do I need to be a biochemist to understand every little thing that is going to happen with that orange when I eat it to get nutrition from it? Or just by eating the orange will I get nutrition from it? By doing the practice, you start getting benefit from it whether you know it or not. How many people do you know who say, "Yoga changed my life"? You come to it for one thing and later you find yourself sitting in a room in Mysore.

What do you think is the essence of Guruji's teaching?
Every person you ask will probably have a different answer to that. The essence is the yoga, the essence is *prana*, the essence is seeking the Self, and this is the great paradox of yoga, of *ashtanga* yoga. You look and at first glance it's all about *asanas*, it's about jumping around, it's about doing this and that, but the paradox is, as David Williams says, the real yoga is what we cannot see. It lies beneath the surface, it's what is happening in that mind, what's happening in our breath, in our energy. Just because we do *asanas*, just because we do *ashtanga* yoga or any system of yoga, doesn't mean we will never get sick. Doesn't mean we won't have problems or difficulties in relationships or money problems or whatever. We will have the same kind of problems. But this yoga as a tool somehow gives us strength of character. Hopefully, if we are using it right, we can deal with it in a different way. We have some kind of a bubble/filter around us, so when some kind of obstacle comes our way, there's a filter so that it doesn't quite hit in the same way.

Guruji has all the great scriptures of the world committed to memory, the great yogic writings and Vedic literature there in his head. He taught Sanskrit in the Sanskrit College for decades. He speaks in very simple English terms, but his English is much better than my Kannada, his language. We have all been too inept to learn his language, to really communicate in that way. So he's had to convey things in very simple terms and with few words, which is part of his great legacy. How did this man, without demonstrating anything, without great command of the English language or any language, how has he inspired so many people around the world? How has he conveyed the essence of this yoga and knowledge without that ability?

Guruji always says 99 percent practice, 1 percent theory. What's your understanding of the theory part?

Theory is what you do the rest of your day, when you are not on your mat. If the theory cannot be woven somehow into the fabric of our every step, of the rest of our day, then it's useless. Theory without application is just mental gymnastics. So the theory is determined by the choices we make. There are all kinds of people who can do amazing *asanas*, and they can be mean, nasty people. They might be really flexible, that doesn't mean they are a yogi. So the philosophy means the choices we make. What is the 1 percent theory? You know what Mahatma Gandhi said when someone asked him what is your religion? His reply was, "You follow me, you live with me for two weeks, you will understand." It can't just be in words, it's everything we do. How does someone walk? How do they sleep? How is their interaction with other people? How do they interact with their other students? How do they interact with people they don't like? Watch someone, every little thing, and you can understand what is their perception of the 1 percent. If it's only about the *asanas*, we've missed the point. The danger is that it can become too much of an elitist program, only for people with two arms, two legs, and a strong, healthy body.

On my first trip here in 1977, I watched Pattabhi Jois work with a quadriplegic boy. His family would carry him into the yoga *shala* and place his body on the floor. Pattabhi Jois would stand over him, take his body, manipulate him, put him in a yoga posture, and just say, "You do breathing one, two," and just count and have him breathe. Then he'd put his body in another posture. He didn't say, you can't do yoga. So we have to be careful we don't limit this to just some physical thing. This is also where the theory comes in: How does it apply? There is a definition of a yogi that I like: a yogi is one who leaves the place a little nicer than when they arrived. So a question each of us can ask is: Is the world a better place by our presence in it? What does it matter if we can do all kinds of yoga *asanas* if the rest of life is a disaster?

Do you see Guruji as a representation of the ideal life?
As students, we have to see that the teacher is one thing and the system is another. The duty of the teacher is to introduce the student to the practice. The true guru is the practice itself. None of us are perfect, or we are perfect—at being ourselves. So Pattabhi Jois has a very clear purpose in this life: to convey the practice of *ashtanga* yoga internationally, to inspire hundreds of thousands of people all over the world to do this yoga. He's like Johnny Appleseed. He taught for so many decades in

one little room. He would still be teaching and dedicating his life to it whether there were hundreds or thousands of students coming to Mysore, as there are now, or if there were just a handful. So his embodiment is that he lives his purpose. He's done what he's supposed to do. Now it's our duty. What are we going to do? Are we going to be an embodiment of this yoga? It is up to each of us to figure out and answer that question: What can we do with the yoga now? Pattabhi Jois had done his duty, he has given this yoga to us, he told us everything he can about it. Now we each have to decide: How can I use this to better the world around me?

It's wonderful to come to Mysore and spend time and unplug and concentrate on our practice, but at some point we each have to take whatever we learned here and go back and become a productive citizen of the world. That was sort of my thought on not coming back here all the time. I thought the greatest respect you can give to a teacher is to take the teachings and go out and teach and do something positive. It doesn't have to be dramatic. You can be a better parent, you can be a better auto mechanic. I think that Pattabhi Jois's embodiment, his purpose, was to inspire us, to bring this to us.

Do you have a sense whether this is a system of yoga that Pattabhi Jois learned from his teacher, or that they developed together, or that Guruji researched?

Because there are no historical factual references we can look at, we can only go by the word of mouth, which is the way knowledge has been transmitted through the ages. And there are different stories about the *Yoga Korunta* and how Krishnamacharya and Pattabhi Jois found this book from Vamana Rishi and how Vamana Rishi said, "Oh yogi, do not practice *asana* without *vinyasa*"—the whole description of the movement/breathing system as we know it today. Pattabhi Jois said, "Look, I'm just teaching what I learned from my teacher. Krishnamacharya taught me this, this is what I am teaching you; I say, does it truly matter if this method of yoga is five thousand years old or five years old?" The true test of any system of yoga is, does it work? Does it help you in life? If it doesn't, do something else! Life is too short. If it is helping you, then carry on doing it. If not, there are many systems of yoga to choose from. So I believe Pattabhi Jois is teaching what he learned from his teacher. Where did Krishnamacharya learn it? Did it come from leaves? Did it come from the Gurkhas in northern India? Was it just for gymnastic teenage boys? I've heard every different theory and philosophy about it. None of it matters. If you practice it and you feel better when you do it, do it again the next day.

How important is family life and integration into society?
I've always felt that the greatest yogi is one who can tread through life and not let it disturb his mind. That means, can they get their kids to the soccer game and go to work and pay their rent and do all of their family duties and everything else as a yogi? A yogi can be many things. Yes, a yogi can be someone who separates and goes off and lives in a cave. But in my mind, an even greater yogi is one who's integrated and woven right into the context of daily life and society without becoming disturbed by it. It's a greater testament to yoga and its beneficial aspects if that person can live as a yogic accountant, as a yogic politician, a yogic piano player, rather than one who separates and is totally removed from society. But both can be valid.

How important was Amma in supporting Guruji and supporting the shala when you were there studying?
Amma is a bright light. Anyone that you ever asked about her, one of the first things they will say is that she laughs, she smiles, she was a bright light. She was always sitting way back there, almost as a way to correct things. She had an incredible presence, almost like a child, but at the same time like a real Buddha. She'd sit back and watch Pattabhi Jois give a talk and sometimes she'd say a little something and he'd change the direction of what he was saying. We used to say, "Guruji, are you coming to America next year?" and he'd say, "You ask Amma." She was an incredibly learned, compassionate, loving woman who lived up to her name: Amma. She was like a mother to all of us, you felt a sort of warmth and caring and love from her presence.

How do you see the transmission of Guruji's teaching passing on to his children and grandchildren?
It certainly is being transmitted through Saraswathi, Manju, Sharath, Sharmila. His family lineage is there and strong and they are all teaching and the things he has taught are being transmitted. But what's fascinating is there's a bloodline family and there's a family of students that are

another type of family. They are certainly different, yet in terms of the yoga itself, there are people around the world who have been doing this yoga for decades and studied intimately with Pattabhi Jois and are also great representatives of his.

What is the value of daily practice, day in, day out, twenty years, thirty years? What kind of inner quality is produced by it?
Well first of all, it's really not a daily practice. If you look at the method of *ashtanga*, it's daily but I wouldn't say it's seven days a week. *Ashtanga* yoga averages out to five days a week. When you take out the moon days and the Saturdays that's nearly six days a month, then invariably there's some holiday, especially when you are in India: it might be Cow Day or some other kind of day and there's "ladies' holiday," so it's not meant to be practiced every single day. You need to have at least one day of rest a week. Sometimes there are two days of rest a week. We are kind of like houseplants. If you deal with them with a regular schedule, they respond more easily. In a healthier, stronger light they grow stronger by this regulation. There is a saying of the alchemists: through repetition the magic is forced to arise. Aristotle said that practice is the strongest teacher of all. It's only through repetition that we can gain depth of understanding. If you want to learn how to play the violin, you just play it the rest of your life, you continue to improve. Doesn't mean you can't play other instruments as well. It's okay for people to practice different systems, you don't have to practice only *ashtanga*, as long as we have the same goal to learn about ourselves. The benefit of regular practice is the strength that comes from that. However, if for some reason, any reason, a health reason, or out of sheer frustration, anyone goes away from the practice, it's okay, don't feel bad. You come back to it and start again. If someone only has twenty minutes twice a week to practice, great, do that. Very few people are going to be able to do it ninety minutes a day for six days a week for the rest of their lives. But many people will be able to say, "I have fifteen, twenty minutes. I could do that Monday, Wednesday, and Friday." Great, do that much. Even Pattabhi Jois has said, minimum daily practice *surya namskara* A, *surya namskara* B, and the final three postures of the closing sequence. So anyone can take benefit from this. Even if you are confined to a wheelchair, whichever part of your body you can move, you can move that and breathe with it.

What do you think the ultimate aim of yoga is, according to Guruji?
Self-realization, understanding our relationship with God, and that perception will be different according to one's particular faith. Yoga is not a
religion. You can be Hindu, Muslim, Jewish, atheist, Christian, and practice yoga. You don't have to take any kind of vows to practice yoga. The
system itself facilitates personal growth. The interesting thing about yoga
is that it's such a universal tool. For some, it's a fitness program. Nothing
wrong with that. Yet that is the surface, that is just what you can see. Underneath the surface it's amazing, it's like an iceberg. What you see above
is just a tiny bit of the iceberg; below is all this other stuff just waiting for
us to dive in there and drink from it. But it's up to the individual to
choose what they want to do about it. It's just waiting to be plucked, like
fruit, you know, fruits that come from the practice.

*Those fruits are not so easily gained. I think often the moral and personal
lessons you learn are through sweat.*
What in life of great value was easy to attain? I mean really, relationships
aren't easy but it's great, right? So certainly there needs to be some endeavor. But here's the other problem or paradox of yoga: yogis shouldn't
be lazy people. Regardless of what it is—is it a business? is it a relationship? our practice on the mat?—we should endeavor fully to do everything we can to make something happen. But what makes it yoga is that
at the last moment you detach from the result of it and now it's out of my
hands. Successful or not, I've done my duty, I've done everything I can.
Now I've got to let it go.

*What do you think is the relationship between teaching yoga and practicing
yoga?*
Just because someone has a great practice doesn't mean they will be a
great teacher. Michael Jordan was a great basketball player but he might
not be a coach. Many times people who have the greatest struggle and
difficulty with the practice become compassionate teachers with a
depth of information because they had to go through so much. It doesn't
mean that someone who also has a strong practice can't be a good
teacher, but they don't always equate. Strong practice doesn't mean
strong teacher.

My question was more about teaching itself. Is it a practice? Guruji is not doing asana *practice anymore but we all acknowledge that he is a great yogi. Has teaching become his practice?*

As long as possible, you have to have some kind of practice. Teaching without practice becomes dry. You won't have anything to say. It will just become a job. Through practice we get some kind of juice, but what we have to do is define practice. Is practice only doing the sun salutations, or is practice the rest of the day also? I'll practice these *asanas* as long as it makes sense to do it. I don't see that the yoga has to be equated to only an *asana* practice. Again, everything comes back to a sort of paradox. Without a practice, it's hard to get depth of understanding. David Williams, who has a lot of one-liners, says that before practice theory is useless, after practice theory is obvious. To gain insight you have to practice. And even to carry on teaching you have to have some kind of practice or it's just a job and you'll be miserable. We gain insight and knowledge and recharge through our practice. As he is getting older, Pattabhi Jois's practice is more involved in *puja* and things like that. You ask, "How long will you practice?" And I'll say, "First define practice." I'll keep doing *asanas* as long as it makes sense in my body. I know that now, when I practice I feel better.

Can you say something about the role of breathing in yoga practice?

Same as the role of breathing in our life: it's the most important thing. Try going through a day without breathing. Our first act of life is to inhale. Last act before death is an exhale. We are one breath from death. Yogis understood this, they created whole systems of *pranayama*. With *ujjayi* breathing, we have resonance of breath, so we continuously turn our meditation back to that. *Asana* practice without breath is gymnastics. Nothing wrong with gymnastics, but it's not yoga. Breath work is the most important part of yoga.

How about food?

Food is an individual choice. When you begin to practice yoga, you become more aware, different foods make you feel different. So rather than telling anyone about their diet, it just makes sense. You try to get into some twisting posture and you're like "Ohh!," you feel the foods that you ate, and so I don't tell people they have to eat a certain way, those choices will evolve.

What do you think is the role of pain?
The role of pain is to signal that we have gone too far. You have to listen to pain. Let's say I'm driving my car and the back tire starts going, *tat tat tat . . .* and I think, "Oh, that's a little weird, I wonder what that is about." I drive faster and it goes TAT TAT TAT . . . "Strange, maybe I should turn the radio on. Ah I can still hear it, maybe I should turn the volume a little louder." Then one day the tire falls off and I say, "Wow, what happened?" So it's like this: my knee says, "David this is your right knee speaking, I feel some discomfort. I just thought you should know." And wow, I think that's groovy! I should sit in lotus. And my knee goes, "David, maybe you didn't hear the first time: Ow! Ouch!" Oh that's weird, maybe I should just do extra practice, I'll just eat some more Tylenol and go through some more practice. Ouch, ouch, ouch! And the knee blows up, and how did this happen? Pain is there as a warning sign. It will tell us if we have gone too far. There are only eight limbs in *ashtanga* yoga and one of them is not injury or pain. If someone is injured or beat up, something has gone wrong, you need to change how you practice.

Why does it take so long to get the message?
There are different ways that people learn. Let's say there is a fire on the floor here between us, and you say to me, "David, if you put your hand in the fire, it's going to burn you, it's going to hurt your hand." And I say, "Thanks for telling me. I'm not putting my hand in that fire." All I had to do is hear it to get the message. There's a rare few like that. Then there's someone else. "David, if you put your hand in that fire, it's going to burn you." And I say, "Really? I don't believe you." Then someone walks by and puts their hand in the fire and goes: "Wah!" And I say, "Wow, that looks like it really hurt. I'm not putting my hand in that fire." I had to hear it, I had to see it happen to somebody else and got the message. Fine, another rare person. Third person: "David, if you put your hand in that fire, it will burn you." Someone walks by, puts their hand in the fire: "Wah!" And I say, "Well, it hurt them, it wouldn't hurt me." I put my hand in and: "Wah! Fire really burns!" I had to hear it, I had to see it, and I still had to do it to believe it. Now there's a fourth person we gotta love. "See that fire over there? Put your hand in, it's going to burn you." "Really? I don't believe it." Somebody walks by, they put their hand in it: "Wah!" "Well looks like it hurt them, it wouldn't hurt me." I put my hand in it: "Wah! It really hurt. Maybe if I turn to the side and try it? Ouch! Well it

really hurt. Maybe if I spin three times and put my hand in it? Ouch! If I stand on my head and put my hand in it? Ouch! What time is it? I'll try it at a different time tomorrow. Ouch!" I go through a thousand combinations and keep putting my hand in the fire and finally I go: "Ouch! Okay, fire burns." All of us learn in different ways. But the good news is that it really doesn't matter if we are person one, two, three, or four as long as we get the message.

Most of us learn the slow way.
It's true.

If I tell you, "You can't," what will happen to you?
How many children won't eat ice cream because their parents said, "Don't eat ice cream?" They want to try. You know what I mean? I know parents who are macrobiotic, who force their children to go to school with bark sandwiches and no television and no sugar. These kids sneak out their windows at night to eat doughnuts and ice cream and to this day won't eat a piece of broccoli. It doesn't really matter which one of those people we are, the duty of the teacher is to present the knowledge. Those who have been on the path for a while can report what they found on the road ahead, but that doesn't mean that everyone will listen.

Can you say something about the bandhas?
First of all, they are highly misunderstood. A misconception about *band-has* is that *bandhas* mean strong abdominal muscles. A lot of people have ripped six-pack abs and don't have a clue about *bandhas*. Just because someone is jumping through doesn't mean they are using their *bandhas*. There are people who don't jump through who understand about *band-has*. *Bandhas* deal with energy. My image for a *bandha* is more like a valve than a lock. You lock the door and no one can enter or leave. A valve, as in the circulatory system where the heart beats and blood flows, is the thing that prevents the blood from sloshing back from where it came. Valves can move energy in one direction but not back. So in specific areas of the body we stimulate and start to draw the energy up. When it tries to fall back down, the door closes and we stimulate more and keep on pushing energy through these valves, through the body. This is it in a nutshell. There is more to be said. There's a book called *Moola Bandha: The Master Key*. It's 140 pages about *mula bandha* alone. They are the

subtle force of the practice. In the beginning, it's about the *asanas*. But *drishti*, breath, *bandhas*, the internal aspects of the practice is where real refinement comes.

If there is one thing that you could identify, that you are grateful for on this whole journey of yoga, what would you say that was?
I am grateful every day for the opportunity to practice this yoga, when we stand on our mat and give appreciation to the teachers who walked the path before us. I give thanks to my brother for introducing me to yoga. I give appreciation to my parents for being so open-minded and compassionate to me, examples of yoga even though they don't know an *asana*. I give appreciation to David Williams and Nancy Gilgoff for introducing me to the system of *ashtanga*, for introducing me to Pattabhi Jois. I give appreciation to Pattabhi Jois for carrying on a system of yoga in a funky little room in Mysore for sixty years with no students. I give appreciation to his whole family. I give appreciation to everybody who walked this path and carried on until today. There is much to be thankful for in every moment. Life is uncertain and fragile, and it's so easy to look and be discouraged by the things we used to be able to do. I used to be able to do this, I used to be able to do that, now I can't do this, I can't do that! We're only human, but if we just look in a slightly different angle, we see that there is much to be appreciative for. And it's not just the system. I say, learn to be appreciative in life. One of the greatest appreciations I have is for the presence of my wife in my life. And the yoga is a tool. It's not the only thing I'm appreciative of, but it supports everything else. It's woven into everything else.

Is there anything you'd like to add?
In the most simple terms, the best advice I can give anyone is enjoy your yoga practice. If you enjoy something, you'll want to do it the next day. How do you enjoy it? Try to achieve the definition of *asana*. One I like is "posture comfortably held." Move through the practice, practice for the rest of your life. Focus on your breath, don't worry if you can do an *asana*. If you can't do an *asana*, if you are feeling beat up, change your practice. Doesn't mean the system is bad, use the tool differently, find a way to do this for the rest of your life. Enjoy your life. Let's all strive to be a yogi, meaning: Is the world a better place by your presence in it?

Mysore, 2009

Ricky Heiman

Ricky Heiman met Guruji in Hawaii in 1979 and made many trips to
Mysore to study with him. Ricky lives and teaches in Maui and has had
the honor of being Guruji's host a number of times.

How did you meet Guruji?
I first met Pattabhi Jois in 1979. It was by accident, actually. I was in
Kihei, on the south side of Maui, and he was at a fruit stand, with
Amma, in the backseat of a car, and I knew the people who were driving
the car and they asked me to meet their guru. So I stuck my head in the
window and saw two of the sweetest people I ever met in my life, and
immediately was drawn to their love and warmth. I felt like they were my
grandparents. And it started right there for me.

What was your impression of him?
It felt like I had known him forever. It was just immediate. You know
when you meet somebody and you just feel that warmth? I just felt naturally drawn to him immediately. I didn't think I was going to study yoga
with him, I just liked him as a person. I had no baggage, nothing to compare him with, I knew nothing about him, it was a pure meeting.

Did you go and study with him right away?
They were doing a workshop on the other side of the island, in an area
called Paia, on their first trip to Maui. I went the next day to watch them
do this practice. I was actually shocked, watching sixty, seventy people
sweating like I never saw people sweat before, and this little gentleman
jumping all over the room helping everybody. So it looked like a party to
me. As I found out later, it wasn't a party—it was hard work.

What persuaded you to take practice with him?
Once I saw the class, I knew it was for me. I really needed some yoga. I was turning thirty-nine, forty, I had a very bad back injury, and for some reason my instincts drew me there. I've always felt lucky that way.

How did you experience Guruji as a teacher?
My first experience of Guruji as a teacher was unbelievable. He was so gentle with me. As soon as I got on the mat, it appeared to me that he knew who I was and knew what I needed. He knew I had some fear because of my back injury. It was a pretty aggressive form, and he just looked me in the eye as I was doing one of the first few postures with him and said, "No fear!" Getting that concept and surrendering was of course half the battle. Immediately I wanted to go to India and study.

So you continued to study with him?
Just briefly. He was only here for a short time. I actually studied with some of his original first teachers, who were quite excellent. I enjoyed their teachings also.

How did you find your way to Mysore?
One day Guruji came up to me in the class. I'm trying to remember the name of the posture where you're standing and you put your foot up and you go to the side [*utthita hasta padangushtasana*]. He said, "You come to Mysore! Three months fixing"—it will take three months to fix this posture. I was on a plane in a few weeks and stayed six months the first time. I loved Mysore. I loved being there with him and his family. It was a very quiet time in Mysore. I enjoyed it very much and I felt actually that I was going to move there, I loved it so much. I would go back year after year. Unfortunately, as Guruji says to me, "Oh, Ricky is a lovely man. Next lifetime—good body!" I'm a beginner still but I love the practice and I love doing it.

Can you describe the yoga shala *in Mysore?*
It was the first time I'd been to India and I was quite frightened. It was a long journey to get there, as you know, and I immediately went to their home. It was around noon. I found my way to this very humble abode and they took me in and they fed me and got me settled in and took me

to their yoga *shala* in the back. It was this little, teeny room. I don't really remember, it's been so long. I think it's been twenty years. I just felt at home. I felt at home in Mysore, I felt at home with them. And I knew I was there to get some serious work done, I had a serious injury.

What was the atmosphere like in the shala?
The atmosphere in the room, in the early years, was very quiet, actually. There weren't many students in there, could be three, four students at a time. And with Guruji, it's such a personal relationship you think you are the only one in the room, and don't really pay much attention [to what else is going on]. In the months and the years that followed, the energy of the other students in the room became overwhelming. I never worked harder, I never sweat more, and I don't know if I could work that deeply anywhere else.

Where there any Indian students?
No Indian students in the Western classes. The Indian students would come earlier. They would come from 4:30 to 6 a.m., and we would start to come at 6:30. And by 8:30, 9:30 it was pretty much over.

How would you describe Guruji's teaching method?
I would describe it as being one of the most sincere messages I've ever received. When you are in there with him, you know he has totally dedicated his heart and his soul to this teaching, so you want to give him the same in return. I've had many teachers of all types throughout the years, from English to basketball, and of course, you meet great teachers along the way. I've never met anybody who loved to teach as much as Guruji. In fact, it seems to me, as he is teaching he seems younger, he's a different person in the room. Out of the room, he's such a beautiful wonderful householder that the combination was overwhelming to me. To me, he is one of the great humans.

Can you relate an incident that characterizes Guruji as a teacher?
The way Guruji teaches is not lazy in any way, shape, or form. He brings the same energy, or more, to every class every day. I would be dragging, it would wear twenty of us out. I think it was the consistency and the genuine love and desire to see you learn this practice and improve your

health. It took me four years in Mysore, off and on, to get into lotus. I remember the day that he finally, after sitting in front of me, got me into lotus. He stopped the whole class and almost started crying with laughter and joy. I think he was more thrilled to see me in that posture than I was. You know, that's just one example. It goes on every day that you are in there. Whatever posture is difficult for you, he never forgets, he always makes you do it, even if you've gone by it. It's his discipline and his tenacity along with the love of the practice that make him unique.

How do you see Guruji as a spiritual teacher?
As far as a spiritual practice goes, Guruji is a teacher by his own example. He's 99 percent practice, 1 percent theory—one of his great, great quotes that we hear year after year. But I think it's the way he is out of the classroom, in his love for his family and the way he goes on with his life, and his simplicity and his religious beliefs—I think that's the hook that takes me.

How important is Guruji's family? Amma in particular—what role did she play?
His family was everything. I think he married Amma when she was fourteen and he was twenty, so they were babies together. They had this beautiful family, and they went through all the normal experiences: the ups, the downs, the heartbreaks and joys of all families. But the love he and Amma had for each other, and the love he has for his children and his grandchildren, is very deep. And the love that he has for his students, for me, is almost equal. When he takes you on, you're his family. He loves you. And sometimes the love is a little tough, but he loves you. It's pretty amazing.

What was it like having Guruji as your guest?
I've had Guruji as a guest in my home in Maui three or four times. I've had hundreds of guests over the twenty-eight years I've lived here, and they all have been quite lovely. Guruji was the most gracious, easiest houseguest I've ever had. He never complained. I never met anybody like him, phenomenal, so sweet, so loving, so easy to be with. I feel honored and blessed to be able to spend so much time with him out of the classroom. And of course, in the classroom, we all have our own experience of him which is so unique, so different.

What would he like to do?
I was with him for a few months when he was in Encinitas and we would take him to Disneyland. Guruji would not leave. He wanted to go on every ride. And he went on the ones I couldn't even begin to go on because I would be dizzy and nauseous. And he would stand in line and he was patient. His zest for life is unbelievable. What a great example.

Why do you think this ashtanga *yoga appeals so much to Westerners?*
The *ashtanga* system, or what we call *ashtanga* yoga—to me, it's all *ashtanga* yoga—but this form that Guruji teaches draws a very energetic kind of person. I think it draws the kind of person who has a lot of drive and a lot of mental energy. And Guruji, he's like a psychiatrist. He knows you immediately when you get on that mat, and he works and goes after your weakest areas within this form, whether it's first series or second series or third series. It's a very stimulating form and the sequence seems to be a very brilliant creation. I've watched people over the years, and it doesn't matter if you have a good body or a bad body, it's very serving.

Do you see Guruji as a healer?
Absolutely, absolutely. I don't know if you want to talk about what kind of healer, because yoga seems to be union between body and mind, but he seems to get in there with you. Boy, he gets right in there, he's right there. And I think he heals himself every day with this teaching. I haven't met anybody who loves to teach as much.

Can you think of a favorite story about Guruji?
Well, I don't know if I can use this language, and I don't know if I'll even quote it properly, but when he was here this last trip, visitors would come to the house sometimes in the afternoon and we'd be hanging around talking, just chatting. I remember one young lady came in and started talking about what was wrong with the world: the world was this and they are killing that . . . Guruji just very casually said to her, "You let God take care of world, you take care your anus." That was brilliant to me, it was brilliant. I don't know if you'll be able to quote that, but maybe you could say: "God takes care of world, you take care of your *mula bandha.*" I love that.

Let me think. There are so many stories. During the first few years that I went to India, I think it was '82 or '83, there weren't many of us there, but he'd always have a dinner for us in the room and he'd always invite us to go places. On the weekends, we would rent a van, and he would take us to some beautiful temple with the family. Sharath and Sharmila were young kids and Saraswathi would come, too. It was very beautiful. They were so gracious, and the way they were enthusiastic about the teaching, they would be just as enthusiastic about the excursion of the day. And you know, on Saturdays we were exhausted. You want to rest, you want to sleep. No matter how advanced you are, he took you a little deeper than you would go on your own. Ah, there are so many stories.

How will ashtanga *yoga continue after Guruji's gone?*
Guruji has set the foundation. It will go on for a long, long time, probably forever. People will try different variations—just like in religions, there's the orthodox and reformed and people will do this. But yes, this form of yoga, I think he has enough foundation and solid teachers throughout the West now who are really terrific and are very dedicated, and he has his son and his daughter who will carry on this tradition and of course he has his grandchildren, Sharath and Sharmila, who have started teaching. I think Sharath will carry on this tradition in a beautiful manner.

I haven't seen Sharmila in a long time but I understand she is teaching, and remembering her as a young girl being very determined and very wonderful, I can't imagine why she wouldn't be a phenomenal teacher also. They were raised by their grandparents and they all lived together in this yoga *shala.* I'm anxious to go back and see the new place once it's built. What a thrill that Joseph Dunham has taken the time and the love and the energy to bring him around the world so many times. We really appreciate that. We never thought we'd see him again here, but he continues to come.

What was Guruji's relationship with his grandchildren like?
In the early years with Sharmila and Sharath, their father was in Bangalore a lot doing his job. They all lived in their house when the father was home. [They lived with Guruji when he was away.] Guruji was the father and Amma was the mother to everybody. Now Saraswathi was certainly the disciplinarian, because all children need some guidelines, but Guruji was absolutely very influential in their lives, very loving. We'd all go for

coffee, usually after class, and everybody would sit around with the kids, and Amma had so much wisdom. Those of us who were fortunate enough to know Amma, she was wonderful in her own way and so patient with all of us and our Western ideas to keep going forward. "You take your time [progressing in practice]." She'd get into all these postures, she'd get her leg up [behind her head]. "Oh look, I can do!" She was great. They are a phenomenal family. They are blessed.

Can you say more about Amma?
The question has often been asked, what was Amma's role in this teaching? By the time I got there, of course, they had been there many, many years. And Amma knew every posture, knew the name of every posture, so obviously Guruji had put her through the same rigor. So she knew everything and she was so dedicated to him and so dedicated to his teaching and who he was—I thought they were one. Amma was always in the room next door, washing some pans or getting coffee ready, and you'd hear her voice going, "Oh good pain, good pain!" She loved everybody. And she was the boss, as most women are, and Guruji was brilliant enough to keep Amma very happy. They were always so beautiful together, it was like being in your grandparents' home.

Is there anything else you would like to say?
There is one last story I remember about Guruji. I think it was 1984 or 1985, and Guruji said, "Oh, you come with me today," and he took three or four of us students, one who could do *asanas* pretty well, and we went to this high school, junior high school. He was to give this little talk and demonstration. So we get to this school and it is packed, I mean there must have been a thousand people, and Guruji makes us come up and sit with him on the dais and we are all very nervous. Guruji proceeds to give this talk in Kannada and this demonstration with a girl named Lea Johnson who was doing some postures from first series. He had the students laughing hysterically for an hour and a half. I don't know what he was saying to them. He was laughing hysterically himself. He loved it so much, I think he would have stayed there for days and days and days. We had to get him out. That's just the same feeling we get all the way through. It was a phenomenon, you had to be there to really appreciate it.

Did you have to do a demonstration?
No, I'm not the best to look at, but the girl who did it, did it very well. Oh, and one other quick one. I remember we were in Encinitas and we were going up to LA to do a one-night class at Ganga and Tracy's place in Hancock Park. It was a very big room and we weren't used to rooms that size. It started at six o'clock at night, and we all had plans at nine, nine thirty to have dinner with friends. There must have been eighty students there and we stayed there from six to eleven at night because he went around the whole room, the whole practice, to make sure he got to every student. It was the most amazing thing. And then we had to drive back three hours for him to get up the next morning to teach at seven thirty or eight. It was unbelievable. So there were incidents like that all along the way. So when he comes, get on the tour! Go.

Maui, 2001

Saraswathi Rangaswamy

Guruji's daughter, Saraswathi, was born in 1941 and practiced daily with her father from the age of ten to twenty-two. She has been teaching continuously since 1971, and cared for Guruji from 1997—when her mother, Amma, died—until his death in 2009. Both of her children, Sharath and Sharmila, became yoga teachers.

You were born and raised in Mysore. Can you share any particular memories or moments that stayed in your mind?

I love Mysore. I was born here, I grew up here. After I was married, I spent a few years living with my husband, Rangaswamy, who was working near Calcutta. But when I was pregnant with Sharath, I came back to Mysore and didn't go anywhere else afterward.

At school, I would practice yoga every day. Once, at a school function when I was fourteen, I did *ganda bherundasana* and the president of the school said, "Stop or something bad may happen." But I didn't care—I was very happy, very flexible. I loved sports in high school. I won so many prizes. I was chosen to go to the maharaja of Mysore's parade for Navaratri [the nine-night festival of the goddess]. I remember the maharaja sitting on a gold chair on the elephant . . . such a special memory.

My father took me to so many places when he was lecturing on yoga. I would do the demonstration of the *asana* as he spoke of the particular benefits. He would call the *vinyasa* and I would demonstrate, say, *kurmasana* [tortoise posture]. My father was a big man, maybe eighty kilos. He stood on my back and then started to lecture, explaining the benefits of the *asana*. Maybe he was talking for one hour while standing on my back. My mother would tell my father, "Don't talk too long." My father would say, "Only five minutes, that's all." But then when we got there, he would do the same—one hour! It didn't hurt; I was very small, very happy, so many people were seeing me.

How has Mysore changed since you were a young girl, particularly since the Western influence is now so strong?

Before, it wasn't crowded. Mysore was a very beautiful place with nice people. You only went to the city at feast times, where there would be many people buying flowers and fruits. Then it would be crowded. But nowadays, every day is a feast and it is crowded all the time. So many factories, so many visitors.

The old traditions were very nice; people had so much energy at those times. At feast time, you would cook a dish at your house for the particular celebration. For Ganesh Chaturthi, you would cook *ladoos*, *payasam*, and *idlis* specially for Ganesh. For Gauri [the divine mother], you would cook sweet *chapatis*. People were interested in the *pujas* and the families would celebrate together at home, eating beautiful food and being very happy. Before, particular days were for particular things. Now everybody has everything, every day. They prepare whatever they want; it's not special anymore. If you want sweet *chapati*, they are already there.

In those days, the man of the house was responsible for everybody in the family, and they respected him. Now, after marriage, people want to live separately. It wasn't like that before. All the family lived together, all the generations in the same house. If one person has a problem, they can be looked after by the others. Not so many headaches for the family. Now everybody is the boss in the house. Before, in the olden days, people liked children, not property. Everybody was very poor, but very happy. It's rare now to want to keep the family together. The traditional way is slowly going, although we have four generations in this house. Now the Western way is coming to India. Before, every house had only one bicycle, but now one house has two scooters and three cars.

Your family is Smarta Brahmin. Can you talk a little about the character and beliefs of this particular Hindu community, and how it affected your life?

My grandfather and great-grandfather on my father's and mother's sides were all Brahmin people. I like these methods—the prayers, the *puja*— not just Smarta but all Brahmin traditions. Smarta Brahmins follow the teachings of Shankaracharya. We don't only worship Shiva; Ganesh and Devi also, but really God is only one. My father's side worships Shiva. When I was married and went to my husband's place, the God I worshipped changed to Venkataramana [Vishnu]. After marriage, you don't follow the father's side; everything follows the husband's side.

Puja brings a love of God into your heart. I love Ganesh. Every morning I wake up with Ganesh in my bedroom, I chant some shlokas to him, and then I go to the shala to teach. Brahmins have many generations of experience in chanting the shlokas correctly, doing the pujas correctly. In the past, Brahmin people were very poor people. They couldn't become engineers or doctors, so they became lawyers or professors, the whole education field. The Brahmin people are very intelligent; it was their work to preserve the traditional wisdom of India. They master Sanskrit, and then all other languages come easily. They would memorize the Rg Veda, the Yajur Veda, the Sama Veda, and the Atharva Veda.

What are some of the important pilgrimage places in Karnataka, and what role do they play in Hindu life here?

If you go to south Karnataka, so many Hindu temples are there: Dharmasthala, Sringeri, Subramanya, Kateel, Mookambika, Udupi. Near Mysore itself is Nanjangud—the oldest temple, a powerful Shiva temple. Tipu Sultan [the ruler of Mysore in the late eighteenth century] had a blind elephant; people told him that the Shiva lingam at Nanjangud could cure the elephant's blindness. Tipu didn't believe it, being a Muslim himself. For forty-one days he took the elephant to the temple and applied mattika [temple mud] to the elephant, and on the forty-second day the elephant could see. So Tipu Sultan made a Paccha lingam [a jade lingam], very rare and costly, and installed it in the temple. It is still there.

Dharmasthala is home to the Manjunatheshwara temple. It is also very powerful. So many people go there to pray when they are sick. Krishna devotees in the area go to Udupi. Subramanya [another name for Shiva's son Skanda, the god of war] is a snake temple. You have to be so careful when you go there. You take a bath. If you have no children, you go there and do Naga pratishta [a snake worship ceremony]. You stay there ten days and on the eleventh day you do puja and maybe you will have a baby. There are three places for Subramanya: Kukke Subramanya; then, near Bangalore, Ghati Subramanya; and in Kudupu, the Sri Anantha Padmanabha Subramanya temple. One is the snake's head, one its stomach, and one its tail. In the Kudupu temple, there is a mirror and in it you can see Narasingha [the lion avatar of Vishnu] reflected. In Horanadu, there is Annapoorneshwari temple, where the goddess gives food. Also a very beautiful place, it is near Sringeri. Gokarna is one of the main places for the Brahmin death ceremony. In Tamil Nadu, you can go to Chidambareswara and see Nataraja. In Murudeshwara [north Karnataka], there is a huge statue of Shiva.

Do ladies have the same religious duties as the men?
The really important person in the family is the mother. If there are ten children in the home, she is controlling them, not father. Father is working for money, but the mother takes care of the morality, food, and education. When she is giving birth, she suffers a lot, but when the baby comes, she is very happy, ready for the next one, so strong. When the mother is managing the house, the whole family is very happy. Ladies also have different texts to learn—*Gauri Puja, Durga Abhisheka, Lalita Sahasranama*. And now, many girls are learning Sanskrit; they are the ones sharing this knowledge.

What relationship did you have with your father's guru, Sri Tirumalai Krishnamacharya, and his family?
Not so much, but I took yoga examinations with Krishnamacharya. I have first class and intermediate, and a certificate from him. A long time back, maybe 1985, I wanted to go to America with my parents, but I didn't get the visa. Sharath and Shammie were so small, and my husband was working in Saudi Arabia. They said, "If you leave your children in India, you can have a visa." But I couldn't leave them; going to America wasn't important, my children were.

At that time, I went to meet Krishnamacharya in Chennai, because Guruji's Western students wanted to meet Guruji's guru. So, I took them. Desikachar [Krishnamacharya's son] and his family have also visited my house, so there is a little relationship coming now.

What is your personal experience with the ashtanga yoga practice, and what have been its benefits in your life?
That is why I am so strong, so many benefits are there. I was a small child when I started the practice; my father started teaching me when I

was five. I was bending nicely, and my grandmother was shouting at me, "Your father is killing you!" But I was happy. From ten years until twenty-two years, I had a daily practice. Sometimes, if my mom wasn't feeling well, I would skip. I wanted to take care of my family while my father was working in the *shala* and in the Sanskrit College, and also because Manju was very small.

I was the first lady to do *ganda bherundasana* alone with no help. I would go to a demonstration with my father; he was so strict. He would tell me to do a certain *asana*, and I would say, "Tomorrow." He would say, "No, you do," and I would do. At that time he was not helping so much, he would just shout, "You do!" My standing *asanas* are very fine, but *baddha konasana* is very difficult for me—too stiff now. So many days I am crying because of that posture.

How did motherhood and marriage affect your relationship to the yoga practice?

I got married in 1967, when I was twenty-six. After marriage I had to move away to be with my husband; that is the rule in India. He was working in Jamshedpur, near Calcutta, for Tata Motors. I didn't know my husband when we got married—in India, arranged marriages are like that. Not much practicing yoga, because my husband didn't like it so much then. But still, I was teaching small children. I won't stop my work. Then in 1975, I left college. I didn't want to go, I wanted to teach yoga. So I stayed at home and my father taught me to teach. Many ladies would come to my father's yoga *shala* and I would teach them. When I was pregnant, I came back to my father's house, where Sharath was delivered.

It was difficult with my husband's family and, since he was always changing jobs, changing places, my mother and father asked, "You have two children, where will you go?" I was thinking about their education—one place talks English, one place Hindi. It is very difficult for children to learn anything if you are moving every six months. My parents said, "If you stay in one place you can go, but otherwise you stay here." That seemed like a good idea, so I stayed at my father's house for fourteen years. My husband was coming and going—when he had holidays he would come.

Finally he went to work in Saudi Arabia for six years. I asked him so many times if I could go, but he didn't want me to go there; that country is very different from India. So I stayed in Mysore. This made my family very strong.

What were your early experiences teaching your own yoga classes?
Because I came back to my mother's house, everybody began teasing me for being back. Every day I was crying.

When Sharath was four years old, I went to Santpur at the top of Karnataka where my husband was working. But there was no good water, no good milk, and Sharath got an infection. I stayed a month there, but he was so sick—fever, headaches—and my husband was so busy working. I was worried, so I came back to Mysore. I took him to the doctor, who said Sharath had glandular fever—very serious, one year of treatment. When the treatment was finished, Guruji started building the yoga *shala* in Lakshmipuram. There were bricks everywhere, and Sharath was jumping over them and fell down and broke his leg. He had to sit down for three weeks; he was only seven. Then his hemoglobin became low, and he developed rheumatic fever. For four months he was in bed, he couldn't move. From ages four through fourteen, one thing after another. At that time I had so many financial problems, so I was thinking, how can I pay for all this treatment? I decided to start teaching my own yoga classes. My father said, no advertising, it is not correct. But he had a student, an American lady, Sally Walker, who had stayed in our house. She put an advertisement in the Hindu newspaper for my class [which was held at a temple], as a presentation, and that day, four students came. I was charging fifty rupees admission and twenty-five rupees monthly fees. That day I will never forget—I had two hundred rupees in my hand, a very good feeling. Then our doctor, J. V. Narayan, took out an advertisement in the *Star of Mysore* for four Sundays as a gift to me, and many people started coming. When more people came, jealousy came also. People complaining about money: "When Guruji started teaching, he charged three rupees, now you charge twenty-five—why?" I said, "In Guruji's time, one kilogram of rice was one rupee, now it is ten rupees." Every few days they would use the room for shaving people's heads like in Tirupati [a Vishnu temple near Chennai], or for making *ladoos*. I said, "Are you going to let me use the room or not?" They had another room at the back of the temple, which was not used in the afternoons. The students liked it very much, and I taught in that room for eleven years. At that time, Guruji and Amma were always going abroad. I wanted to stay at home and take care of the house, and I also took care of Guruji's students. After eleven years, jealousy started again. Someone wrote on the wall "Don't teach here." My mom had come with me that day and said, "Don't teach here anymore." When things go well, people start to discourage you, when they should be encouraging.

I built a house in Gokulam. My husband was back from Saudi Arabia, but then he moved for five years to Bangalore. I took my children and moved into the new house in Gokulam. Many of the students followed, some who had been practicing with my family for thirty years.

You were the first woman to be educated in the Sanskrit College in Mysore. Then you were the first woman to teach yoga to men and women together. What were your experiences?
The Sanskrit College had no ladies—it was very conservative at that time. People didn't like men and women being educated together. I was the first lady to be admitted, and for three years I studied kavya, primary Sanskrit. I would practice my yoga at the Sanskrit College—me and all these boys. When I left college to take care of my family, many ladies started coming. In the temple, I only taught ladies. This was what my family wanted, the traditional way. But after I went to America, where boys and girls learn together, I thought, "Why don't I teach them together? What is the difference? All are the same, I don't care." So I started. I wanted to see what would happen, for if my mind and heart were strong, where is the problem? I had many boys in my class then. In India, if they see you talking to boys, they automatically think of you badly. But I didn't care what people thought.

How did your mother influence your life? I hear she was a very special, loving lady.
She was a very funny lady, jokes and everything. She loved all the students. She would feed the Western students food, coffee. My mom liked to look after people. She took care of my father, who was very poor. He left all his things in Kowshika [his hometown] and went to Mysore with only two rupees. After marriage, my father's salary was only fourteen rupees, but my mom was very happy to stay with him. Out of the fourteen rupees, four rupees was for rent, one rupee for electricity, and nine rupees left for everything else for the whole month. But it was fine for her. Sometimes for a few days we wouldn't eat . . . only one or two papayas

from the tree at the back of the house. When my brother and I were very small, my father would bring rice sometimes when he had some money. There was nothing, just small things for *uta* [lunch]. Later my father started making some money, but my mother always remembered how it was before. Money didn't change her. Even though their horoscopes didn't match, she loved my father, and he also [loved her]. For sixty-three years they were very happy together.

She was always teasing my father. One day he bought a scooter. After seventy years old, Guruji started riding a scooter and every day he would fall off it. He could have broken something, and my mom was always scolding him, "Send back this scooter." My father said, "No, you sit on the back." She said, "I will never sit on that thing! You will have to find other ladies for that! If I fall off, who will take care of me? If you fall down, I take care of you. I will never sit on that thing." My father was always falling off. She was a clever lady.

Sharath is now a father and a yoga teacher himself. How has it been watching his development, and what advice have you given him?

When Sharath was a little boy, he played at yoga a little bit, but he didn't like it. He preferred cricket. But the first time I went to America in 1989—just Guruji, me, and Amma—at the Seattle Airport, Guruji got food poisoning from a fruit juice and was very sick. When we got home, the doctor said, "Guruji needs rest, he is working too hard." At that time, he didn't have an assistant; he taught in the morning and evening alone. I said to Sharath, "Guruji took care of my family, but no one is helping him teach *ashtanga.*" When Guruji would go abroad, one of his students would teach the class. I scolded Sharath, "What will happen to *ashtanga* if no one is helping Guruji?" The next day Sharath said he wanted to go to the class. After that he would never miss a class. His interest started growing and the number of Western students coming was growing also. My children want to spread the *ashtanga* method like my father did. It is the family project. In my last moment, I want to teach yoga. Nowadays, I want to teach and look after my family and me . . . that's all.

Your daughter, Shammie, is teaching ashtanga *yoga in Bangalore, which is a busy Westernized industrial city. How are the Bangaloreans taking to the* ashtanga *yoga practice?*

Guruji told her to start teaching in her house. Many people are teaching yoga in Bangalore, but not the correct method like her grandfather. So she thought, "Why don't I teach people the correct way?" And Guruji gave his blessings. Now some students are coming, Western students also. People who have come from abroad to work there are coming now, too. People are beginning to hear that Pattabhi Jois's granddaughter is teaching there, and they are excited, because she is his granddaughter, and that is important.

As a woman and teacher, what advice can you give to pregnant women who want to practice ashtanga *yoga?*
It is good for pregnant women to take practice—the breathing brings oxygen to the blood and to the baby. The baby gets exercise, too, and the mothers are very flexible at this time. Women should take three days' rest during their periods, but many Western ladies keep practicing. That is very bad. The ladies' holiday is a time for rest. In the old days, Brahmin ladies would work all the time, but during their ladies' holidays, they rest and the rest of the family cooks and cares for them. After the delivery of a baby, the mother should take three months' rest from the practice and the first three months of the pregnancy also; you can do a little bit, but no jumping. Sitting and breathing is best. I have one girl who comes to my class who is four-and-a-half months pregnant and she practices intermediate and advanced, no problem. It depends on the person. Sometimes it is good to check with a doctor, too.

What advice can you give to ashtanga *yoga teachers who want to teach this method over a long period of time, as you have done?*
You don't want to change the method. What you learn in Mysore with us is what you should teach in your place. Guruji has told us so many things; you can't go changing it. If you follow Guruji's method, definitely everything is becoming spiritual. It will change minds; everything will change. People like it the way it is—that's why it is spreading everywhere. For forty years nobody has taught like him. But in old age—seventy years, eighty years—you keep a few *asanas* and make them your regular practice. Just do primary, that's enough, but don't stop. You look at the people and see what is suitable for them. You can choose what their practice should be. Even a very big man can do *surya namaskara* with correct breathing—you can make him try. Soon it will be much easier for him. If you can't do *surya namaskara*, you can do simple *asanas*,

with breathing and *mula bandha* and *drishti*. Even sick people can do the breathing. Eventually they will feel happy and their bodies will become light. So many people tell us Guruji has changed their lives with *ashtanga* yoga. Westerners are very strong people—when they start, they keep going. Indian people are not doing yoga. They are scared. They go to the hospital and they are told not to work, just rest and eat.

How do you see ashtanga *growing in the future? How can the traditional aspect of the practice best be preserved?*
The teachers should preserve the traditional method . . . it is so precious.

I like this yoga, not the others, only this one. The breathing, the *bandha*, and the *drishti* is a very special thing. Now people are changing the yoga, mixing it up, but that is not *ashtanga*. You want to practice with our old students, not the others who don't know the correct method. The teachers who practice with us in Mysore are very honest, we know them; they have asked for permission to teach. But there are so many people teaching *ashtanga* who have not come to see us—this is not honest. They are not recognized by us. It is not our property, but it is important to go the correct way, then it will spread everywhere very happily.

First you want to respect the teachers who brought this yoga to you. Guru—that is *mula* [root, base]. If you don't give that respect there is not coming God. That is very important. Some people change it, but it is just their ego. Think who is the best teacher, and go there. If you keep changing teachers, it is not correct. You will get confused. When your mind is strong, you stay with one teacher. You go everywhere and try, then when you find one, you follow that one person. When you meet the right one, you will know in your heart.

Mysore, 2008

Mysore Residents

·

N. V. Anantha Ramaiah

N. V. Anantha Ramaiah is a highly regarded scholar of Sanskrit and Sanskrit drama in Karnataka State. He was a student at the Maharaja Sanskrit College in the 1940s, where he became a friend and yoga student of Guruji. The road where he lives in Bangalore is named in his honor.

How did you first become friends with Pattabhi Jois?
I first met him because he was teaching me yoga—yoga shikshana—at the Sanskrit College. Later, his brother-in-law, Puttava [Amma's brother], was my roommate, in room number 29; we were opposite each other [Guruji was in room 31]. Pattabhi Jois and I became very close because of him.

We used to do many things together. In the town hall we had acted in a Sanskrit drama, written by Bhatta Narayana, called *Veni Samhara*—it was a part of the *Mahabharata*. In it there was a competition between Duryodhana, Karna, and Aswattama to become the chief of the army. I was Kripa, Pattabhi Jois was Aswattama. Krishnappa, another student, who passed away recently, was Karna. The role of Karna is a very heroic role. Whatever he was reciting and whatever Pattabhi Jois was reciting, I am remembering now clearly. I was Kripa, the maternal uncle to Aswattama. In the town hall there were big audiences. Like K. T. Bhashyam [a famous bodybuilder], Pattabhi Jois's body was so strong and manly with his regular exercises. He was a very good actor. We had three performances, but had only acted in one drama [play]. I bet in the name of God that none had enacted a play before like this, and no one will repeat it in the future. It was in 1949.

So Guruji was already married?
Yes, at that time Guruji was already married. Savitramma was his wife's name. She cooked very nicely and sweetly. She used to prepare Mysore *pak* that was so tasty. In that time, our guru was very poor in his financial condition, he was getting maybe only fifteen rupees salary, but he was always content. He had only two sets of clothes—dhotis—that Amma was washing and pressing, fresh and neat every day. She was a model in keeping things fresh and neat. Those were *khadi* cloths [cotton]. Guruji was using snuff also, but Amma made him throw it away. Pattabhi Jois and Savitramma had a very good family life, and they were very friendly, and used to tease each other—Amma used to call him Joisre [Mr. Jois]. They always had smiling faces. They used to feed us very well, and it was such nice food. That was Savitramma.

Can you say a little about the Sanskrit College and its reputation in south India in those days?
It was very famous. Krishnamacharya used to teach yoga and people even from Germany used to come, and also from the northern part of India. I used to study the Shakuntala drama in Sanskrit. A German scholar came and asked me, "What are you reading?" I told him, "I am reading Shakuntala *nataka* [drama]," and he said, "Do not call it Shakuntala *nataka*, it is Shakuntala *nataka ratna* [jewel]." Afterward, from America two or three scholars came.

Can you say a little bit about what Guruji was teaching and how he was teaching you?
We used to do a lot of *asanas* like *shirshasana, sarvangasana, mayurasana, kukkutasana, garbha pindasana*. When we were very tired we would plead with him, "Mr. Jois, it is enough of all this, please allow us to do *shavasana*!" *Shavasana* means lying down silently, without any movement—like a dead body. He would laugh: "Oh, do you want *shavasana*?" "We want rest—very tired!" He was very strict, but also he used to have very soft words. Even now from all that yoga I am very healthy, with my hearing, with my vision, even at my age, no sugar complaint—eighty-three years and running.

Very good—I hope it works for me, too.
Guruji, Puttava, Ramaswami, and myself used to get together every

evening to chat. Guruji used to talk about his experiences, how he grew up, his college days, and chat about general things. He would talk to us for an hour or so every evening. He used to talk about the dramas he had seen and sing the dialogues, in Ananda Bhairavi raga [Anantha Ramaiah sings some lines in Sanskrit].

He had a very good knowledge of music, and used to tell a lot of jokes. We would all laugh and tease each other. He was like any other boy that way, too, not always completely serious. We had a stove in the room, and we used to make coffee every day. If Guruji did not come and talk with us, our day was not complete, we would not feel content without seeing him for that hour.

Can you speak about Guruji's reputation as a yoga teacher and as a scholar?
He was an ordinary man, with his children Saraswathi and Swami [Manju], but that ordinary Pattabhi Jois became very, very rich in the days to come. That is his good fortune. He became very popular in America and other countries, and then all of them came to Lakshmipuram to learn yoga. Previously he was in an ordinary rented house there behind the *patashala*. But then, Lakshmi blessed him. The knowledge of yoga attracted all the foreigners to him, then later Guruji settled in Gokulam. Not just foreigners, the whole world came. If God blesses, anything can happen. It is his guru *bhakti*, his devotion to his guru, it is Bhagavata *anugrahah*—the blessings of God—and it is also the *punya* [good merit] of Savitramma.

I was interested in how he was seen by local people. He was a very fine philosopher and he knew a lot of shastras, *many people had a lot of admiration for him.*
Generally, we don't become famous in our own place. There is a proverb in Kannada: The herb that is grown in the backyard is not valuable, only when the doctor recommends it will we know the value of it. It also happened to Kalidasa and to Shankaracharya in their respective places because people used to see them every day, they never knew the importance of their teachings. There is a good quote in Sanskrit which means the one who doesn't know the value of sandalwood uses that as fuel to cook at home. Only when the foreigners started coming and identified him as precious, then the local people started recognizing him. An ordinary person gets recognized only when he wins the lottery.

When Guruji speaks about yoga, he always relates it to shastra. *His knowledge of* shastra *is very great. Can you say something about that?*
He has learned yoga according to the *shastra* very well, I know less about yoga, just some *asanas*, and that's all. He was very close to Krishnamacharya. Pattabhi Jois was the only person who was very famous in the field of yoga and knew so many *shastras*.

What was the influence of Shankaracharya on Guruji's yoga teaching?
He studied Advaita Vedanta and was learning from Palghat Narayana *shastras*, studying Shankara's philosophy.

I did not study Vedanta, I studied only Alankara *shastra* [poetical grammar, decorational language]. There are only two real *shastra*—Vedanta and Vyakarana [grammar]. I studied Sanskrit thirteen years, Vyakarana, and studied *Ṛg Veda*. Patanjali's yoga is *chitta vritti nirodhaha*—mind control. The *Amara kosha* [dictionary] gives five meanings of yoga: *Yoga sangha mano'paya dhyana sangati*. All of these are the synonyms of yoga according to the *Amara kosha*—which I know by heart. Yoga is *upaya* [means], *dhyana* [meditation], *sangati* [connecting], *yukti* [union with *paramatman*]—yoga brings *chitta ekagrata* [one-pointedness of mind]. By doing *dhyana* or contemplation on God, we can control our mind.

Once Animandavya was being hung, he was unaware what was being done to him. It is concentration to that level, that is what happens with yoga.

Did you know about Guruji's relationship with the maharaja, or did he ever tell you about it?
Sometimes he used to go to the palace, and I would go with him. We used to meet Maharaja Jayachamaraja Wodeyar because we would perform his father's yearly death-anniversary rites. We were court pandits, so there was no big relationship between the king and Guruji that I saw.

Can you speak about his character?
Even though he didn't have much money he was very generous, as was Amma. If anybody visited his house, they would feed them very well. They were generous, whatever they had they would share with their friends and family as well.

What is it that gives Guruji happiness, what does he enjoy most in life?
A friendship used to give him pleasure. He was very happy with friends like us. He used to derive pleasure from his students' progress. He used to also make some yoga demonstrations to show his students, and he was always happy when his students met with success. He was a contented man. He did not have much greed, he was happy with whatever he had. He was not concerned about the future. When he listened to music, he would completely forget himself in its enjoyment. Once he was made the chairman for a music concert at Purnaya Chhatra [an auditorium]— which is now gone. There is a small temple there.

We never knew he would become such a great man, and neither did he. In the Sanskrit College no scholar could earn so much. Like flying in airplanes. With all this change, he still used to be so good to us, not changing his behavior with his friends. He used to invite us for every event, like marriages.

Do you have any favorite stories about your friendship with him?
I have told everything there is. A few people were very jealous of him, of his wealth, of what he accomplished. He had no enemies, though, no enemies.

Bangalore, 2008

T. S. Krishnamurthi

T. S. Krishnamurthi, a renowned astrologer, resides in Mysore. He met Guruji in 1947 while a student at the Maharaja Sanskrit College and became his student and lifelong friend.

Tell us about your days as a student with Pattabhi Jois. Where did you meet him for the first time and how did your friendship grow?
Pattabhi Jois is older than me. By the time I could join the Sanskrit College he had already been a student of Advaita Vedanta and had completed the eight-year course of Sahitya literature. I came from a little village near Hassan and joined the Sanskrit College *patashala* in 1942, by which time Pattabhi Jois had already become a senior student.

Initially I did not have any association with him. That happened in 1947, when he became a yoga teacher in the *patashala* after completing his studies. He began to teach yoga to the students in the morning as well as the evening. I wanted to try my hand at yoga. I was very enthusiastic about it. That's how I came in contact with him. I was a devoted student and my focus was honed by Pattabhi Jois, who taught with a great deal of commitment and sincerity. I could easily see that he was keen to teach us all that he knew. So I consider him more of a guru than a friend.

I continued to study yoga under him for about four years. He would even take me with him to listen to speeches on yoga. Not far from the maharaja's palace was the other royal residence known as the Jaganmohan Palace. Nearby was a man named Krishnamacharya, a renowned yogi who had been appointed by the maharaja to teach yoga. Pattabhi Jois would take a few of us to him for yoga examinations that Krishnamacharya would conduct. I passed three of them and was awarded a certificate signed by the maharaja.

What kind of a man was Pattabhi Jois? What kind of a guru was he? What were his teaching methods and how did he interact with his students?
In those days, teachers in the Sanskrit College took a great deal of pride in their students and taught them with total devotion. The students, even if they had learned only a few basic lessons from them, would consider them wholeheartedly as their guru. Such was the culture. The guru/*shishya* relationship was based on mutual trust and respect. Not once in the history of the college was there a difference of opinion or disagreement between the two. Obedience came first, and remained. Moreover, money never played a role in either the guru teaching or the students learning from him. Salaries were laughably small. I am sure even Pattabhi Jois's salary was meager, perhaps fifteen rupees per month. We could all sense that he was struggling in his life. We knew he was forced to change residences frequently. But not once did he express frustration or undue anger in front of his students. He had a pleasant disposition at all times. I don't remember him falling sick or abstaining from class for any reason. He is old now, but I can tell you his personality has never changed. He is the same man now he was then. I sometimes think, "How can a man show this sense of equipoise, not letting anything, either good or bad, affect him?" Pattabhi Jois is still the same person, even at the age of ninety-two, that I met for the first time so many years ago, it's just he can't move around with agility now. The only thing that has caught up with him is age.

Do you mean that he is not changed in his mental makeup or his behavior?
First of all, there's his health. For virtually many decades, until recently, his health was always in perfect order. He maintained that level of robustness. Secondly, there's his manner of conducting himself, not only with his students but with anyone he comes across. Even to this day, he shows such affection toward friends even though we don't meet often. I am so happy about that.

Coming back to his early days, he got married and it turned out that his wife, too, was an extraordinarily warm person. I would visit him often as a student, and each time I was greeted by his wife with a delicious cup of coffee. Such was the understanding between the couple that we looked forward to spending time with them. As the years rolled by, some of us became his pet students. Krishna Bhat, who is now in Mangalore, and Shankaranarayana Jois, who lives in Mysore, were two other students who went on to not only practice diligently but also achieved an impressive grasp of yoga *shastra*.

What did you and the other students find most impressive about him?
Well, straightaway let me tell you that he was extremely concerned about and connected to his students. The manner in which he went about teaching us showed that he had faith and pride in us all. And not once did he let poverty and its attendant problems get in the way of discharging his duties. As young boys, we really didn't have a complete understanding of the trials and tribulations of life. But now, as an old man, when I sit back and think, I realize the enormous social suffering that Pattabhi Jois encountered.

There was not a hint of the tensions of family life on Pattabhi Jois's face the moment he entered the class. He had this great ability to swallow hardships within himself. He never let them come in the way of his teaching.

Pattabhi Jois began to have more students and eventually moved to Lakshmipuram in Mysore, where he built a house and named it Ashtanga Yoga Nilayam. The door of fortune opened a little for him after he began to travel abroad and teach yoga in various countries. I would visit him often and he would excitedly tell me about his experiences abroad and show pictures of his trips. We have always maintained a good relationship since then. Jois has gone on to acquire a legion of students, riches have come his way, God has been kind to him, and he has honestly offered his knowledge of yoga to all who have shown a desire to learn. Jois has followed the dictum of the *shastras* that says, "*Vamshodvita vidyaya janmana cha*," which means that you have to pass on your knowledge and legacy to others down the ages.

It's sad he lost his wife, but the rest of the family, including his daughter and grandson, have taken care of him well. I am happy that Jois doesn't forget my family and myself on occasions, be it a wedding, a thread ceremony, or a birthday.

Tell us about the relationship between astrology and yoga.
All the *shastras* in this world have been devised for the benefit of
mankind. "*Shubham va shubham va nityena krtikena va pumsam enu
pratishyeta tat shastra abhidiyate.*" Each *shastra* has its own use. There is a
distinct link between the earth and the sky. The interplay of celestial
forces and the movement of planets have a bearing on the weather and
the temperature, not to mention the daily passage from daylight to darkness. The *shastras* suggest that all our daily actions should be done in accordance with the movement and the placement of the stars and the
planets high above. This, the *shastras* say, has a direct bearing on the ful-
fillment or futility of our actions. Surely there is a link. This is clearly
stated in Jyotish [astrology] *shastra*. Nothing should be done without con-
sulting the astrological charts. There are many divisions or departments
in this, and to master them all is daunting. Mostly they are based on
mathematical calculations aimed at ascertaining the effects planets have
on life on earth at various times. Yoga, too, is a full-fledged *shastra* which
has to be followed meticulously. Since yoga aims to bring about a harmonious confluence between the mind and the body, I am sure its practice
has to be in accordance with planetary movements.

*Is yoga just a method to seek better health, or is it aimed at cleansing the
mind and soul?*
As I said earlier, all *shastras* were written with a view to helping mankind
attain peace. The sole aim of every living being should be to still the
mind and focus it in the direction of the force that may be called
Brahma. Yoga *shastra* tells us that the mind can be controlled and commanded through the constant practice of the various *asanas* that are explained in the yogic texts.

What is the sole aim of Jyotish shastra?
It is unknown to mankind why or how life came to be created. But it is
widely believed that there is a force that is acting upon us all, not only on
the face of this planet but also beyond. We can see there is only one sun
for the whole world. The sun's power is virtually unfathomable. Likewise,
various other planets that exist also have their own power that is quite
impossible to quantify. These planets, it is said, have an impact not only
on human beings but also on plant life. So all actions have to be done at

·designated times, as enunciated in the *shastra*. It's only Jyotish *shastra* that has the answers for the emergence of a particular star on a particular day or the precise movement of a particular planet at any given point in time. All this is aimed at minimizing suffering and offsetting the malevolence that may be wrought on humankind by the deleterious effects of certain planetary movements at certain times. For example, *yagnas* [sacrifice in the form of fire ceremonies] in the past were done only at that precise time clearly recommended in Jyotish *shastra*. This was done to maximize the effect of the *yagna*.

Why is it said that the practice of yoga shouldn't be done on certain days, for example the new and full moons?
Let me explain. The *shastras* have marked certain days as days on which no study, or *adhyana*, should be done. It is also understood that the moon has a great impact on human thought. For example on the new-moon day the light of the moon would be in a completely diminished state, thereby diminishing the power of your own mind to reflect good and powerful thoughts. Also, on a full-moon day, when the moon is shining at his brightest, a situation or scenario exists where there could be a state of severe agitation of the mind, which again is not conducive for any kind of meditative or contemplative activity, like yoga. Any planetary extremity should be taken note of and acted upon so that the pursuit of an intellectual practice is not affected.

Does the knowledge of a teacher who teaches on these two days decrease?
Indeed, there is a Sanskrit *shloka* that hints at the teacher being affected as well as students being subjected to a sense of ill will. The intellectual growth of the *shishya* could become stunted if he were to take lessons on these two days. His mind could become dull and unresponsive. Even while we were students at the Sanskrit College, these two days, and also the first three days after, were considered unsuitable for any form of serious study. These things have been concluded in the *shastras* since time immemorial. It is not for us to ask why but just to follow. We all have been following the same lineage laid down by the *rishis* of the past. The dharma *shastras* are the cornerstone around which is built everything in our culture. Adherence to the *shastra* will lead to peace and prosperity, the flouting of [the *shastra*] would result in chaos.

We all do a lot of surya namaskara. *Why is* surya *so important for yoga?*
The *shastras* say that every god has to be propitiated in a particular manner. "*Namaskara priyo Bhanuh, abhisheka priya Sivah, alankara priyo Vishnuh, stotra priya Devi, Brahmano bhojana priyah.*" Bhanuh, or the sun god, it is said, can be pleased through salutations. Shiva on the other hand can be pleased through *abhishekam*. Vishnu, it is said, is fond of *alankara*, or dressing and adornment. Brahmanas for that matter can be pleased by *naivedya*, or food offerings. The goddess is pleased by *stotra*, or praises. So the more salutations you offer to the sun god, the more pleased he will be. Perhaps in yoga *shastra* this could be the method to seek his power while going through the entire gamut of *asanas*.

Any final thoughts on Guruji?
I recall a passage from the *Ramayana* where King Dasharatha summons his son Rama and tells him to assume the throne and later, through a quirk of circumstances, orders him to go into exile to the forest. The passage wonderfully illustrates the level of equanimity that Rama showed on both the occasions. Apparently, he was unmoved, untouched, and completely bereft of any excessive emotion. I would like to say that Pattabhi Jois's attitude toward life, his successes and failures, his poverty and riches is similar to what is said in the *Ramayana* about Rama's sense of maturity in thought and action.

It says that Rama's face not once betrayed even a hint of anger or animosity when he was ordered by his father to forfeit his kingdom. His face was as calm as the day he was asked to ascend ceremonially to the throne. I can see that in Pattabhi Jois as well.

Mysore, 2008

Norman Allen

Norman Allen commenced his studies with Guruji in 1972. He settled in Mysore for ten years, becoming integrated into the local culture. He taught for Guruji when Guruji was away from Mysore traveling, and assisted him on lecture/demonstration tours. He has settled on the Big Island in Hawaii where he lives "off the grid."

After my daughter was born in Malaysia, we stayed there a little while to get her in traveling order, then took the ship across to Madras. We were heading to Pondicherry because I had got word of Dr. Gitananda's ashram. There it was basically yoga 101. You don't know about this man particularly, but he had a broad-scale perspective on Indian culture.

Who he was and where he came from was a little bit unknown, but he was a real showman. He had the litany and he had the stories and there he was four miles from Aurobindo's great ashram. David [Williams] was there, I was there. It was the first wave of people who kind of made that pilgrimage from the West, in one manner or another: in a British double-decker cargo ship to Kathmandu, or to hitchhike, take the bus, go this way or that way. That was the road, those were the days—'68, '69. There was not yet Goa to hang out in, seasonal places to hang out in, that was not happening.

But we checked out India, touring. It was wild. I was always on my way to the East, but slowly. I was born in Hollywood, California. And I went east to New York and then to London and Greece and then Kosovo, all through Yugoslavia, Istanbul, Iran, Kabul, got married, went up to Kathmandu, and ended up in India in this yoga 101 ashram where Swami Gitananda was going to give you the whole works. He had astrologers, he had Vedantic scholars come and give lectures, we did *asanas, pranayamas, laya* yoga, *kriyas*, we did levitation, visualization, we did coffee enemas, we fasted and then ate *dosas*, we did everything that you could see in any yoga book. He had a big menu and we had a taste of this and that.

Then the swami organized an all-India yoga conference. In that part of the world you give an invitation and a first-class rail ticket to the participants, because that is the way it's done. B. K. S. Iyengar got an invitation, Sri K. Pattabhi Jois got an invitation. Some of them were adept at certain procedures that were known in southern India only locally. They could do a *nauli kriya*, or some special aspect of a *nauli kriya*.

One man was a yoga *acharya* who had the ability to create *soma*, and he would do that in *nirvikalpa samadhi* while entombed. And you can go to certain authorities and they will give you the dimensions for a proper burial to make sure no ants will come in. I think it was David who dug the hole.

Iyengar didn't come. He sent a paper to be read. A *nauli kriya* expert came and spun his belly around nicely. The yogi came to be buried and the hole was dug. The police came out and would not allow us to put him in the hole to bury him. Instead, the yogi demonstrated what *soma* is and how you make *soma*. He declared that you have to do the *khechari mudra*, you have to catch that *soma* by secreting it. *Soma* was something from inside, not from a plant, not from outside, not from a mushroom but made through certain physical adaptations.

Pattabhi Jois, he came with his wife and his daughter and cousin and nephew, who was lean and really spiffy and he came to demonstrate. Pattabhi Jois came to discuss, the cousin to translate, Amma to take care of him . . . I'm not sure whether Saraswathi was there.

A month or two before the conference, two young Indians from Mysore showed up at the ashram selling saris and little sarongs. Basaraju and Manju. Manju demonstrated some yoga postures that he had learned from his father. Oh man!

So I saw Manju and Basaraju and then a month or two later saw Manju's father and then saw Vishvanath demonstrate, and I said, "Okay, this I want to learn."

Had you seen anything like that before?
No. I had seen the Iyengar book and that was interesting and what we did was kind of nice, a little bit of a mix with some Sivananda stuff. But not like that.

I wanted to study with Jois, no question. I asked, and they said, "No, he does not want to take any foreign students." One of the reasons was that he had had a bad experience.

He didn't want to have you as a student?
No, he didn't. But I would bring them everything that they needed, water and coffee, I'd go to town for almonds and *badami*. I had my beautiful daughter with me and my wife, and my daughter had her one-year Hindu initiation with a great scholar in the ashram in Pondicherry. She was a little baby, and you know in the East, they like babies.

How did you persuade him?
Well, I didn't keep on, but I'm a nice guy and Ammaji asked him to give it a chance. So because of her . . . otherwise he wouldn't have taken us. There was no need. In those days he was teaching at the Sanskrit *patashala* making fifty rupees a month, and he would have his *chetty* merchants who were his patrons, and they'd come and he had a room where the locals would come [for yoga classes].

So, he agreed to take me on as a student, and in a month or so I moved to Mysore. At first, I stayed upstairs, where they reside still, unless they got a new house.

Was Guruji teaching non-Brahmins or only Brahmins?
He would teach some non-Brahmins, not too many. But in the later years it started to happen more. You have to understand the culture. You grow up in south India in a rural setting as a Brahmin. That's conservatism and conservatism means fundamentalism, that's it. It's hard and long before you make a transformation from that. What do you call that? Evolution?

He certainly got thrown into the forces of a movement of society, and I saw which way he was going, and I saw which way I was going, and they were opposite. But there was a meeting. If you go to eternity, you get off the wheel. What can I say?

So I went to Mysore and I used to go to the market for him on my bicycle. I had brought a ten-speed bike. I'd bike around, shop quite extensively, go to markets, get the *puja* flowers, do all kinds of things, anything I could, and go to class. In the beginning, I'd wait until everybody was done, until about seven thirty in the morning, then get a private lesson. Then I graduated into the five o'clock period. I used to go five o'clock in the morning and five o'clock in the afternoon: two sessions. Later on, between those I would go to the university. I did that for a number of years.

After I practiced, I sat and watched. Most of what was being said I never understood. I would talk with people like Kokoraju and Shanta, I would socialize with them and go to their villages and learn about their culture. I probably know more about the Iyengar community than anybody. My first wife became a Bharatnatyam dancer. Her dance master studied with Krishnamacharya's father. Living with these great men of a very fine scholarship—you know, very sweet *bhakti*—I got the whole infusion.

David went to America and started to teach. He was teaching in California, in Encinitas. He wrote and asked if Guruji would come to Encinitas, and Guruji wanted to go. Guruji talked to me about it and asked me to sponsor him. I said, "No problem."

On several occasions when I had gone back to America, to show the grandparents my baby, I taught. One of my students was a lawyer. His name was Friedman. Mr. Friedman sponsored Guruji legally. I went with Guruji on the train to Madras to the American consulate to get the paperwork done. We got his visa. The problem was with Manju, because Manju had asked me if I would get him a visa as well. They said, "We ain't gonna give you a visa—you ain't gonna come back." And he hardly ever came back!

When Guruji went to Encinitas I stayed in India. By that time, I had been there a few years and was one of the men who would go talk in universities or give demonstrations, just like Sharath might do now. Guruji would talk and I would demonstrate the postures.

Would he stand on you the way Krishnamacharya used to stand on Guruji while Guruji performed an asana *and proceed to give a lecture?*
Well, it depends. In class, sometimes he would do something like that. In conferences, it would depend where it was. In a university it was different, more sophisticated than that! Because you see, it's a class thing. Even though Guruji is a *vidwan* or even maybe a double *vidwan*, there is still a class consciousness of some type inside Brahminical orders. At that time he was just working his way up into a position. He was recognized as a great man, a scholar, a pukka Brahmin, but when he would mix with the academic people or with rich people, you would feel a little bit aside. But he was cool as long as he was in his language. The Kan-

nada language is so beautiful, it's like a cross-blend. It's like Italian, it's a mixture of Sanskrit and Dravidian, so nice!

Bellowing through the streets of Mysore [you would hear] this very beautiful Carnatic music. I used to listen to many dozens of concerts with Guruji and Ammaji. You could sit and eat *dosa* and listen. The lyrics of all the songs that you hear—this is eighteenth-century Carnatic rap, man! Spiritual rap to the utmost! To Vedanta, to *namarupa* . . . that's where it's at, this is their heart, that's Mysore. The music is spellbinding. You can bring the dead back to life with this music. Guruji, he knew every one of those songs. That's where the culture is. Right there.

Can you say a little bit about the character of the man himself, his teaching?
Well, I went in there and trusted him right away. I was ready to let him do it to me, to submit to that kind of practice. First, I lived in the house and used to crawl upstairs and crawl back downstairs. I was laid up, disabled from time to time. Most of the time! My body was a hard body, I had been a bit of an athlete, played football. I couldn't do *baddha konasana*, couldn't do anything! I had some idea of form and the ability to use my body, but I wasn't trained. So I could see I was in for it. It was like having a drill instructor. I was a good student, I showed up, I was determined, and I submitted to it. Sometimes, if you're not a natural, it's good to go through the whole cycle of events, and I most certainly went through the whole cycle of events. I know how you can transform and get a new body if you want, if you persist.

One day I could hardly move. I said, "Guruji, can we just take it a little easy, you know, I have time, I'm not going back, I'm here and I'm digging everything. Do we have to do it so hard?" Six days a week, double sessions, I did that for so long. But you didn't have to do it that way. Many people in class with me never did it that way. They were the merchants with different motivations, and had a whole other kind of criteria for the practice. The personalities are different, the events in their time are different. That's what I liked about his room. You knew who came in there because they needed their regularity or had too many *dosas* in their belly. This person comes because they gotta come. They're never gonna be jumping around but they can do something else. Maybe they are going to have to stand on their head for thirty minutes against the wall and all these different things, depending.

Guruji was very beautiful in the way he could speak about the flowers and gems of the Vedanta of Shankaracharya, his guru and his Advaita philosophy. He was nimble and anecdotal in Kannada and Sanskrit, and was known as a very erudite, perceptive, and humorous man, if you knew his language. I started to pick up on this language and enjoy it. In the room you could have—you can't use the word "serious"—but you could have people who did the form explicitly and those who did it inexplicitly to the max but with different accents, and this was going on simultaneously. If you saw the class that I taught this morning, I kind of do it like that because that's the way I saw it and that's the way I learned it.

I've never seen a group class. He started teaching group classes at the Ayurvedic College with Basaraju, where they did them in batches, but that's not the way I learned. I learned to look at the body and see these things and go like that [give an adjustment] and that's what he had done to me.

Sometimes you would get a prescription from the doctor at the Ayurvedic College and then work one-on-one. I used to work with him or watch him work on a polio victim or stroke victim. It was wonderful to do that kind of work. And so I learned and watched and learned and watched. I never saw any kind of big classes, and I always wondered how you could see what was going on.

So he broke me in, he took me all the way, I was there and integrated there and studied *ashtanga* yoga.

How far do you think the physical practice can take you?
In most cases probably nowhere, without taking other steps.

Without the right intentions?
Without the right intentions, without the right diet, without *yama* and *niyama* it ain't happenin'. You gotta make sure that you dissolve the ego, get rid of the ego. If practice becomes sensational and competitive, it becomes *tamasic*. You gotta become *sattvic* in potential, in means, and in intent, or you don't have a chance.

You don't think that practice destroys the ego?
Practice often amplifies the ego, depending where the intent comes. The warnings are out there, it's in the songs, it's all over the place.

Do you think Pattabhi Jois makes some kind of provision for helping people destroy that: the ego?
What I'm talking about is common Vedanta. Everybody knows it.

Do you think the physical practice can lead to liberation?
Without real consideration? No. You might get a kundalini flash, an ah! ooh! Or some ecstasy or euphoria or something like that. Until you know you are not the body, what are you going to do? So if you associate with the body when you are doing the practice, you've got some traveling to do.

You don't think that the obstacles that you encounter when you are practicing can produce a sort of sudden self-knowledge and understanding of your self?
Yeah, you can say, "What am I doing with this compost, this carcass here, this heavy weight? I wanna be light! I wanna rid myself of it!"

But to rid yourself of it, you gotta culivate that thing that you don't get rid of, and that's the Self. That's what you cultivate. If you cultivate the shell, the carcass, this compost pile—you shouldn't get enamored with it—you are really going to suffer, really very much, when it goes. And it's gonna go. And the sooner that you can develop your Self, you don't have to worry about it going anymore. You are more free.

The *asanas* take you out of the body and into the *prana*. You gotta go deep. You have to go to the next level. Forget *yama* and *niyama*. *Prana's* where it's at. It has to be cultivated, purified, and considered. That's much more subtle. The practice has to lead you to *prana*.

If you died right now—and this is what they do in Mysore—they'd tie you up into *padmasana* real nice, you'd sit good! So I could put you in any posture right now if you were dead. You wouldn't moan or groan, but I couldn't give you the *prana* back. The body would look fine, the statue would look fine, but the *prana* is not there. *Prana* is really the next level. Everybody that has been doing this practice for so many years, if they are not into *prana* in every kind of consideration, I think that they have some nice things to look forward to. [*Laughter*]

I've heard some people say that they see the practice as incorporating all eight of the aspects of ashtanga *yoga. For instance, if you have a violent attitude and you exert that on your body, you experience suffering and pain*

and so you learn how to develop ahimsa. *With the breathing you are work-*
ing already with pranayama, *with the* drishti *you are already introverting*
your senses, and so on. The practice somehow contains the whole ashtanga
yoga in itself. What do you think about that?
Not much! [*Laughter*] The fine art of disposition. You can develop any
kind of argument nicely and debate anything to justify positions, but it
wouldn't stand in any council of Vedantists. You can say that it would be
something like that, but you would have to look to see: Is that potentially
there? No big deal, it does a lot of things. It can do everything.

If you wanna be a *hatha* yogi, then you are going to put it into that
perspective. The way people use that word *hatha* yoga is worse than *ash-*
tanga yoga—much worse, to use generically *ashtanga* yoga as a system
when there are only a few postures even mentioned in Patanjali's *Yoga*
Sutras. Just get the equanimity from body pain and suffering, if that can
be accomplished.

Hatha yogis had different ideas about what to do: using the body as
an instrument for emancipation. They wanted to have the pure crystal
body. They wanted to use this to transmute the soul and use it as a
real vehicle. They are the ones who cut the little ligament under the
tongue to catch this *soma*, which we saw take place with that man
in Pondicherry. He had to have extreme vows of *brahmacharya*. They
couldn't go and take their intestines out and wash them without conti-
nence. That's *hatha* yoga, the commingling of the sun and the moon, the
Shiva/Shakti is where it's all at. They would not be prepared to do *hatha*
yoga if they knew what *hatha* yoga was.

So you think that this is some kind of fantasy? People think that they prac-
tice what we call ashtanga, *that somehow they will achieve emancipation*
without paying attention to the yamas *and* niyamas *and having instruction*
in pranayama.
That's only the beginning. You've got a lot of other things to consider,
even in *samadhi*, before you are going to be happening. You have so many
stages and things to consider—*samadhi* with seed and without seed—
you have to bring it on up. It's serious work. One in twenty million. It's
not suited for everybody, this yoga or any yoga.

Except we gotta watch it roll: everybody on the road, you know
Richard Alpert; the whole lot of them tramped across to the East some
years ago and came back with the good stuff. We went into their box and

took the jewels. They are available to us. So many choices we get as dilettantes in the West. I'm afraid we are still looking for Ponce de León's treasure! You know what that was? The Fountain of Youth! But you know, this practice has many other auxiliaries. It depends on how it's approached.

Don't get me wrong, it's beautiful, it's a whole trip, but it's all kinds of integrated things. But here, we just want the gems because somehow we deserve it. It's the same reason we find ourselves in problems again and again in the world.

You gotta know the *gunas*. How can you do anything and not know the *gunas*? You gotta study something. He used to say, and I was the first one to hear it, "99 percent perspiration and 1 percent theory." But that 1 percent theory is a lot of theory, and you have to know *some* theory. To have a practice that locks you into a format and a discipline that calls you to attention. It will teach you that if you get afflicted in the body, what means you can use to un-afflict yourself. That's all there. That's precise and glorious if you can deal with it. It's too late to dig the well when the house is on fire. "Oh, man, I gotta go do some yoga!" No, man! You learn it early and practice it and then when you are in trouble you can call on it, because then it's appropriate.

Be established in it. It takes a few years of regular practice to get to be intimate with your body. Then you know when it's out of humor, and you can invoke some relief for it.

Do you have any idea where the system came from originally? Do you have a sense that this is something very ancient?
I became very friendly with a guy who was my Sanskrit teacher for a while. I studied *The Yoga Sutras* with him. You know Norman?

Norman Sjoman, author of The Yoga Tradition of the Mysore Palace?
Yeah. He's my very good friend. Norman was one of the earliest students of B. K. S. Iyengar. When he took his Sanskrit PhD from Pune all those years ago, he was being beaten by Iyengar heavy duty! [*Laughter*] Broke ribs there doing backbends. I got to hear all his stories. Norman came to Mysore. Norman is a brilliant man. He has to be the most brilliant "Sanskritist" in the world today outside of India. I would lay a bet on that. The court astrologer at the Mysore palace even wanted him to be his stu-

dent, that's why he got in and got those photos. He's brilliant. He has a few flaws but other than that . . . ! [*Laughter*]

He didn't study with Guruji, did he?
No, Norman used to give Guruji a hard time, but he didn't study with him. The man on the cover of Norman's book, Dattatreya, he was Norman's student. When he had to go away, I taught Dattatreya Pattabhi Jois style.

Norman had his theories and I would listen, and Norman always wanted to see the document [*Yoga Korunta*], because he would be able to [verify it].

Yeah, so that question, you asked me [about the origins of the system]. First of all, so what? This whole practice is to go beyond authority and to experience. In my opinion you can't trace it back to some thousand-year-old document, and you have to know the nature of Krishnamacharya to understand how he first presented it. It's not too hard to investigate. But investigating is really not reaching out spiritually. Unless it's for an academic approach, that somebody like Norman tried to present, it's moot. I won't even discuss it too much. It [*ashtanga* yoga] turned out to be a nice system.

No, I don't know. It's moot in terms of its origin. But its development can be isolated. Mainly, practice and experience is where it's at. So you enjoy it, you watch your trip, and see how you develop in that trip. You got to continue, forget *yama* and *niyama*, you gotta do everything eventually.

Big Island, 2001

S. L. Bhyrappa

S. L. Bhyrappa is one of south India's most famous authors of both fiction and nonfiction. His books have been translated into almost every Indian language and several are translated into English. A distant relative of Guruji, he began practicing yoga with him in the 1970s.

Where do you live?
I live in Mysore. I was educated here, but after getting my MA from Mysore University, I worked in north India for about twelve years. Then I got a transfer to Mysore in 1971 and worked here for twenty years, and then retired in 1991.

What were you doing in north India?
I was a lecturer in Sadar Patel University in Gujarat, and also I was a reader in Delhi, National Council of Educational Research and Training, then I came to Mysore as professor of philosophy in the Regional College of Education.

How did you meet Guruji for the first time?
I wanted to practice yoga. I had heard about Guruji, and my home at that time was near Guruji's house in Lakshmipuram. So I used to go there and practice and learn.

Was there a particular reason that led you to want to practice yoga?
General health and well-being. I had heard that Guruji not only teaches yoga but he had studied the philosophy of yoga. He knows Sanskrit and had studied the Sanskrit texts on yoga and the Vedas. He was teaching

yoga in the Sanskrit *patashala*, the traditional school. So I went to him. Later on I discovered that he was my distant relation.

Being a philosopher and a teacher yourself, were you interested to learn yoga from someone who was not just teaching one part of yoga?
Yes, I was interested in knowing its philosophy also. I think I was interested more in its philosophy than actually practicing it, though of course I learned the practice for more than a year. Every day in the evening I used to go to him, and then I used to practice under his guidance.

Would you speak of philosophy with him?
Sometimes, yes.

What were your first impressions of Guruji?
He was a very simple man, and he knew the philosophy of yoga. He would answer any question I asked. He was a very friendly person.

What questions would you ask?
I used to ask more about Patanjali's yoga—*yama, niyama, asana, pranayama, pratyahara, dharana, dhyana,* and *samadhi*—the eight concepts and the details of these eight concepts. I used to ask about these, and he would answer.

What were your impressions of the yoga practice when you started?
I had studied a bit of yoga theoretically, but when I started practicing I realized that it really gives peace of mind and a sense of well-being. That means you feel physically your body is light and your mind is calm, and after practicing yoga for an hour or a little more, I used to feel a kind of peace.

So you would see that the yoga is not simply a physical practice.
Yoga is not merely physical exercise, it is a philosophy in the sense that the first two steps of yoga, namely *yama* and *niyama*, are moral precepts, and without practicing these moral precepts, just to go to the physical exercises part, is not yoga. You see, *asana* is the third step in yoga according to Patanjali. *Yama* and *niyama* are important, that means *ahimsa: satya, asteya, brahmacharya, aparigraha*—*yama*. And the *niyama: shaucha, san-*

tosha, tapas, svadhyaya, ishvarapranidhana—they are also moral principles. We must practice them, or at least be aware of them, in our daily
life. Then we should do *asanas*. In fact, the purpose of *asana* is to tune
our body in such a way that we can sit for long hours in meditation. It's
not for pure physical exercise.

How does yoga fit into all the different spiritual traditions of India?
I think that there are philosophical differences—Shankara, Ramanuja,
Madhva. It's only when you go to the highest point of yoga that these differences arise, like whether at the end the individual soul dissolves itself
in the universal soul or retains its identity. They are the end stage. For a
practitioner of yoga on the day-to-day level, these differences will not
matter. They are more theoretical than practical.

Do you think these differences mattered to Guruji?
By his birth, Guruji belongs to the Shankaracharya tradition; he tends
more toward that. It does not mean that he rejects other traditions.

*Many academics feel there is a conflict between Shankara and yoga. Guruji
never felt that. Did you ever discuss this with Guruji?*
No, I have never discussed this with Guruji. But as far as my understanding goes, there is no clash. Take Vivekananda for example. Vivekananda is a proponent of Shankara's philosophy. He is an important
person in modern times to popularize Shankara's philosophy. But
Vivekananda himself is a great yogi. He has also explained the important
tenets of yoga, and has written books and given lectures with so many insights about yoga. Therefore, I think there is no conflict between the
two. In fact, if there is any conflict, it can be with the philosophy of Ramanuja and Madhvacharya. They also speak of yoga, but Shankara's
philosophy is more in tune with yoga than the other philosophies. Krishnamacharya had two important *shishyas*—B. K. S. Iyengar and Guruji.
Iyengar belongs to Sri Vaishnav, the same tradition as Krishnamacharya.
And Guruji belongs to Shankara. There is no conflict. When they study
Vedanta, theoretically there may be differences. But when they practice
yoga, there are no differences.

*What did the practice reveal to you in your own mind, perhaps about un-
derstanding yourself? You are a very prolific writer. You have written in En-*

glish, Kannada, and several other Indian languages. Your mind is very sharp and you are a disciplined person. Was there anything special that the practice revealed to you?

When I started with Guruji, the first question I asked him was, "I am basically a fiction writer. Will practicing yoga affect my creativity?" The mind works through the imagination for a fiction writer. It may be good, bad, indifferent. I create villainous characters, I create good characters, I create normal characters, and when I create villainous characters I identify myself with the villainous also. Now, if yoga insists on my thinking only good things in life, to that extent my creativity will be limited. So, I asked this question: Does it? He said no, your imagination is your imagination. Yoga will discipline your mind for your practical life. But for your creativity it doesn't interfere. It didn't interfere actually. After all, my practice of yoga is not at a higher level. I practice only some physical exercise part of the yoga, about one hour in the morning, and then I do *pranayama* for half an hour. I don't go so deep in *dhyana* or anything, I don't go so deep practicing the moral precepts also. If there is any moral dimension to my thinking, or in my day-to-day activities, it was there before I started practicing yoga. My personal subject is philosophy. I have studied Western ethics, Indian ethics, what is good, what is bad, moral analysis of the situation, and I have been practicing it—that's all. But when my imagination works, it tries to understand even bad characters. Goodness of life, badness of life, it doesn't interfere.

At the very end of Vamsha Vruksha *[one of Bhyrappa's novels], when the boy who became a* sannyasi *is walking down the street in pouring rain in Lakshmipuram, in my mind I completely saw him walking down First Cross toward Guruji's house!*

[Laughter]

I know you had a very personal relationship with Guruji, as you used to write letters for him, and used to translate some of his writing.

Because Guruji's English is not that good, I used to assist him. If he wanted to write some letters—he was very clear in expressing his thoughts in Kannada—I would translate them into English. That's all. I have translated some of his articles also. In the process of translation I tried to make his writing more communicable because, you know, writing is an art that you develop by practice, and Guruji has not developed that. Even in his own subject, yoga, he has not developed it. So I used to assist him. When he would write in Kannada, I would read and ask him questions, "Is it what you mean, is it what you mean?" and only when it was clear in my mind, would I translate it.

That must have been a nice experience, to work with him like that.
Yes, it was.

Could you tell us about your relationship with Amma? I know you were very dear to her.
Amma was a very pleasant, very generous-minded lady, and she had all the qualities of an Indian woman, mother, wife. She was fond of cooking, of feeding people, and she had a very good sense of humor. She took everything in a humorous way. She took a special liking to me, maybe because of my novels, or maybe because I was a distant relation. She was close to many people, and she was a very hospitable person, a good host.

Guruji and Amma had a way of bringing all the students into their family, making everyone feel welcome. In what ways did she have a good sense of humor?
She used to create jokes out of any ordinary situation. She used to make jokes about Guruji, oh so many! Whenever she was present, there were smiles and humor. She would make people smile, she had that nature.

Guruji was strict. Did she bring out good humor in him, too?
To create humor requires a certain attitude. Guruji was too serious-minded to create humor, but he would enjoy Amma's humor. He was never displeased by the humor of Amma, but he himself would not create humor.

Much later, when we became students, he would surprise us by how he would make jokes.

Did you know Ramesh very well?
Ramesh leaned even more toward worship, God, rituals. It is understandable if an old man is much given to worship, God, and ritual practices, but at such a young age, for Ramesh to be taking to such things,

was strange to me. I had a feeling that he would become a *sannyasi*—I had a feeling about it.

What was the common thinking about yoga thirty or forty years back? How was yoga seen? Now it has become so popular. Before, it was not so popular in India.

Even in India, the real benefit of yoga was not that much known forty or fifty years ago. It is a recent phenomenon that yoga has become popular. Not only Guruji but other teachers are making it popular in India and in the West. These days, yoga is looked at from the point of view of modern therapy, even allopathic therapy. It releases tension, it is a treatment for the mind, it's a kind of holistic approach to life. Its philosophy is gradually being spread. It is becoming popular. There are various other trends, not only in India but in the West. Vegetarianism—it is connected with yoga. Then, eating foodstuffs without chemicals—organic—this movement is connected, not that it is a by-product but it is within yoga. So there are various movements which are taking place in the world, and yoga is connected with them. ISKCON movement [International Society for Krishna Consciousness]—yoga is connected. Naturopathy—yoga is connected. All these trends accept yoga in some form or the other.

In the olden days, Guruji and Amma used to say that people were afraid of doing yoga, that it was only for the sannyasis *and saints. What is your view about this?*

It is a wrong notion. Now all those wrong notions have almost vanished. For a healthy person, whatever his vocation, whether he is *brahmacharya* or married man, whether he does intellectual work or any other job, yoga helps him. Doing some yoga and meditation start the day. And, you know, another thing—this Japanese influence, Zen Buddhism, it is an offshoot of yoga. When we speak of yoga, we should not think that only Patanjali yoga is yoga. Patanjali is not the creator of yoga. Yogic practices were in India from Vedic times. In some of the *Upanishads*, like the *Shvetasvatara Upanishad*, the different steps of yoga are already described. Patanjali only systematized. Buddhists, Jains, they all developed their own systems of yoga, giving it a twist depending on their beliefs. The Buddhist practices went to China and Japan, and they developed their own system of yoga, absorbing some local practices. Japan and China have been good influences on the Western countries. Nalanda was a center of Buddhist studies. Students came to Nalanda from all over Asia, from all over India. Many kings, most of the kings in India supported Nalanda, including Hindu kings. Just as in modern universities there are different departments, they were teaching Veda, Sankhya, Nyaya, and many of the kings were supporting it financially. Not only Hindu but Buddhist temples as well. Practiced and taught in almost every village. Any house is a school, wherever the guru lives. He may live in an ashram in the middle of the forest or in his own house. Students will come, stay in his own house, eat with him. Later on they would go, settle in their own place, and teach there. This was the case of the Hindu. But in the case of the Buddhist, they would live in centers, monasteries—and they were big. All these centers were destroyed by the Muslims. Nalanda was destroyed by a Muslim named Bakhtiar Khan. Even now if you go near Nalanda, near Patna, there is a railway station called Bakhtiar Pura. Bakhtiar Khan went with his soldiers and butchered these monks. All of them were Buddhist teachers. He butchered nearly ten thousand Buddhist monks, and the remaining ran away from there, carrying their manuscripts. They went to Tibet, and because Tibet was on the other side of the Himalayas, the Muslims did not follow them. This is why Tibet is a center of Buddhism—was, until the Chinese came and occupied Tibet and destroyed Buddhism, and the Dalai Lama left and came to India. Even today it is known as Tibetan Buddhism and Tibetan yoga also. Tibetan yoga is another type of yoga—*vipassana* yoga. Its purpose is to remove *dukha*. What is the difference between removing the *dukha*, and positively getting the *sukha*? It is a matter of philosophical niceties. What I mean to say is there are different styles of yoga, but all these styles of yoga resemble each other. The difference is only a matter of details, therefore. Yoga had been there in India in all schools, not only Patanjali yoga. Yoga was in China and Japan. In modern times, all these schools have influenced the West. In the West, Buddhism is an important religious influence.

Basically, there are no differences between the Buddhist yoga and Patanjali yoga. The differences are only in the final philosophical interpretations, at the ultimate level of *samadhi*; what kind of *samadhi* do you have—*nirvikalpa* or *savikalpa*? The Buddhist style of *samadhi* is different. But there is not much basic difference. The church has become rather apprehensive about the influence of yoga in the West because if people turn toward yoga they desert Christianity, because yoga, in whatever form, the basic idea is to look inward, search inward, in order to find the truth.

Is it a valid fear? If you do yoga and are a Christian, it can increase your faith in Jesus. Jesus said, "I and my father are one." This is a yogic teaching. In the Gita, *Krishna says, "In whatever form you worship me, in that form I come to you."*

No. Krishna says in the *Gita*, "Whatever the way you worship, ultimately it comes to me." If the church accepts that, then there is no ground for the church to go on converting the whole world. That's why they are apprehensive. A real yogi will not go proselytizing. That is why the Semitic religions are afraid of yoga, because if they accept the basic tenets of yoga there is no ground for them to go and convert.

It appears that yoga is able to cross boundaries.

Whatever I say as an answer to this is only theoretical. I have not practiced up to that level, but I have read biographies of yogis, some yoga texts. Like, for example, in the *Shvetasvatara Upanishad*, there is a verse that says a person practicing yoga feels light, water, air, etc. coming to his experience in an elemental way, and if he thinks that he has got the Parabrahma [Supreme Consciousness], he is misled because he has to go beyond it. And to understand it, he needs a guru. Most of our yoga teachers cannot be a guru at this level, because a guru is one who has himself experienced that, like Ramana Maharshi or Ramakrishna or Vivekananda. There may be some in modern times, but only those who have experienced this can personally guide. They can say, "This is this, now go beyond, practice further." Therefore, just to say up to this and beyond is Parabrahma, it is only theoretical, but I have no qualification to say anything about it.

But Guruji also said, "Don't ask too many questions, just practice, because the knowledge will reveal itself." So it is hard to ask questions in interviews like this because I have become accustomed to not asking questions. And what answers are there to the higher questions anyway? If there is something like self-realization, then it's not an answer, there is not a question that is answered, but that realization is the melting away of all doubts. It is an absence of questioning, not an answer to a question.

Whatever we do in yoga has a mental component, whereas other exercises do not have that mental component. Because this breathing is a very important component of any exercise in yoga, without breathing, any of the exercises are not yogic. Earlier, I would get a lot of dreams. Several dreams would come in a row—no connection, no continuity of theme. But after I started doing yoga, the dreams disappeared, and I get a deep sleep. I think it is because of the *pranayama* and yoga. It is not from the physical exercises, it is more from the *pranayama*. One can explain, when you say the *makara* [sound of "M" at the end of *om*], it has a resonance to the brain, and it soothes the brain. It can be explained physiologically.

If you have to keep the breath smooth and steady, only the mind can make that control. The body will not control the breath. You can only do it through the mind.
In Sanskrit breath is called *prana*. *Prana* is both breath and vitality. It means breath also is vitality. So controlling your breath means controlling your vital power also.

Mysore, 2009

Mark and Joanne Darby

Mark and Joanne Darby met in Mysore in 1979 while studying with Guruji. They settled in India to study with him for four years. Two of their three children were born there. They live in Montreal and travel and teach internationally.

How did you become interested in yoga and start to practice?
JOANNE: I finished university and wanted to travel. In the back of my mind was the idea to go to India but I was too scared, I was traveling alone. At university I read those Hindu books, Eastern philosophy.

I was a pharmacist, so it was not my field of study. But I was one of the only people interested. But when I finished university I decided to work for a full year and then my idea was to go to Europe and see what happens, so I left everything behind. I left my money with my mother and said, "I'm probably going to be gone for six months and when I need money just send it to me." I arrived in Paris in 1976. On the plane there I met two girls who were going to Greece, so after Paris I ended up in Greece and after Greece I met some people who were going to Israel so I ended up working on a kibbutz. Then I met some other people going to Africa and so I ended up in Kenya for a few months. I met somebody who wanted to go to Pakistan and India so I'm like, okay, that was basically where I wanted to go. Took me about a year and a half to get there.

In India, I arrived in Delhi and went to Varanasi and thought, this is a mad, mad place. In the '70s, you could see cremations, and when you are not used to that, total shock, so I left for Nepal, did some trekking, went to Dharamsala and saw all these Tibetan monks. At that stage in my life that's all I was doing, traveling.

The Tibetan monks left a big impression on me, and then I went to

Sri Lanka and Thailand and Indonesia and then I read *Siddhartha* [by Hermann Hesse], and the moment I read the book I thought, that's it, I'm going back to Dharamsala. Somehow the depth of that very simple book was enough to hit the right spot. I went to Dharamsala again and met the Dalai Lama. In those days he was teaching with a small group of people. I studied with him for three months, but there was a lot of hepatitis going around, people were not so healthy, and the rain was coming. A guy was doing some yoga on a rooftop, and I said, "Where did you learn that?" And he said, "Oh, from Pondicherry." So then I had a choice because I had a friend who was going to Pondicherry. So I went to a Buddhist monk and said, "You decide for me," and he said, "Make up your own mind," so I decided to go down south to the Gitananda ashram. And that was a shock, because I was free up to then—a couple of years traveling on my own—and when I arrived there Gitananda says, "What's your date of birth? Okay, eight days of fasting." I'm like, what? Eight days of water cleansing, the water fast and salt, and I'm like, wow! So okay, I'm here, I gotta do it so. That was rough, eight days on water—I'd never done that in my life. Some people had one day, some people two, but for me it was eight. And I did it and it was very, very positive, because I did a lot of cleansing, got very sick after—high fever and all. I stayed for the course, for three months. And after that I said, "Do I leave or do I stay?" I used to play *I Ching* and it said, you got to stay in there, stay in there, and I was "Ugh, I had enough!" And I said, okay, I'll stay another three months, another eight days of fasting. Then Vishvanath, Guruji's nephew, came and did a demonstration. That was the first time I had ever seen *ashtanga*, and I found it interesting.

During the fifth month, an old Indian who had a scooter asked me, "Do you want to go to Bangalore? I can't, I'm too afraid to drive. If you drive it, we can go to Bangalore and you can see Vishvanath"—because he knew I liked him. In those days there were just fields of rice along the road, and no traffic.

After two or three days, [we] end up at Vishvanath's. All he did was teach me *surya namaskara*, because I had not much strength. That was it, every day a half-hour *surya namaskara*, a few standing poses, hardly anything. After two weeks he said, "Why don't you meet my uncle in Mysore?" I took the scooter and drove down to Mysore with the old guy because he wanted to see the city. So we go and see Guruji and I remember they sat on the front porch and Guruji saw me arrive on the scooter with the old Indian guy behind me. He accepted me, offered me a coffee and said, "You come to see the class tomorrow." I was staying at Kaveri Lodge. I think you [Darby] were there, Gabe—with a real weirdo look, like an old bundle on his hair—and a French couple.

I had a plane ticket for Montreal one month later. I came back the next day [to watch] but I didn't have money. I told Guruji, "I have no money but I want to take class." And he said, "Those French people will give you money, they are leaving anyway so you can have their house." They were living behind [the *shala*] in the attached house, so he told them to move. I didn't know them, they didn't know me, but Guruji asked them to give me $100 and their house because I wanted to study and didn't have the money. So that was pretty amazing. So I decided to stay. When people say, "Why did you decide to take yoga?" it's hard to explain. It's that magnificent manner Guruji has, you certainly want to study this practice, and things worked out like that. I had a house to stay in, somebody gave me money, and the plane ticket ended up in the garbage can. That's how I ended up with Guruji, and from that day on I never stopped. I put the motorbike back on the train and told the old guy, "I'm sorry, I'm staying in Mysore."

How about you, Darby?
DARBY: I was traveling to Europe from Australia, taking the hippie trail from Indonesia to Malaysia and Thailand through India, and when I got to India a whole new feeling came across me. I considered myself to be a *bhakti* yogi in those days. I was a very devoted Catholic as a young child and as I got older, got disenchanted with the Catholic religion. India fired up that devotion, that *bhakti* in me. I spent three months in India, headed to Africa, and then back to Australia. Decided I wanted to go back to India. I had no idea what yoga was, I just said for some reason I'm going to do yoga while I'm there.

I surfed in Sri Lanka for five months and went to Goa to spend Christmas smoking chillums and stuff like that. Chillums had more or less become *Om Namah Shivaya* [I bow to Shiva], so in that aspect I became very devoted to Shiva. I wanted to do a pilgrimage. I wanted to become very Indian and walk to a holy center, and the holy center was Gokarna, in the north of Karnakata. Nobody wanted to do it with me so I ended up walking alone.

I would get up and find a place to have breakfast, walk until lunchtime, buy food to cook in the evening, then take a little siesta and walk until sunset. Wherever I was at sunset, I would cook my food and sleep. If I happened to like a place, I would stay a couple of extra days. I ended up in Gokarna a few weeks before Shivaratri [Night of Shiva festival]. Every day I would do the rounds of the temples. Still, in the back of my mind I was going to do yoga. Someone had given me *Light on Yoga* by Mr. Iyengar, so I started to do some postures. Eventually Shivaratri came. It was very special thing to do, to go in [to the temple] and touch this lingam.

So here I am coming out, and somebody who I met in Goa came up to me and said, "I'm going to Mysore." This guy was going to lend me money to travel back to Mysore. All my possessions, my passport, and my money, I had left in Mysore.

When I arrived back there I felt, "Now I'm ready to do yoga, where's my teacher?" Some of Guruji's students were staying in [my] hotel. Cliff Barber, or as we called him then, "Old Cliff"—he was forty-eight years old—said, "Come and meet my teacher." So I went with him and Guruji let me watch and at the end of the class, I said, "I'd like to do this yoga. How much is it?" And he said, "$100," and I'm going, "I just lived in Goa for a whole month on $100." I didn't go to Iyengar because I thought he was going to cost a lot of money, so it was kind of an ironic situation. Anyway I said, "*Baba*, this is too much."

Baba, that's respect when speaking to Indians. I said, "How about $75?" and he said no. A day passed and I went back and I said I was going to practice, and he gave me a discount. All I did was *surya namaskara* A, B, *padangushtasana, padahastasana, trikonasansa, parshvakonasana*, and then the finishing sitting postures. I had started on a Thursday but Guruji wanted me to do three days in a row, so he asked me on Friday, "You come in tomorrow, do Saturday"—traditionally the day off. So I came in the afternoon and he gave me a little class and I came back the next day. I did those three days plus the next week. By the next Saturday I was so thankful—I was so sore, so beaten up—to get a day off after a week and a half of practice. Then it continued basically for the next three months, continuous pain in different parts of my body. And Old Cliff Barber, he was a mentor. I could ask about practice and tell how my body was feeling, and [he would] tell me, "It's normal: no pain, no gain." Joanne came one week after I started. After three months, I'd had it. I needed to get out of there. I took a month off. Coming back,

I had no pain and I'm all ready to go again and three days later my shoulder popped and here we go again.

JOANNE: I had done five months of internal cleansing with some easy yoga [Sivananda style] so my body was ready, it was no problem for me. But for [Darby], it was every day something was going on with him, it was just unbelievable: if it was not the knee, the hip, the back . . . at one stage he was walking with a cane. I was just plugging along, one posture [at a time], and in three months did the whole primary series.

Why do you think one keeps going in spite of the pain?
DARBY: I guess it's belief in Pattabhi Jois. In this period I read *Autobiography of a Yogi* and also the atmosphere in India was starting to fuel an understanding about the teacher/disciple relationship. So Guruji is going to be my teacher, he is my guru, whatever he says to do I'll do, I have complete faith in what he teaches and wants me to do. And that was it, I just went with that belief. And it worked. I went away and after a month everything healed, the whole body healed by not being pushed. Where he had pushed me, I could now go to—I just needed to relax afterward. When I came back it was a different pain, more from getting stretched out, it wasn't that intense breaking down, so it did change.

You had a very strong devotional attitude toward Guruji. Can you speak about that?
JOANNE: The first time I looked at him I had a magnificent, strong attraction. Nothing would make me go back to Montreal. And when I got pregnant, nothing would stop me from doing my practice.

He would always say something pulls us there, some past [incident] that we don't know about.

When I was studying with him, it was so personal. There were two of us in the room and he was sitting in the back on this little chair and you knew that his eyes were on you whenever you did something. If you needed help, he was there. He had a very strong presence and you just did whatever he said. Even in our life, he made decisions for us very easy. Like when Darby came back, he asked Guruji for a place to stay because he was sick of walking from the hotel to the *shala*, and I am living right in the back of the house. So Guruji comes to me the next day and says, "Oh, Joanne, Darby's a good man." And then he says Darby has no money and he says, "Well, you let him stay in your house." My jaw dropped, because how can an Indian man ask a woman to have a man living in the house which is one big room and no separate bedroom? I couldn't say no even if I was not 100 percent sure of this decision because he is my guru; if he is asking me, there is a reason. Darby moved in the next day and eventually we got a relationship going, but did [Guruji] know that from before? He was charging me two hundred rupees for the room, so is it a financial thing or he had an intuition that we would make a good match because we were both very devoted to him? And then he put some French girls in there after a month.

DARBY: I remember he said to me, "One woman, problem!" And he looked at me and said, "Two women, *big* problem!" I'm in the house with three.

JOANNE: He was always there, almost like a driving force, you know?

[After] two years we went to Australia for a year then came back and stayed another two years.

And you were studying with Guruji during that time?
JOANNE: Nonstop.

DARBY: I asked Shiva for a guru, a yoga teacher. And I just feel that Shiva or God or whatever you want to call that said, "Okay he's the one."

He was having me come into the *shala* to assist him for one of the evening classes. I'd be trying to assist an Indian and I would adjust an Indian the way Guruji would adjust me and he would look at me and go, "No, no, no, not like that." His adjustments to Indians were different from the way he adjusted Westerners.

Westerners were there to do yoga, that was all. Life for us revolved around practice and getting ready for the next day's practice. Whereas the Indians were just like Westerners now taking yoga: they work during the day, they come and take a yoga class. You couldn't push those people the same way. I didn't know this, and my first teaching stint as a professional teacher in Australia was a catastrophe because I [taught] just like Guruji taught me. I was given a class with thirty people, and after one month I had four.

When he went to America, he asked me to look after the *shala*. But he also asked an Indian person to look after the *shala* as well. There weren't that many students, and because he was Indian and understood the language, he was doing the adjusting, so I became bored. But when I helped a couple of them do drop backs they accepted me as a teacher.

You said that your whole mind and whole day were focused on the practice for four years.
JOANNE: Yeah, you should have seen us. Even when we went to Australia in between. I got pregnant and didn't want to stop because my whole focus was on doing my practice, in the morning or afternoon, depending, and I felt so good doing this practice that when I got pregnant I just kept going. By the time I told Guruji I was pregnant, I was almost five months.

DARBY: At first she thought she was constipated.

JOANNE: I had a period, some blood, not very much, but I thought it was my period.

DARBY: By this time I had done a five-month stint and was having a problem with my knee. By the end of my third month my knee hadn't healed. Guruji said, "Stay another month and see how your knee is." I stayed another month and it still hadn't healed properly and he said stay one more month so I stayed another month, and in that month it was very, very nice. At the end of the class I managed to sit and get into *padmasana*. And Guruji was in the front and he put his hands together in prayer position and said thank you. After that month I said, "That's it, I'm going home."

JOANNE: He couldn't take it anymore, but me, I couldn't leave.
   I wasn't in pain, I wanted to learn more. We were completely the turtle and the hare. I just plow along in my practice.

You went at the same pace?
JOANNE: Yeah. But he was going through injuries so by the time he came back I'd be a bit further and then he would catch up.

DARBY: It changed when Jo got pregnant. Suddenly I'd get all these arm-balance postures, lifting up, so there would be more strength postures. Then after the baby came Joanne did all the same postures as well.

Did Guruji change the practice for you?
JOANNE: No, he kept on going, and even for him it was something totally new, because he never had a woman who was pregnant taking yoga to start with, and somebody who was willing to do yoga while they were pregnant.

Presumably he was changing the postures to some extent.
JOANNE: Not at all until the fifth month and Amma saw me doing this and he was forcing me into it.

DARBY: Amma saw it, and she said to Guruji, "No, no, don't do that."

JOANNE: I broke my rib and the baby's head was against my rib. I must have been more than five months because—

He actually broke your rib?
DARBY: We had an X-ray taken when we went to Australia and it was a hairline fracture.

And you had pain that time with Guruji?
JOANNE: Not that time but that day. I couldn't breathe for about three days because every time I breathed, pain was there. After that, he was starting to be more careful.

DARBY: What's interesting for people who are pregnant to know is that the person who is having the baby will break before the baby.

JOANNE: Guruji used to make me do scorpion with him.

To the very last day?
JOANNE: Yes, the day before.

Without any adaptation?
JOANNE: Yeah.

And did you do marichyasana *D?*

JOANNE: No, he didn't make me do what was not possible. He would add some new advanced postures which were good, like *siddhasana*. And he would make me keep doing headstand for one hour. And we were reading that is a thing a pregnant woman should not do.

He told you to do a one-hour headstand?

JOANNE: That is an interesting story. I would do headstand and after ten breaths he would come over and lift my feet so I would learn how to lift my head. So I would not come down from headstand until he would lift me. At the beginning ten breaths, then fifteen, then five minutes, then ten minutes, [then] I'd be there for half an hour, for a long time. And one day I was already up for almost half an hour and I hear the phone ring and Amma talking in the background and Saraswathi and everybody excited and I was wondering what's happening. They had a big call from America. He forgot about me completely. So I'm there, stubborn as I am, not coming down until Guruji comes back. So he comes back and sees me and looks at the time and says, "One hour! Wonderful! From now on you do one hour."

Are you still doing one hour?

JOANNE: No, I don't have time. When I went back in 2000, I did half an hour.

Can you say you experienced some special result from such a long headstand?

JOANNE: I would say especially when we were doing long practice, like three-hour practice. We started with a fifteen-minute practice, but after some years we were doing primary, intermediate, advanced A and B almost, and then headstand, so it was a three-hour practice.

DARBY: We had to do primary, intermediate—

JOANNE: Well we started primary, intermediate; then primary, intermediate, advanced; then he cut off primary and it was intermediate, advanced, and more and more advanced.

DARBY: The first two years we never took away a posture; primary, intermediate, advanced—and it's not the same advanced that they are doing now. It's a series I think he adapted to us because there were different advanced [series] at that period. Joanne's was almost a four-hour practice and I had a three-hour practice.

So you had no time for anything else.
JOANNE: Especially [after] Shankara was born. By that time the baby was starving [because] I was breast-feeding.

One-hour headstand was very beneficial. It was so relaxing. That is why I never had pain, because being on my head for one hour just relaxed everything, your mind becomes almost blank.

How was the birth?
JOANNE: It was pretty good. We were in Mysore so I did my practice the day before, and it was interesting because when I got the first pain—

DARBY: It was eleven o'clock at night. Too late to go to the hospital and I said, "Well, I'm going to deliver the baby." At two o'clock in the morning I had second thoughts. Saraswathi and Amma came and—

JOANNE: We took a rickshaw to a private clinic. The doors were not even open and then once they opened the doors—

DARBY: The cleaners had to get out from sleeping underneath the operating table.

JOANNE: But otherwise it went very well. When they said, "Push," I pushed so strong the baby just flew out.

DARBY: I was sitting outside in the waiting room with Saraswathi and the baby started to cry.

JOANNE: The birth was very easy. But quite an experience for us and for the family, too, I guess. Western lady doing yoga in their *shala*—at that point in time, it was an event for them, too, I'm sure.

How soon after giving birth did you go back to practice?
JOANNE: By myself, quite fast, I was a maniac, in those days nothing could stop me. Guruji had to go to America. I think he didn't want to see

me for another month or two, so I could not go back to the *shala* for a couple of months.

And pretty soon you and Darby were—
JOANNE: On the same racetrack.

DARBY: Four years [in Mysore] then one year in Australia, and somehow we got money to get back again.

JOANNE: Saraswathi kept telling Darby that we needed a second child. Shankara was a handful to start with, but anyway—

DARBY: Saraswathi said he needed someone to play with.

JOANNE: We kept asking Guruji, and Guruji would not answer. He would not approve or disapprove but only say it was our problem, not his. But Darby decided to have another one and I got pregnant straightaway when he decided. Guruji knew from day one I was pregnant. The moment my period didn't come, I told Guruji, "I'm pregnant," and he said, "Nah, nah, you have to wait." Because in India, you don't say you are pregnant unless you are three months pregnant. So he knew and I kept doing my practice. That's why when I read later for pregnant woman not to practice the first three months I was confused because I know that he let me practice from day one. That's when my mother told me, "You have no more money in the bank, it's time to come back." I left for six months and it was seven and a half years [that I'd been gone] by then. My money had run to zero.

DARBY: We couldn't afford to pay fees to Guruji so we went to Gokarna and were basically living in a mud hut in the jungle.

JOANNE: That was in 1984. I was doing an intense practice in Gokarna because there was nothing else to do. I was reading the *Shiva Purana* all day long and doing practice and going to the beach. We stayed for Shivaratri, so it was a very beautiful place to be. It was risky to have a child there because there was nothing, but we thought it was paradise. And we both had so much faith that nothing wrong could happen, and it was a beautiful birth.

And you went back to see Guruji with the baby?
JOANNE: Never, we went straight from Gokarna to Bombay, and we went back to Canada and for fifteen years Guruji never heard from us.

We arrived home at my mother's house without a penny, with a husband and two children, and say, "Hi, Mom, haven't seen you for eight years but now you have to look after me."

It must have been quite difficult, too, for you to leave the hippie lifestyle.
DARBY: Well, I had to work.

JOANNE: It was easy. My brother-in-law called him to work the next morning.

DARBY: He was president of the company and had a job for me, and when good positions came up, I was given priority, so I began to make money and became more of a businessman. I started playing golf instead of doing yoga.

How long did it take before you stopped practicing yoga?
DARBY: It was a gradual thing. I would do my practice when I would be working. I stopped doing advanced, then I stopped doing intermediate, and I wouldn't practice every day. I didn't feel confident enough to teach. I did a demonstration at the Hare Krishna Center. Shandor, who was pretty established, heard about it. He was going to India, so he said, "Look after my school while I go to India."

So yes, after a month of teaching thirty students I had just four left. He actually came back early because I think somebody had told him I was relieving him of his students.

JOANNE: We went to see some schools in Canada and they were all Sivananda style. They didn't want to hear about it, they were saying, "You just want to show off," so it was not very good. It was too early for Canada to do this. Even in America it took a long time.

Did you continue to practice?
JOANNE: Longer than Darby because I was home looking after the children. I kept it up a little more than Darby, but within three years, there was less and less time to practice.

And it was another twelve years until you met Guruji again?

DARBY: In 1997 I got fired, which meant I got a six-month severance and a year's unemployment. So the very next day I started my yoga practice. If you don't keep contact with the guru you sort of lose touch with it [the practice]. And it might have been a blessing in a way. We were so intense with that practice that we probably would have broken our bodies. By the time we got into yoga again there was much more awareness of alignment. In fact, I remember when I first started, I felt a conflict between Iyengar, who had alignment, and Pattabhi Jois, whose method was *vinyasa* yoga. It was that kind of thing, where we don't associate with alignment and they don't associate with us. As the time went on, both parties started to take from each other. I think that's what saved us. I took a workshop with Richard Freeman and he talked about alignment, something we never heard about. I decided to go to Colorado. I spent a month with Richard in Colorado. After that I had a person who came from an Iyengar background and we worked together and started to combine, and I think that's what really saved me afterward.

If we just bend in one spot all the time while doing the postures, eventually that's going to break. If you keep bending it like a coat hanger in one place that's what is going to happen, and that's probably what would have happened to my body.

JOANNE: When we were in Gokarna you had a hernia I'm sure. He couldn't even get up. He was walking on his knees and couldn't bend.

DARBY: And that healed and I was fine again. I blew my knee out in Mysore but it had nothing to do with Guruji. I was just learning to do *janu shirshasana* C and I'm looking at my friend Old Cliff Barber and he's doing *viranchyasana* B, which is taking the foot right over. I'm just a beginner and I took my foot right over and this is how I wrecked my knee. Fortunately, Guruji was there hearing it pop. I wasn't going to stop. My knee was popping out every day. Third day he said that's it, no more, you don't do any more knee-bending postures. That's when he asked me to stay until my knee healed.

You talk about pushing yourself, but how was it to be pushed by Guruji?

DARBY: Guruji's method, from what I can gather, and I've seen this in my own teaching, is that the first time you give someone a new posture, the person's body has no idea what is happening, so the body stays very relaxed. He pushes you into that posture to where your body can go, as far as you can go. The next day he knows your body can go there, but by this time your body is saying, "I don't want to go there because that was scary." He will still take you there, he will still take you to that point even though your body has had that reaction, and in that resistance you get the pain. If you didn't have that resistance, you could keep going. And he'll push you until the body gives up and then you can do the posture. I believe that's his method.

Do you understand why that happens?
DARBY: The body says, "I didn't want to do that."

JOANNE: But is it mental or physical?

DARBY: The body has stretched and then it needs to soften and relax. If someone pushes you down and you didn't do it for another month you'd have to be pushed down again. So if you get pushed down every day, like in Guruji's method, eventually the body will soften into that place where it's already been.

JOANNE: Yes, but if it's easy to do the first time, why would it be difficult the second time?

DARBY: Because you actually stretched stuff further than it is used to going and it needs time to heal. And if you don't give it time to heal it's going to resist that stretching.

So the body is really not fully open to do the posture, but there is no resistance, then when the body is pushed to that point, then the body reacts and it tries to protect itself from opening too much.
DARBY: Yes. I've helped students the first time, the next day they are not able to do it. Guruji's method is he would make you do it. In the West people kind of back off a bit, whereas the best method is to try and keep doing it.

Do you have a different take on it?
JOANNE: My main problem was always my strength, but Guruji never

worried about it and it built up by itself. Darby always said my arm balances where better than his, Darby's, because for me it was just a balance point. It's not even strength, it's balance. Guruji trained me. He would just hold on to my toe and make me get the perfect balance point. And the rest is just getting up there and doing it. In those days they were not concerned with *chaturanga vinyasa*, holding it for fifteen, twenty breaths. We were going a fast flow, basically.

DARBY: Pain was there as a beginner. The pain changed as I got into advanced. Even doing advanced there was pain, but it was just more a soreness from new postures. It wasn't the pain of a beginner, breaking and getting stretched out.

When I was teaching they would ask me, "How long did it take you to learn *eka pada* [*shirshasana*]?" And I said, "Guruji came up and we did it." So Guruji's method in the beginning is to push, and in the end he was giving us postures that we were ready to do. It wasn't so much learning them; it was more when we were ready, we could do it.

It's key as a teacher to know when a student is ready.
JOANNE: None of us learned the same advanced. Now it's a very A, B, C, or one, two, three, but in those days I think he would see what were your good points and he would just give us the postures.

Today people get so obsessed about the sequence that he taught you in such an individualized way.
DARBY: I think now when you transition to intermediate you have to be able to stand up from *urdhva dhanurasana*. We learned primary and intermediate and when you got into advanced, then we did *urdhva dhanurasana*, and we didn't even have to stand up from it.

And I think it's because of the number of people who are going. They don't have the time, so they made it more difficult and shortened the breaths from eight to five. Some of the postures we held for five breaths are not there, they would just be in the transition.

JOANNE: There were just a few of us in those days. Now it's 350 people.

Were primary and intermediate different in those days, too?
JOANNE: There is a slight difference, mostly the standing postures.

DARBY: We didn't learn the reversed triangle or reversed *parshvakonasana* as beginners. *Utthita hasta padangushtasana* and then *ardha baddha padmottanasana* were at the end of primary instead of the beginning—after *setu bandhasana*—then we did *utthita hasta*, which made sense because you don't have the strength as a beginner to stand on one leg and take the leg to one side. It's easier to learn it in *supta padangushtasana*. Even *ardha baddha padmottanasana*, to stand up on one leg and bend, is quite dangerous. First you learned primary and you had the strength of ten, eleven, twelve weeks' practice before the postures were introduced.

If the precise sequencing is not the most important thing—
DARBY: The sequencing is there, just the details are a little different. Like standing *trikonasana* with the side twist is not a beginner's posture. That was given as we got more into intermediate. If you are a beginner watching an advanced student and you copy the person . . . I think what happened, with so many people doing that coming to Mysore, Guruji gave up and said, "Okay, everybody does it now," and put it in the beginner series.

JOANNE: Besides those minor changes, the only one I remember in intermediate is the scorpion. We used to do *pincha mayurasana*, *karandavasana*, and scorpion. Other than that, intermediate has not changed; primary has not changed, either. So primary and intermediate are 90 percent the same.

How was going back to Mysore?
DARBY: In 2000 we arrived, and Eddie took us to Guruji, and one of the first things I asked him was, "Can you certify us?" And he said, "No, I want to see you practice."

JOANNE: First he said, "Why not calling?" Fifteen years we never gave him a call. Never. He didn't know where we were, he never heard from us, he was totally upset with us.

DARBY: I think the first time we called him was the death of Amma. We read on the Internet that Amma had died and called him.

JOANNE: And he said, "You come to Mysore." But then our finances were not the greatest, so we said, "Oh, not so possible." He said, "You come."

DARBY: Money came and we ended up in Mysore.

JOANNE: Guruji never gave us led classes. All the time in Mysore I never heard of it.

DARBY: I think he gave us one or two when he came back from America and we did it one day and said, "Oh, that's fun." And we did it the second day and thought, "That's enough, Guruji. Let's go back to Mysore practice."

When you went back to Mysore how did you feel?
JOANNE: It was interesting because we saw how many people were waiting in line.

DARBY: Quite funny, actually.

Was he still at the old shala?
DARBY: The old *shala* the first time. He said, "You come at nine o'clock." We came and did our practice, and after our practice we said, "Well, how does this system work, Guruji?" He said, "First batch fixed. After, queuing system." We said, "Okay, let's get to the front of the queue." We just joined the line not knowing it was a system. And the next thing you know Guruji calls us in to practice. I think when people saw us practice we had a little bit of respect. It wasn't very long before we were in the first batch.

JOANNE: The whole family was supposed to be there for two months. But after a month I thought maybe I'd love to stay longer, so we found a place to stay, a pretty nice house in Lakshmipuram. And the younger son said—

DARBY: "How can I stay in India? I have no school! What's going to happen to my life?"

JOANNE: We found him a school, so I end up staying there another five years.

DARBY: And I would come twice a year. At Christmas I would spend two or three months, and in July I'd come again.

JOANNE: And I would go to Canada in April, May.

How was it to get into the same level of practice after all those years of a break?
JOANNE: A bit of a shock because we thought it would have been easy. We've done it before, we can do it all again. But that wasn't our experience because our bodies didn't want to respond like twenty years back.

So what was your program?
JOANNE: We started back with primary, which was fine.

DARBY: Then gradually intermediate—

JOANNE: But intermediate, already I could feel that *kapotasana* was not like it used to be, and *eka pada shirshasana*, the legs did not want to get there as fast. I realized that this is not as easy as it used to be.

Looking back, I wish I had taken longer because I got really injured and that's when I ended up with sore back, shoulders, sleepless nights with lots of pain which I didn't have in the past.

But now it's stopped. How long did that take?
JOANNE: It took years. I had a lot of work to do on my shoulders. I had been working many years on computers. I would put all my strain on my lower back so then I had to learn to open up other parts of the body when I got some lower back pain.

DARBY: You know the flexibility has never been the same as it was.

JOANNE: Of course. Fifty-six years old and he's still upset by it—

DARBY: It's a different practice.

JOANNE: Yes I know, but you wish sometimes—

DARBY: I wish I could put my feet on my head. The practice is more internal. Before it was more, let's do the posture, whatever posture, whatever backbend. Now I'm starting to want to understand what I feel inside a posture and how can I get an energy going from one end of my body and continue that energy to the other. So it's more watching *nadis* or meridians and understanding how there is a connection from the big toe to the front of the perineum. When I take the little toe, the connection goes up the other side of the leg and comes to the back of that area. So knowing that, I know when I stretch my feet I'm going to connect to the perineum by using my toes. This kind of connection.

This is experiential, something you've explored.
DARBY: Talking to people, reading a little bit, and then just feeling it in my own body. If you want to lift the arm and connect and get the full extension, better make sure you lift from the baby finger even though you want to connect to the whole hand. If you lift from the baby finger you can feel the connection coming from the back into the shoulder blades. But when you lift from the first finger or the thumbs, it comes to the front of the shoulders, it's a different way. But a lot of people don't know that. By lifting the arm they get these tight shoulders. And I know, I've done this in classes, lift by the baby finger and the connection comes to the back. So it is experimenting in the postures, watching and saying, "Okay, where is energy going this time?" It's a long process.

So it's become more subtle.
DARBY: More subtle once you get more into the *bandhas* and how the *bandhas* work. I was looking at qigong and the kind of postures in qigong, which my son is working on. In the class we had everybody do qigong and trying to use those muscles in understanding *uddiyana bandha* in the physical aspect. And there is still that spiritual aspect of working more with chakras, and sounds of chakras, and vibrations in the chakras—using that also in the *ashtanga* practice. Lots of times when I'm doing my practice I inhale and I'm repeating [chanting] and using a very long *om* and feel those vibrations in the body and it opens the body up. It lets the body soften. It changes all the time, it's always something useful. I'm just enjoying it so much, just loving this practice.

I've always had Guruji as a teacher, always as a kind of a father figure as well. This is an interesting story. One time he went to Madras to get a visa, so he was gone for a few days and we were left to do self-practice, and I think Brad Ramsey and Gary [Lopedota] and I were practicing and I was having problems with my knee. Guruji wasn't going to be there the next day and so I decided to take the day off. And what happened was, Guruji came back and I had not gone to class. He sent somebody over to get me to class. I couldn't get away with anything with this guy.

He was only pretending to go away.
DARBY: Yes, and my son, who came to practice many years later, didn't feel like practicing so he thought, "I'm just going to do half primary," and Guruji said that's fine, so his attitude is so different now from what it was then.

JOANNE: The time I was there from 2001 to 2006 I thought he was really strict with me, because I could see all of his newcomers would do whatever they wanted. If they didn't feel well, they went home. And me, God! I would arrive with fever and he would touch me: "No fever, you do!" and I would have to do advanced four days a week. Why me—the oldest one there—work harder than any of those newcomers? He always was tough on us.

Because he loved you.
DARBY: That's exactly what I mean. He was tough in that loving way.

JOANNE: He would never let us get away with anything.

DARBY: He was the teacher.
Sometimes I just felt dead. Out of respect, you do, you never question. You never even said, "Well, Guruji, I don't feel well today." There was only one time he let me do something else. I had a cold. I couldn't breathe, and at this stage he taught Gary full *vinyasa*. I said, "Guruji, I have a cold, I don't feel well, perhaps today I could do full *vinyasa*?" He was very much for that, and worse, he made me do full *vinyasa* with everything.

Did he just do the full vinyasa *for Gary because Gary was so energetic and Guruji felt he needed something more?*

DARBY: I think Gary had heard about it and I was kind of watching and I thought, "But I won't dare to ask Guruji." It's only when I got this heavy cold and couldn't breathe that I asked him if I could do it. He was very happy and said, "Oh yeah, you do." He wanted to teach it.

JOANNE: But afterward we heard in 2000 that he told people not to do full *vinyasa* because it was hard on the heart. I guess it was good for young kids who were learning.

DARBY: I got very strong quickly from doing it.

Did Guruji ever teach you philosophy?

JOANNE: No. It seemed like his purpose was to teach us *asanas* and the rest was up to us. He often mentions dharma, *yamas*, *niyamas*. He definitely wants us to know all those matters, but sometimes I get the impression he gave up on us because he sees so much stuff happening in Mysore. The way people live in the West, the way they behave, it's like, "Do your practice and eventually in time you might understand what *yamas* and *niyamas* are all about." It makes him sad, in a way, because he's teaching all these people that wonderful gift. He's giving it to all of us, like a key to a treasure, but nobody uses it correctly. He teaches us what he has to teach, but he leaves it up to us. As he says, a father has kids, but the kids are all wild and they go drinking in bars and the father is not happy, but what can you do? He does his best. He never taught us, but he always mentioned the *Bhagavad Gita*, Patanjali's *Yoga Sutras*. He would give us some teaching on those, very little, enough to get you interested. I can remember at one stage he told us, "You learn the *Bhagavad Gita* by heart." It was a bit of a trend in 2000. You spend a year learning one chapter, you give up after that. So he wants us to be interested.

DARBY: The saddest thing about him is that he's not teaching anymore. I remember a year ago when we were here and he was sitting in the chair and he wanted to get up. He was always trying to get up and assist someone. They would say, "Stay there, you can't do that." In fact, they wouldn't let him in the *shala* because he was always wanting to teach. He just loves to be around and pass on that knowledge. I know every time I go to Mysore and come back I feel I have part of that love in me. I have renewed enthusiasm to be with students and help them more with that kind of kindness and love in trying to adjust. It's just a wonderful thing.

JOANNE: That's what Sharath says about him. He's got a love, an aura around him, that just engulfs us. You can't help it, you want to study.

DARBY: Do your best, 110 percent just to get a little more approval, and then he doesn't give you that much approval.

What do you think he's teaching beyond the asanas? *What is being expressed in his teaching?*
JOANNE: *Ashtanga* for him is not just a name. He has told us in simple words, "Do your *yamas* and *niyamas*." It's very simple for him, it's part of life, you know. Family life for him is very important. You have to deal with that first, then the *asana*. *Pranayama* is also a strong part of the teaching, but it's only for a few with Guruji, when they are doing advanced and he knows that they can do it. To be able to do *pranayama* and to sit there for half an hour and to be able to hold your breath and *bandhas* . . . I'm sure if you are able to do this practice, these five levels—*yamas, niyamas, asana, pranayama, bandha*—that you are going to be ready for the next stage. But most of us fall off so we can't even get to *pranayama*. So this name, *ashtanga* yoga, is more than just a name. Get to the core of the practice of *ashtanga*, don't just concentrate on the *asana*. The *asana* is the foundation. You can stay healthy, at least. If you are screwing up on the *yamas* and *niyamas*, you can get back to your feet again. Your body will be strong and if you work hard at it you will eventually go to a higher level. *Asanas* are important but it's not the whole thing.

DARBY: Especially this practice. It's a practice. At the beginning, it's fun. But if you have to keep doing it every day, you start to have to face yourself. Some days you don't feel like doing it, other days you feel energetic, but if you do it every day you are going to break through those barriers. Guruji tells us to have that faith—belief in God, follow the *yamas* and *niyamas*, have that devotion to believe and then practice—then he says, things are going to happen.

JOANNE: Serious students who are in it for many years have no choice, you have to evolve.

DARBY: You have to start looking at yourself, looking inside. Taking out those emotions that are there, those deep-seated fears. You have beliefs or concepts you have to give up, and so you come into spiritual power.

JOANNE: Well you have to, or there is no point in doing these *asanas* every morning. It's not easy. Nobody I know likes to get up every morning at five or six to do an hour, an hour and a half. You need a strong discipline. It's very strengthening.

DARBY: Much easier to get up and play golf.

JOANNE: Or bicycling. It's more interesting to go bicycling for an hour than doing this practice.

You are always doing the same thing.
JOANNE: We are constantly discovering new things. When we started, we hardly heard about *mula bandha*.

DARBY: I keep discovering *bandhas*. I discovered *mula bandha* three times in one month. I think I had *mula bandha*, but now I have *mula bandha*, and I thought I had . . . *now* I have *mula bandha*.

What is it about doing the same thing day in, day out that helps you to understand and know yourself better?
JOANNE: You don't have to worry about what you are doing every day. This is fixed. It's like entering a door. Every day you enter into your little internal room and you discover new things all the time. You don't have to worry about the outside look of the practice. But we are lucky because we have primary, intermediate, or advanced. We have a choice.

DARBY: Variety. I remember being in Mysore on a Thursday practice, drinking our coconuts and going, "Oh! Thank God it's Friday and only primary," and people would look at us and say, "We do primary every day."

　　If you are doing it year after year, you have to look at something else besides the practice. Something comes from doing it. There's purification in it.

JOANNE: Oh yeah, definitely, it's a constant purification because you bring so much junk up all the time. It's like a daily cleanup, almost like brushing your teeth every day.

Can you say something about Amma, Guruji's relationship with Amma, and how important she was for you and for the students at that time?
DARBY: It brings tears to my eyes thinking about her. She was very special.

JOANNE: She used to cook on special holidays and sometimes there were only two of us in Mysore and she would invite us as part of the family for a feast and always a smile: "Coffee?"

DARBY: Very special, and always behind: the woman behind the man.

JOANNE: Her whole life was devoted to Guruji and to the family. A perfect Indian wife. He probably couldn't live without her.

DARBY: When she died, we made contact again with Guruji. She was always smiling, happy, happiness. He loved her very much, was devoted to her.

What about yama *and* niyama?
JOANNE: If you put so much importance on *asana* and forget about the other parts of yoga, I find it sad. The whole purpose is not a show just to impress or whatever. You do it for yourself: you want to change something in your life and be a better person, you want to improve, you want to reach some kind of higher level of consciousness through this practice. In the West sometimes you find people putting too much importance on the *asanas* and wanting a fit, nice-looking body and forgetting about the rest.

DARBY: A lot of time all that's taught is the *asana*.

JOANNE: In fitness centers that's all that's taught.

DARBY: People who start yoga at yoga centers, not fitness centers, come in with the intention of wanting to learn more. So the *asana* can help you when you start, and if you have good intentions then those intentions start to get better. You can read philosophy or *The Yoga Sutras* and start to understand. I think everybody knows what's good or bad.

JOANNE: It's true, too, that as much as it's important to know philosophy, it's the practice that will calm your mind. Basically, you want to calm your mind. The more you try to intellectualize, instead of calming the mind and stop thinking, you will think three times more.

Is there anything else you'd like to say?
DARBY/JOANNE: Have faith.

DARBY: For me, it's *bhakti*, believing in Shiva, and sometimes in my own mind I ask Shiva for things—

JOANNE: Your famous quote: Be careful of what you ask for.

DARBY: Shiva will give it to you. You go, "Oh-oh, I didn't really want that!" But have devotion, have belief. Have a spiritual life. Believe in God or whatever you want to call God, a belief in a higher power. Do your practice.

JOANNE: And let go sometimes.

DARBY: Do your practice with that belief and whatever you want through your practice will be given to you. You don't have to worry about anything else. God will find a way of giving it to you. But don't ask for too much.

JOANNE: And also believe that things will happen. We try to be too rational sometimes; we want results. We forget that God is there to look after us. There is nothing to worry about. Things will happen in their own time in their own way. We are just here, it's not even us sometimes.

DARBY: Just have faith and be with the practice. When I'm ready for something, it seems to open up; something opens up.

JOANNE: As they say, when you are ready for a guru, the guru appears. When you are ready to go to a different level, something will happen. You'll find the road that will lead you to that place. We didn't know, when we started, what we wanted. Why do yoga? But suddenly Guruji appeared. The best example is Arjuna with the arrow. You try to keep focus on what you want. Eventually the arrow will hit the target. The path is not ours to decide. It's just going to happen.

What is the one thing above all else that you appreciate on your path of yoga? What do you have to be thankful for?
JOANNE: Wow. Everything. Guruji gave us the key to the treasure. He was sent by God to give us that and it's like a piece of gold. It's up to us to do what we want with it. Depends on how hard we work on it and how much intention and with how much intensity we want to discover. It's like a map almost. Here is Pattabhi Jois to teach you *asana*, now from there you can look at other things and it opens up the doors, whether it's books to read or people to meet and talk to. I feel that. Even the time in between the practice, ten, fifteen years, it was maybe our dharma to be having a family life, working as a family to understand other people.

DARBY: *Asana* practice seemed so easy for me when I first started, that when I was first teaching, I didn't understand that people couldn't do things. Stopping and starting again helped me get that realization. And it made me realize—

JOANNE: Wow, that was something precious, I don't want to lose that again.

Cologne, 2008

R. Sharath Jois

Guruji's grandson, R. Sharath Jois, was his assistant for nineteen years. He started experimenting with yoga at the age of seven and began formal practice when he was fourteen. He is now the director of the Sri K. Pattabhi Jois Ashtanga Yoga Institute in Mysore. He also travels and teaches internationally.

The last time I spoke to Guruji about the difference between Advaita Vedanta, of which he was a professor, and yoga, he said, "They are the same, no difference. Advaita Vedanta is the internal aspect; yoga is the external aspect." Can you tell us about the ashtanga *yoga view of yoga?*
First I would like to say that *ashtanga* yoga is totally unique. In *ashtanga* the main thing is not only posture but also correct breathing, that means *ujjayi* breathing and *vinyasa krama*. This is a very powerful practice, which came from Krishnamacharya, and it's unique in its effect on the body. So this I think is totally different. It energizes your whole body through practice. You can feel the difference. In the philosophy also, if you take Shankaracharya's books, they always say that you have to do *mula bandha* with the *asanas*.

Asana is the foundation from which we build up to self-realization. When you do *asanas* correctly, then only will your mind and body transform, you will see them change, you can make out the difference.

It's very difficult for someone to practice the *yamas* and *niyamas*, but through the *asana* practice I think you'll be able to understand what is *yama*, what is *niyama*, and all the other limbs of *ashtanga* yoga.

Even if you are not able to do many postures—in Guruji's and Krishnamacharya's method we do lots of *asanas* as a way to change—you may still be able to understand what yoga is through correct practice.

In the *Hatha Yoga Pradipika*, it says without having a healthy mind and healthy body it is very difficult to understand what is Brahma *jnana*, to realize what is God or to realize what is the divine, which is within us; this is only possible through practice. You can read many books, but without practical experience it will be very difficult to understand what it is. Many people, they read many books and they have lots of knowledge about yoga, but they don't have practical experience, so their knowledge is of no use.

How does asana *practice create transformation? It seems like a big jump from doing* asanas *to knowledge of brahman. What happens in between?*
There are two types of practitioners. First, you can see yoga as a sport just to be healthy, but there is a limitation in that. When you see yoga in a big way, in a different way, if you see it as a spiritual practice, there is a lot of transformation that will happen within you.

When you start learning *asanas* you say, "Okay, I'm learning *asanas* now so I need to know more about this. I need to know about the philosophy or I need to know what is real yoga." Yoga is beyond *asana* and *asana* is one limb of yoga.

Yoga is *chitta vritti nirodhah*, that means to control your sense organs and realize what the divine is, that is Brahma *jnana*. So you have that thirst in you: "What is that?" We are not all yogis, we are trying to become yogis.

There are many people who practice yoga in India also who think of it as a sport. They do competitions. They think it is just to perform better than the other guy. That is not yoga. Yoga has a different meaning. It's a way of worshipping God. Nobody can compete with worshipping God.

In a practical sense, what is making the change happen? Can you give an example? You have been practicing twenty, twenty-five, thirty years—I don't know how long you've been practicing.
I think your whole personality will change and you become softer.

Is it a mechanical thing in the sense of a physical process, or is it how you are using your mind in relation to your practice?
It is the practice. For example, if you take a small piece of gold from the earth, it is impure. You take that gold and then you have to heat it up and when you heat it up all the impurities, all the bad particles in the gold,

will go and you get the pure gold. Yoga is also like that. When you start, you have lots of impurities in you, and slowly, by practicing, practicing, practicing *asanas*, all this time reading philosophy—but mostly it's the practical experience that you have to go through—then, slowly, it's like the gold. Our body becomes more purified and so you get more and more understanding.

It still seems to me that the way practice transforms you is really a mystery.
As I told you, if you follow the *yamas* and *niyamas* in your daily life you won't get lost. Some people practice for many years but they don't understand what is yoga because they don't understand what is *yama* and *niyama*. You see, everything is connected: *yamas*, *niyamas*, then *asana* comes next. If you don't understand those things, I think you won't be able to understand what is yoga. So that is why they put these first.

Ahimsa, that is nonviolence. Even thinking badly toward someone is also *himsa* [violence]. Not only should you not do it physically but also when thinking. When the mind doesn't think bad things, then you won't act, you don't do it physically.

Yoga practitioners should practice *yama* and *niyama*, practice *ahimsa* in themselves. They should be an example to other people like Mahatma Gandhi. He said, "*Ahimsa* is my first dharma [duty]." He said, "I'm going to follow *ahimsa*, I'll be nonviolent." Many people were inspired by Gandhiji, he had lots of followers.

So each person should be like Gandhiji. It's very difficult to be like him; not everyone can be like him. But you have to try, that is the real yogi. No matter if you read all the texts, if you are a big scholar, if you had read all these things, but if you don't follow this in your daily life what is the use of reading so many books and getting so many degrees, becoming a scholar? It's useless. Yoga practitioners should at least try to follow this.

What do you think are the biggest obstacles for most people in practice?
There're lots of obstacles. Westerners have lots of choice in their life, and if they don't want they can leave this and do something else. They are not committed to one thing.

I'm not talking only about practice. I mean, practice is one thing. It should help you to commit to one thing. It can be anything—your family or your job or your dharma—what you *have* to do. You have lots of choices.

Your duty?
Your duty toward society, or even teaching yoga is like social work. You're giving this knowledge to many people and many people are getting the benefit from this. And then, the yogi or teacher, his dharma or his duty is to teach his students properly what he has learned from his teacher. Everybody has his own field: one is a yogi, one is an engineer—in that he has to commit himself. Whatever his work is, he has to commit to that. His intention, his work, should be to serve people.

From the point of view of the physical asana *practice, most students coming here are interested in that. Do you see one obstacle especially? Could it be lifestyle or work or diet or lack of* brahmacharya? *Is there one thing you think is strongest in terms of its negative impact on the Westerners?*
I think the main thing is *brahmacharya*: committing to one person. That is very important. I think that is reduced in the Western student. That is very important in life. When the mind gets distracted, then it also becomes weak. You should be committed to one thing. It can be your family, to your wife and to your children and that's all. You shouldn't get distracted by other things.

What you're saying is mental distractions are the most problematic.
Yeah, mentally you have to be strong. The strong mind is committed to one thing. The yoga should help the individual to go in a straight direction, which goal you should be reaching.

Can you tell us about the importance of lineage, or parampara?
First of all, yoga should come from *parampara*, from a teacher or guru to his student, *shishya*. The tradition that he has learned from his guru for many years, and should pass to his students, that is called *parampara*. And the relationship between the guru and the *shishya*, the bond between them: the longer you spend with your guru, the more you understand him and his knowledge and his teaching. So it becomes like a father-and-son relationship. The more you understand your guru, and the more you believe him, that trust you have with him, I think the more knowledge will pass to you, and you will be able to understand more what he is saying. If you go for one month or two months and just be with him, your knowledge and understanding is only limited. Since I have spent so many years, I would say seventeen years—for past two

years Guruji is very sick, he is not able to teach me—but all those seventeen years I have seen, I have learned from him and his knowledge and his experience, what he learned from Krishnamacharya. The way of his teaching, only the people who know the knowledge can teach, this method of yoga we are doing. Nowadays people do not know about *parampara*, they do not know about lineage, they do not know about that relationship between guru and *shishya*. Everyone wants to have instant things: in one month they should get certificate, in one month they want to become yoga teachers. Before becoming a student, they want to become a teacher. It is not possible! Yoga is like a science, every step you take is learning, every practice is learning, so how can anyone become a teacher in one month or two months? It's very important to understand the practice, understand your teacher, and understand what he is teaching. That takes a long time, you have to put lots of energy, and even your teacher will put lots of energy. What I have seen in Guruji, he has presented yoga exactly the same way that he has learned from his guru, Krishnamacharya. I mean, there must be some little changes here and there, but the original practice that he learned, Guruji is representing the same thing. See, *that* is *parampara*: what he has learned, he is teaching the same thing. He could have done his own yoga, called it Pattabhi Jois yoga, or Jois yoga, or something, and he could have created his own method of teaching, but he didn't. The same thing that he learned from Krishnamacharya, he taught his students, and most of his students are teaching the same thing. Like that, that is *parampara*, that is the lineage that we should follow. Nowadays not many people understand yoga. They think it might be very physical, or some people are creating their own thing. It's a lie, misrepresenting yoga to the world. The real meaning of yoga is to get self-knowledge about our inner Self, realizing what we are. So if that is not there, it is more physical, you know, and everybody has their own system which does not come from *parampara*. Only a few people are there that are teaching from *parampara*.

When you mention Guruji, Krishnamacharya, and parampara, *and whoever came before Krishnamacharya, are you basically pointing out that everything that Guruji has been teaching to you and your students goes back in a link that is endlessly long behind him, that he is trying to keep carrying it forward, to not break any link in the chain?*
Yes, that is the essence of *parampara*.

So if you try to create your own yoga, you are breaking the link.
You are breaking the link. You know in India we have *gotra* [clan]. I am Gautamasya *gotra*, it has been from many forefathers, it has come from there, I can't change that suddenly, I can't say tomorrow, "I am not Gautamasya *gotra*." I cannot be whatever-I-want *gotra*. You can't do that. Is it possible to do that? It is not. *Parampara* should also go like that.

And *parampara* means the bond with the teacher also, the more you spend your time with him, the more energy he has got, the more that will come to you, his experience will come to you. *Parampara* means that sometimes you have to research also, like you can't stop at what you have learned from your guru, you can still advance your knowledge, but the fundamentals are the same.

Describe a way that Guruji has given energy to you, put energy into you for your practice, and how that has helped mold you.
When I started, it was difficult to understand, like anyone who first comes to do yoga. But in that time when Guruji was helping me do *asanas*, teaching me *asanas*, and I was doing the *asanas* with him helping, the body and mind and everything started changing. I was not the same as I had been before, your thinking will change. That is one part in learning that got very advanced. When your mind is stronger, the body also gets stronger. The other part is the teaching part. I did both things, I learned as well as helping Guruji. So, helping I used to observe him, how he used to help his students, and he used to teach his students. That is also something I got to see, after my practice, I used to see how he would help. His teaching method was very good, he used to put lots of effort. It takes a lot of physical energy to teach, its not just talking, you have to help many students, go there and lift so many students. Before I went there to teach he was teaching alone, and he was almost seventy years old, more than seventy years, when he was teaching, and he was lifting all the students.

Do you think that Guruji has a special way of looking at people?
Yes. For a teacher, it is very important to understand your students. Not all students are the same. They have different bodies. One student may be very flexible but another student may be very stiff. So you have to understand the student, how to teach him, how to help him, so that he can improve his *asana*, that is very important. I think Guruji had that tech-

nique because of his experience, he knew how to adjust each student, he used to read the student so that he could help him in a certain way and help him improve in his daily practice. That is the main thing that I have learned from Guruji, how he used to see the students and teach them.

He seems to be able to read people's faces very well, too.
Yes, everything is involved. When you see the student, it is not only their body, it is also their mind, their way of thinking. When you see a student, you tell him many times, but he doesn't understand what we are telling, his grasping power is very limited. Some other students, you tell one or two times and he will understand, within two times he will understand. You have to have the patience to tell the student and make him understand. Guruji has that quality, that patience. He used to be strict. Strict is also important. That is the Indian tradition, the teachers used to be very strict so that [students] would have that fear and then they would learn it.

Yesterday I was talking with Manju about the perspective that people have of yoga. In the West we have a limited perspective because we have been practicing yoga in the West for a relatively short time. What have you seen from yourself and Guruji, what is the big perspective of yoga, where do you look at it from? For example, in the West a lot of the perspective is from our yoga mat, that is where the focus is. Where do you, and where does Guruji, see it from?
Yes, understanding of yoga is not only your mat, two and a half feet by six and a half feet, that is a part of it. The *asana* that we do is a part of yoga. Yoga, Patanjali yoga that is, says that *yama* and *niyama* are very important, the first two steps of *ashtanga* yoga. *Ahimsa*, etc. . . . . *shaucha*, etc. . . . . all this we should practice in our life. If you see Guruji, he is a very simple man, he is like a child. He does not even know how famous he is. He is very simple. Whoever comes, he talks to them, he is very lively, always smiling. They say bad things, also he smiles. I have seen some students asking him silly questions, and he laughs. I think in his mind he thinks that we should do more practice to understand yoga, but the guy who has asked the question, he thinks that he has mastered yoga! But Guruji gives a smile. I think he thinks that what the student doesn't know is that he has to practice more. The Indian practitioner's understanding of yoga and the Western practitioner's understanding of yoga is totally different, especially those who have learned from the *parampara*.

In the West what I see, since I have been going for the past eight or nine years, their way of thinking is totally different, mostly like marketing themselves I would say. Yoga has become like that, it has become more commercial. But if I talk from Guruji's part, because right now in India he is one of the leading yoga gurus, I think in the world, but for him it doesn't matter whether he is rich or poor, his state of mind is equal, especially in the past two years, what I am seeing. He has gone to the hospital many times. When he went to the hospital, his state of mind was even, he never panicked, he never got fear. He didn't have any fear when he was going for his operation. That is yoga, his mind is always still because of his yoga practice, his mind doesn't change. Yoga means *yama* and *niyama* in our daily life, but if that is not there, what is the use of *asana* practice?

What have you observed Guruji going through over the past year and a half, now that his life is radically different? He seems to be continually positive about returning to health.
He has got belief in yoga and what he has done previously, those many years of practice. He has in his mind that "Nothing will happen to me. Yoga will take care, God will take care of me." That is in his mind. The thing is, he doesn't think anything. When you think that something might happen to me, then the fear will start inside of you, but he lives in the moment—"This moment I am fine, next moment also I'll be fine"— so I think this was there in him for many years, and this has kept him strong. Once we have fear, we mentally make ourselves ill, when you get fear you get ill, then you get the diseases in the body. He was mentally very strong from before, and he is mentally strong now. He has got that willpower. Now also if somebody wants to hold him while he is walking, he doesn't like that, he says, "Don't hold my hand, I can walk fine on my own!" He is scolding Kiran [his attendant], "Don't touch me, I can walk on my own." That willpower he has got.

How about the importance of faith, then? Would you say that shraddha *is faith, or something more than faith?*
Shraddha is more than faith. It is also surrendering your sense organs, your body, your everything, surrendering to the practice. When I was doing all the advanced postures for more than two hours every day, my

body used to get lots of pain. Some days I couldn't even get up. Guruji used to say, "Go ahead and practice, nothing will happen," and I used to go and do that, and that day I wouldn't get any pain. Many times I injured my back doing yoga, and Guruji used to say, "Nothing will happen, don't worry. Do primary for one or two days and then do your regular practice," and he would help me. As soon as he used to help me in certain *asanas*, the pain used to go away. That is surrendering, that is very important. In the olden days, parents used to send their children to *gurukula*, and they used to go there and serve the guru and do whatever he says and learn from him. It is not that easy. That is surrendering to the guru. See how many scholars were there. For example, you met Krishnamurthi. He left his village, he came here and he stayed here and he trusted in the Sanskrit College and he trusted in his guru and he wanted to learn Jyotish, so he went, learned. Guruji also, he left his family and everything. In his mind he wanted to learn Advaita, so he came to Mysore and he had to go through so many difficulties, but he had faith. In learning from Krishnamacharya, too. Krishnamacharya used to hurt his students. So many of them. When he started, he had one hundred students, but in the end there were only three or four students. I don't say or know what happened to them or what difficulty they had, but the amount of *shraddha* that Guruji had to learn yoga was immense. He went there, learned, surrendered himself, and see how he has become now.

Without having that faith first, the knowledge—
It won't come to you, it won't transfer to you.

Some people think that whatever practice they are doing has to prove itself to them first, and after, they will get faith in it. What you are saying is: first have faith.
Yes, first have faith. I don't say that everybody should be doing advanced postures, doing all the six series. It depends on their body, mind, not everyone is the same. But for the foundation to be strong you should do *asanas*, they will change your mind and everything. But that is not the only thing that you should learn from your guru. You should learn all these things: simplicity, *yama*, *niyama* . . . What your guru tells you to follow in your daily life, that will change your attitude. It will change your whole life.

Do you see a clash of cultures here? Apart from the physical aspects, is there a difficulty in making the Western student understand the importance of yama *and* niyama?

I don't say that Western students are totally wrong. There are so many things we can learn from them also, it is not that they have only to learn from us. They are very polite. In general, we see that not many of us are polite. That is also a part of yoga. The person has to have the simplicity. That I see in the West also. From their part, when they come to Mysore, they like this culture very much. It is very different. Many of them do not have family bonds, they don't live together with the family, as soon as they turn eighteen they have to go out from the family and find their own way.

Have you ever felt that the Western view on yoga is from a mainly physical point of view?

Maybe 60 percent or more, they think is physical, a workout. But it is not only there; in India it is getting spoiled, too. In India, there are many yoga teachers who are not doing it in a traditional way. They are just bending their bodies. If it is only for bending bodies, we can just go to the circus.

How do you try to ensure that the students imbibe the yogic way of life so that they do not just see it as purely physical?

It is only during the weekly talks. Then we can tell these things. We can't go to their daily life and see what they do. I have so many students and I can't go to each student and look and see. The teacher can only guide you, you know, this is the way to Bangalore, you can go this way, it is a beautiful city, if you go there you can see lots of things . . . Teacher will show you the way, but you have to find Bangalore. I can't come with you to Bangalore and show you all of it! The interaction between teacher and student is very important. I have spent so much time with my grandfather, I have learned so many good things from him, his daily life, his *puja*, his way of thinking which has impressed me, and I am trying to follow that *svadhyaya*. We have to do our own homework, we have to do our own work. There are so many things that I have to learn, there are so many things, it is just beginning. Each step is like a yoga practice.

What are some of the things that you have observed in Guruji's life, the way he lives, that you have tried to do also that have made things helpful for you and work better for you?

All the basics are the same, his fundamentals are the same. He is like a child, he doesn't have jealousy toward anything. He is always normal no matter what. He never has bad thoughts toward anyone. That is very important. Especially for a yoga practitioner, you should not have any bad thoughts toward anyone, and even if you do, it should not stay for a long time, it should go away quickly. He doesn't keep anything in his mind, or inside him. Some people, they keep inside and they do bad things to others, just keep it inside. He is not like that, it comes in and goes out very quickly. If he gets mad, it comes here and goes away—he scolds right away, and then it is gone, it doesn't stay there. So his mind is very clear. When your mind is clear you don't have any bad thoughts, you don't have bad energy in you, and that is very important for a yoga teacher and a yoga practitioner. That I see in him.

Anything else you might want to say that I have not thought to ask?

I would say that it is my good karma from I don't know how many lives that I was able to study with my grandfather and have such a strong relationship, and learn for so many years. It is more than you can imagine, especially when my grandmother was here. Her energy was even more than Guruji's. Guruji used to teach me *asanas* and all those things, but her energy was even stronger.

How so?

Because she is the one who supported my grandfather, she supported the whole family. She was a very powerful woman, though she looked very simple. Without her energy I don't think I would have learned so much from Guruji. It is not just trying to do yoga, but it is the energy around you, too. She used to tell Guruji, "You have to make him learn all the *asanas*, you must make him great." She used to support me so much. She would say, "You have to learn, you have to perfect this art in you, so that the *parampara* will be there." She used to tell all these things. I spent time with Guruji, but I spent even more time with my grandmother. She also was a great yogi. She had so many good ideas. She was a very wise woman, she was not ordinary, her thinking was so wise.

When I was young I was very sick. I had a hernia, rheumatic fever. It was a challenging thing to do yoga because of this, certain parts were very stiff for me. Through Guruji I had to change not only my body but my lifestyle. I had so many friends, and they used to call for parties, and I had to say no, and I slowly got more serious about yoga practice. My mind totally changed, my focus changed. After five in the evening my mind would go to tomorrow morning's practice. When that is there, you don't think about other things, you don't have distractions.

Mysore, 2008

Practice, Practice

◆

Ashtanga *Spreads*

Chuck Miller

Chuck Miller started practicing yoga in 1971, met Guruji in 1980 on one of his trips to the United States, and began visiting Mysore to study in 1983. He lived and taught in Los Angeles for sixteen years, building up a large school called YogaWorks with his partner, Maty Ezraty. Yoga-Works was sold in 2004, and Chuck and Maty moved to the Big Island in Hawaii. He continues to teach internationally.

How did you come to meet Guruji and become his student?
I had been living in Vermont and had been doing yoga practice on my own for quite a while. I had fallen out of it and was really looking to get back into it. I was driving around North America for about two years. My car broke down north of San Francisco and I ended up meeting some-body who had studied with David Williams in Hawaii, who told me that this Indian man was coming to America to teach a couple of towns over from where we were staying.

I really wasn't interested. I had my little book that I was practicing with, *Light on Yoga* by B. K. S. Iyengar, and I was quite content with that, just working through the course of study in the back of the book. But he kept bugging me and saying, "You got to check this out. This guy studied with the same man as B. K. S. Iyengar [T. Krishnamacharya]," and that caught my attention. I thought Krishnamacharya was pretty cool, and anybody who was there at that same time would be worth meeting. But I still wasn't really interested in spending $200—that is what the six-week course cost at that time.

I was sleeping outside on this hill, and it was a full-moon night, the night before Guruji was going to start teaching, and I had this image in my mind of a brown-skinned man with a bald head, a little bit round, smiling, saying, "Come and see, come down, come watch." I walked down the hill the next day, and he had just finished teaching second series and was standing in the doorway with a big smile on his face saying goodbye to the students, some of whom he had known for a while, as this was his third trip to the States, I think.

And he saw me. It was the first day of the class, so a lot people were new, but he made a comment: "Oh, you new student!" And I don't know if I was just a little bit proud, telling him that I wasn't a new student, that I had been practicing yoga for eight years. He said, "Who is teaching?" And I said, "Book—learning from book," and he just laughed. He thought that was really funny. He said, "What book?" and I said, "*Light on Yoga.*" I didn't have a clue about any of the history or any of that stuff. He got a big kick out of that, and labeled me a B. K. S. Iyengar student. He told me to sit down and watch the first day—very much like my vision.

So I sat there and watched and realized quickly that what I had been doing for practice was a whole different level, and what was going on in this room was pretty extraordinary, and I had a lot to learn. I had no problem coming back the next day and forking over my two hundred bucks.

What was your first impression of Guruji?
My first impression of Guruji was when I saw him standing in the doorway between classes that he was teaching in 1980 in Fairfax—he had a big smile on his face, had a sense of power and was at the same time funny, you know, humorous and friendly—I was intrigued. And when he started teaching, he had a similar feeling about him. He was very demanding and at the same time cracked jokes and made people laugh. He brought a lot of humor into this very intense, serious practice.

So let's talk about ashtanga *yoga not being a purely physical practice and about some of the subtle aspects of* ashtanga *yoga practice.*
My first impression, as I sat on the bench watching that first day, was that this was a very strong physical practice. There were a couple of guys at the back of the room who were doing above and beyond the normal pick-it-up-and-jump-back that Guruji was asking for. They were going into full handstands and holding the handstands and coming down slowly with a lot of control and going into the next pose. It was Gary Lopedota and Stan Hafner.

It wasn't what I was looking for in a yoga practice. I wasn't looking for something so gymnastic or hard physically. I was much more into philosophy. That's really what drew me into yoga in the first place, and my understanding was that yoga was more of a spiritual practice. But there was something about seeing Guruji teaching in the room that drew me back and made me feel that this wasn't just a physical practice, that yes, it was definitely very physical, but there was a lot more than that going on. I'm not sure I knew exactly what that was at the time, or why, and I think it was just a sense I had of his depth of knowledge. To be in the room with somebody who had been so immersed in yoga—you could feel it from him—somebody who had obviously both studied and practiced, was really intriguing to me. All I'd had prior to this was books, and a few Western teachers, and a lot of practice on my own.

You started off by feeling that this was a very physical practice, and that kind of put you off a little bit. Could you say something about how you began to understand the more subtle aspects of the practice?

If anybody watches *ashtanga* yoga they are going to see a very strong physical practice, as I did that first day. When I came back the next day and paid my money, I was thrown to the wolves. I did the whole first series the first day, as you do when you start with a conducted class, rather than how you would start if you went to Mysore. Very powerful.

I had been traveling around and needed to find work in order to stay in the area. So the day after I watched class, I was walking home and saw a huge pile of shingles in front of this house. I was a carpenter, so I stopped and it turned out they needed help shingling this house—something I knew how to do very well. They agreed to hire me and I was going to start the next day at nine o'clock, after my first yoga class with Guruji.

I went down the next day, did my yoga class at seven o'clock, and was done at eight thirty, so I decided to go home and get a little breakfast and lie down for a second, take a little nap. I woke up at one o'clock! I was dead—I was completely exhausted! And in a panic because I needed the job. I ran down the hill, and luckily, the people were really cool.

I got to work. I was up on the roof in the hot sun nailing shingles all day long, put in a full day, got home about eight o'clock, and collapsed, went to bed. I went down the hill the next day to class—the same thing happened. I came home, just needed a short rest, woke up at one o'clock again. It went on for three or four days, until I finally started to get my rhythm and catch my breath. It was physically exhausting.

How does that speak about a spiritual practice? I think that's not obvious in the beginning. After a week or two of practice, I asked Guruji about *pranayama* and meditation because I had been doing those things on my own, and he kind of chuckled and basically gave me the impression that it was a waste of time. I later heard David Williams's transcription, if you will, of Guruji's comment about meditation. David translated what Guruji said as "mad attention," that what most people are doing as meditation is "mad attention." And I had to agree. It was really challenging for me to sit still, it was physically demanding, mentally impossible, and the message I got from Guruji was just to do this physical practice for a while.

And I tried that, and committed to doing the physical practice. Learned first [series], a month later learned second. Went home for two years and practiced on my own. After about five years, I had an opportunity through a certain meditation that was organized at a church nearby to sit. I hadn't really sat in the whole time since. It was amazing to me, the ability to sit quietly, to have the comfort and strength in the body, to just be still in your body, to have the channels that the energy in your body moves through and your breath moves through be clear and open.

It was a whole different experience for me. I found meditation accessible in a way that it had never been for me prior to that. I saw the wisdom of doing the groundwork, which really felt different now, studying with Guruji, than it had with other yogas I had been doing. It was strongly grounded, it was really rooted, it was strength-oriented; put your feet on the ground to stand up on your own and do your practice. And through that experience, the deeper aspects of yoga are possible.

I don't necessarily think that it is automatically something that unfolds for a student. I think it is quite possible to get out of this something particular you have in mind—like you want to get stronger, or you want to get flexible—and you just go for that. You could focus on that and get only that, but it would really be a shame. For me, it wasn't what I was interested in. I wasn't even interested in getting strong or flexible and doing wild postures. I was interested in yoga philosophy, and found the strong physical practice really enhanced that a lot.

Did the practice reveal something to you over a period of time? Or did deeper understanding come to you as a result of your pursuit of philosophy and traveling to India?
You learn that there is a wisdom contained within the practice, if you are paying attention. Learning to listen is key. The form of the practice and the method of the practice contain a teaching. I believe that if you are paying attention, if you can look below the surface and ask: Why do we start where we start? What do we do first? What do we do next? How do things link one-to-one through the sequence? There is something informative that teaches you something. You learn how one pose will teach you about another. You work from the outside to the inside. You are basically working on clearing the way and clearing the physical blocks in the body, which are related to clearing mental blocks in the mind.

Yoga philosophy teaches that what we are doing is uncovering, cleaning, and Guruji said over and over again, if you listen, "This is not physical practice, this is mental cleaning." He talks about cleaning the *nadis*, clearing the tubes that energy flows through. I really do feel—maybe this is not unique to *ashtanga* yoga, maybe any yoga practice has the ability to clear the way—but Guruji's method does it so methodically, so systematically, with the sequence set for us, and not relying on just doing postures as you choose. This, I think, is really difficult. It's hard not to fall into biases, taking a practice where you just do whatever it is you want to do, or what the teacher wants to do at that point in time. It's hard not to fall into tendencies for what your preferences might be, or for staying away from things that you don't like. You have a sequence that is set, and whether you like it or not, you are going to do *navasana* and *marichyasana* D, *janu shirshasana* C and *supta kurmasana*. There is something about putting yourself up against that which challenges you in a way that I don't think you would challenge yourself normally.

I remember seeing poses in the first class I watched like *janu shirshasana* C—I swore in this lifetime that I would never do that pose. It just looked impossible to me. *Kukkutasana* I was convinced, literally, never in this lifetime would I do that posture, and within a couple of weeks I was doing it. It is a tremendous thing for a person to get, to realize, that the things that we set as extreme limits for ourselves are just in our mind, and we have to be careful of the limits that we impose on ourselves. As human beings it's amazing how prevalent this is in our society.

How much of a motivator do you think Guruji is in helping people pass through those preconceptions about our limitations?

Guruji is tremendous, he is amazing at getting people to go beyond where they think their limits are. It's a little scary sometimes. I've seen looks of panic and complete terror on people's faces and also tremendous breakthroughs. As a teacher—I've been teaching for thirteen years—watching Guruji is amazing. I don't feel confident to do the same thing that he does. He's got sixty years of experience teaching—he's seen a lot of bodies, he's put a lot of bodies through this practice—and I feel like I need to be much more conservative than him. I've seen him put people in full lotus, and get them into *garbha pindasana, kukkutasana* that I would have never believed possible. And what it gives them is tremendous and you can take that and from that develop the discipline and love for doing the practice, which is something that does happen through that sense of accomplishment. It's interesting.

What are the challenges and the benefits of this daily practice?

As I mentioned before, when I watched the first time, *ashtanga* yoga has a very gymnastic or acrobatic look to it from the outside, and I think that there are certain people who are drawn to that, who are intrigued by the sense of power and extremity of the practice. Some people are drawn to the bizarre just for the sake of the bizarre. Some people are just interested in doing strange poses because it looks cool or it's weird. I think that's a challenge, it's a danger in this practice.

Some people, maybe especially in this Western culture, in Western cultures in general, maybe more in America than in others, tend to drive themselves really hard and not be particularly in touch with their bodies. This is a very powerful practice. And I think that if you do that, the practice will put you face-to-face with what you need to see eventually. You will see yourself. You will see your aggression, if you are aggressive. But some people have tremendous ability to ignore that and just go and push and push.

Personally that is a challenge and a risk in this practice—the challenge being not to push yourself, not to push yourself to that extreme. It's a touchy subject. It's controversial, actually. I think challenge is important—we need to challenge ourselves—but that we need to learn to be conscious and intelligent in how we challenge ourselves.

If you take the time to do the 1 or 5 percent theory that Guruji talks about—95 percent practice and 5 percent theory or 99 percent practice 1 percent theory, I've heard it both ways—but if you take the time to spend 1 or 5 percent of your effort to study the eight limbs of *ashtanga* yoga, it's informative for how the practice can unfold for you better. Rock bottom is *yama*—the first *anga*, the first limb. And the first *yama* is *ahimsa*—nonviolence, noninjury. And personally I think that is really important, that eventually we are going to come in contact with that or we are going to destroy ourselves. And I think that is also true of the human race, that we have to learn to listen.

I think that the practice is a tremendous metaphor not just for an individual human but for all humanity in general. And that is personally what I see as one of the huge benefits of it. So much damage has been done from people trying to change other people but this gives you a chance to work on yourself and change yourself, come face-to-face with yourself, with your own aggression, to see how you treat yourself. And that is going to influence how you treat other people. I do think that is something that inevitably comes through the practice. It's gonna hit you, you are going to come up against it.

So you're saying that this physical practice actually contains within it the seeds of the yamas *and* niyamas?
I do think that this practice does contain the seeds of the *yamas* and *niyamas*. It's actually a brilliantly designed practice. As I've looked at other yoga practices, I don't really see anything that has the sophistication of the method that this has. There are some great methods, there are some other great practices that people do, but there is something about the pattern of the sequencing in this method, and what I get is that *ashtanga* yoga is the sequence that we do—the first series, the second series, the third series, etc. And the idea of *vinyasa*, which Guruji describes as the breathing/movement system—*ekam, dve, trini*, inhale/exhale specific breath with specific movement—and the eight limbs. And you take those three things: the practice, which is the sequence and the method; the idea of *vinyasa*, which means something like he says: one by one you take it, I mean that's really *vinyasa*, it's a step-by-step progression from somewhere to somewhere else, with breath and movement linked together; and the philosophy of Patanjali, the eight limbs or the *Bhagavad Gita*. It's a very old philosophy—it's not just a modern thing.

I do believe that the practice was designed to show us that philosophy. That starting with *samasthiti*—standing straight and still, coming together within yourself, quieting your mind, giving thanks, invoking, acknowledging the teaching contained in the practice—is what we are doing in the beginning of class. And then starting with sun salutes and basic standing poses which work from the outside in—gross physical movements that are relatively safe: you've only got your feet on the floor, learning to develop that sense of rooting through the feet and strengthening the legs which is really important in the practice. Those things teach you something: there is something about the patterns that are revealed in the practice, from the physical practice, that are the same as the practice of *pranayama*, and later on of meditation. There are things that we learn in the physical practice about how to treat ourselves that are important if you are going to go on to more subtle practice.

It's important to come face-to-face with your personality and how you work with your body before you start to do subtle work with the breath. And until the student can mature and reflect through the feedback of the practice—having something to push against like the practice is really important in the sense that we need to be challenged, we are trying to find our way, trying to clear the way, to penetrate who we are—and then from that place of greater understanding of who we are, be ourselves, be true to ourselves in the world. The practice challenges us to do that. It knocks us around. It says can you maintain your cool and do *utthita hasta padangushtasana* or *janu shirshasana* C or *bhuja dandasana* or whatever it is later on down the road. It continues to challenge that sense of being able to maintain your equilibrium and objectivity and calm in the midst of the storm. I think that is all contained in there.

Perhaps you can tell us a little bit about how it was to be practicing in Mysore all those years ago.
It's interesting looking back at the first trip to India in 1983. I got there in October. There were about twelve or fifteen Western students there. He had a good gang of Indian students—they practiced until about six thirty in the morning and then the Western students came in. In a funny way it wasn't that much different. Guruji sat on his stool, occasionally fell asleep, but he would always wake up right when you didn't want him to—he would be right over there, nailing you in the pose you didn't want him to help you in. And I think that is still pretty much the same. It's

amazing how he seems to just zero in on that, he smells it. There was a lot more time with Guruji back then. His whole family lived in the house in Lakshmipuram and he wasn't worked as hard. It's amazing how hard he is working now in his late years—it's just staggering to me. I teach three hours a day in the morning and I'm exhausted. And he's teaching six or seven hours on some days when it's really busy, and he's eighty-six—I mean it blows me away!

After class Guruji would be upstairs at his desk, reading his news-paper. We'd go upstairs and say goodbye, then there was usually some talk—hanging out with him, which could extend to hours in the morning.

Did you discuss yoga philosophy?
Guruji was always willing to talk about whatever people wanted to talk about. If somebody was there who wanted to talk about yoga philosophy, he lit up, he loved it. If people were talking about more casual things, he'd get a little bit bored after a while. It doesn't take that much to get him to talk about philosophy. If he thinks you have the slightest interest, he'll just go on and on and on . . . rattle off his Sanskrit *shlokas* and his broken-English translations, which take time to penetrate.

I had this question about teaching and whether that was actually a kind of yoga practice in itself. Guruji is not doing his asana *practice anymore. Do you see him as a great yoga practitioner still?*
It's clear from watching Guruji teach that he's still very much a yoga practitioner in his own way. What he does every morning is very de-manding physically, the amount of strength it takes. And watching him get up and down and off the floor and how many times, bending over and lifting people and pulling people into poses . . . Yeah, I definitely see that he is still in touch with the yoga practice. It has never been broken for him. He has continued to teach constantly throughout his life. I don't think he has ever stopped for more than a week or two in sixty years.

He had a monthlong break when Amma died and he aged visibly during that time. I see that when he doesn't teach, he seems to age and he just wants to get back to it right away.
Well, you see him when he gets off the plane, when he first comes some-where to teach, and he just looks older, and as soon as he gets in the yoga

room he sheds ten years. He looks great right now. I'm amazed at how good he looks, how little he has changed. It's been four years since I have seen him. I really don't see much change.

How would you characterize Guruji as a teacher?
One of Guruji's real strengths as a teacher is that he obviously practiced strong yoga. He was clearly challenged by Krishnamacharya, and at the same time he was also a scholar and I think that is unique. A lot of people were just yoga practitioners or they were scholars. Guruji has been both, and he brings that into the room. He obviously embodies the yoga teaching, the philosophy, the lifestyle, as well as having done the practice.

As a teacher one of the things that is great about Guruji is he brings a sense of that tradition and power of the ancient teaching of India—yoga teaching that goes way back, he's really in touch with that. I think it has been an interest for him and he has explored it deeply, and at the same time he has explored the *asana* practice and he feels that that is the place for us to work. He makes it fun and at the same time he is really demanding and he is deep and he's tied into the tradition. He is really strong and heavy. He's got that power of guru: it's just boom! "You do!" And you are going to do it the best you can, you are going to make an ef-fort to do it. And then he will make you laugh! I think that is tremen-dous. As a teacher it's been a real challenge for me to find that kind of balance.

Can you think of an incident that would illustrate that?
For me personally, learning the first posture in fourth series, *mula bandha-sana*, was a terrifying experience. I was in Maui—I can't remember what year it was, 1985 or 1987—and we were doing third series and he was throwing in that fourth-series posture at the end of third, which is appropriate: you are getting ready for fourth, it is coming up. And I was positive that my knees were going to blow out. I was positive that I was not going to be able to walk again if I did that pose, and he wasn't back-ing down. It was probably the first time that I ever really tried to refuse him. I was like: "No, I'm not doing this . . . I'm going to die . . . some-thing bad is going to happen . . ." And he just sat there—he wasn't letting me go—and he grabbed my heels, put his feet on my knees, and just pulled my heels down toward the floor. And I was fine! It was perfectly

okay, he knew I could do it and he laughed—and I don't know if I laughed or what but we got through it.

I'm sure you've asked Guruji about the origin of the ashtanga *system. Has he given you a satisfying answer?*
No, no satisfying answer. When I first started practicing the talk was about this book the Yoga Korunta being rediscovered in a library in Calcutta by Krishnamacharya and of Krishnamacharya and Guruji recreating this practice. I can't say that I know what was in the *Yoga Korunta*—I've never seen it. I've heard little snips from Guruji of different quotes. That's great, a lot of good stuff. I wish that book was available but apparently it is not. I don't feel like I have ever gotten a great answer from Guruji. I've asked him a number of times and it's always a little bit vague, you know. Clearly, *ashtanga* yoga is an ancient method, that's clear. What do we mean by that? Do we mean Patanjali's eight limbs is ancient? Definitely. What is contained in *Yoga Korunta*? I don't know. I've never been able to get whether these sequences are contained in *Yoga Korunta* or whether principles of practice like *vinyasa* and certain groups of *asanas* are contained in *Yoga Korunta*. It's all speculation for me and I really don't know—it remains a mystery.

On that same subject, do you think Guruji has put a strong personal stamp on the system, whether it came from somewhere else or not?
To say whether Guruji has put a strong personal stamp on the system or not is difficult for me to say. I never met Krishnamacharya. I tried to meet him just before he died and was unsuccessful. Guruji said over and over again that Krishnamacharya told him to teach this method and not change it, and I believe that that is what he has done. It is really hard as a teacher not to put your personal stamp on what we teach. We need to teach what is real for us. I think that probably what he had done is to take what he learned from Krishnamacharya—I'm speculating, I don't know—and practiced it himself, and through his own experience, what he found to be true based on what he practiced and from what he learned from his teacher, that is what he is teaching us. And that is what I try to do as well.

What I learn from Guruji, I practice, and what I learn from my experience, from my practice, I teach. And so I think in that way, of course, we all put our personal stamp on what we teach, but at the same time

Guruji has been very careful to keep the method pure and to continue to teach it the way that it was taught to him. And our intention with making those videos [primary and intermediate series videos] was to preserve the way he taught it because I was seeing that a lot of people were bringing a lot of personality into their teaching. And it's going to be like the old Chinese telephone game—in a few generations there is going to be no resemblance to the original method and that would really be a shame. And so I think that at least some of us, not necessarily all of us, but at least some of us as teachers have a responsibility to try to maintain that and to pass that on. I see that happening, it's getting stronger and stronger. At one point I was worried about it fading, but I don't think that is going to happen.

I was going to ask you about Guruji's legacy after he is gone.
What we are seeing with the growth of *ashtanga* yoga is really looking favorable for the continuation of *ashtanga* yoga after Guruji passes on. I'm happy to see Sharath being so interested, really enthusiastic about his practice and teaching. I think he is interested in keeping it going. And there are so many teachers, actually, who have been practicing for a long time and who are continuing to practice and teach. It's a really positive thing. There are probably at least a dozen teachers who have been practicing with him for twenty years or more who are continuing to practice and teach, and the number of people they have taught is growing. There has been some great stuff. I think getting the *Yoga Mala* translated and what you are doing here with this documentary—it's beautiful.

Is there anything you would like to add?
We take the method that we are taught and it has a certain structure. Guruji doesn't say a lot when he teaches class. He basically says, "*Samasthiti!*" then the prayer, and then counts *surya namaskara*: "*Ekam* inhale, *dve* exhale," and so on. You learn what that means and it's just little points of information and you've got all this room to fill in.

One of the things that has interested me as a student and as a teacher is to try to find the things that are true all the time, the things that are at the core of the practice, the things that really are essential. And clearly the breath is one of those things, one of those instructions that is prevalent. He says, "Breathe!" "Breathe freely!" "Free breathing!" "Don't hold your breath!" For me that seems to be the primary focus of the practice: the breath. If nothing else, you are focusing on your breath, you breathe with sound and listen to your breath.

The first thing that I teach somebody in a Mysore class is to get them up to speed and to become self-reliant with knowing the sequence, get them to focus on their breath and continue to keep breathing. That's mental training right there: you are training the mind. It's *dharana*, the sixth *anga* of *ashtanga* yoga—concentration: bring your attention back to your breath over and over again. So you are learning a principle of meditation just as we were saying before—the practice contains the teaching. You are learning, you are developing the power so that when you finally do go to sit you'll have the ability to concentrate. At the same time as you are breathing, you are challenging yourself: you are being knocked around, you are being knocked off balance and being challenged to come back to balance, being challenged to remember to breathe, it's all right there.

Sometimes I'd like to have more instruction. When I learned third series, I was upside down on my head and he's saying, "Do this and that," and I was thinking, "What is that?" You don't have a clue. He's talking in Sanskrit and I've never heard this word before. He says, "Put your leg there," and you are upside down and you don't even know where "there" is. But there is something about going through that process that gives you something: you work it out, you find your way, and you have a sense that you have done it yourself. I think that is really great for people. So it interests me to pare it down so that it's not so complicated. And I do think that is what Guruji has done by not giving a lot of elaborate instruction.

New York City, 2000

Graeme Northfield

Graeme Northfield began yoga in Australia after learning that he had a rare spinal condition. After completing his training as a nurse, he went to Sri Lanka, where he met Heather Troud's mother, who asked him to look in on her daughter in Mysore. In Mysore, Graeme met Gary Lopedota, who introduced him to Guruji.

How did you become interested in yoga, and when was that?
I met some Tibetan Buddhist monks when I was still at school—[I was] probably about sixteen or seventeen—who were giving an introduction to meditation. I went along to that. What they were talking about sounded familiar and I was interested, so I started doing the meditation that they prescribed. Then it was some time, maybe a couple of years after that, I was training as a registered nurse, and I came across an Indian sect who were, actually, Ananda Margas.

They had meditation and chanting and I was really interested in that, and started looking at their way of life. But at the same time, I was still looking at other Christian religions, and Catholicism, and sort of exploring for myself. I guess what started me questioning was that my father died quite suddenly when I was fourteen. This hit me with a lot of questions: What's it all about? What's the purpose? Why do we die? What does it mean? So that's what set me off questioning: What's going on?

Around the same time I met the Buddhist monks, I had pneumonia, and when they did the X-rays, it showed that I had a certain condition in my spine that, they said, there was nothing they could do about. Basically [they told me] to sort of give up. As a teenager, it was like, "Sure, I'm going to give up everything!" And then later on, around the same time I was nursing, I experienced a lot of back pain from that condition. So I started exploring, and got into chiropractors, acupuncture, etc. I soon realized that this wasn't the way, and that I had to look at this myself, and what I could possibly do. So I started exploring exercises for strengthening and ways to go about it. I'd always been physical and enjoyed working my body. So I was working at that stage on how to strengthen and work my back so I didn't have the pain.

Getting to India was interesting. I was finished with my nurse training and was working in a hospice where people go when there's no more effective treatment for them. They're going there for the purpose of dying. And that whole scenario brought up much more of that feeling and questioning and "What's going on?" One of the patients there had a picture of Swami Muktananda in her locker. I was really drawn to it. I started asking questions, and it so happens that the nephew of this elderly lady was a journalist who had sent her that picture because he had been assigned to interview Swami Muktananda during his tour of Australia. A few weeks later he came to the hospital and I spoke to him, and he sent me some books and literature on *siddha* yoga. In those books they were doing some *asanas*, but it was very simple, preparation for sitting meditation. So I started doing those but also, at the same time, started having this intense longing to go to India to see Swami Muktananda. I finished working in the place and got some money together and took off.

That was the beginning of 1982. I felt a little bit afraid to go to India, being the first time I had traveled at all, so I thought I'd go to Sri Lanka first and have a look around. In Sri Lanka I met some people, some American women, a mother and daughter, who'd come from Hawaii. The mother had another daughter, Heather, who had had a diving accident and was a quadriplegic. They had brought Heather to live in Mysore and they were staying there for twelve months so that Guruji could work with her. The mother and the other daughter were having a holiday in Sri Lanka when I met them and [they] said they were doing *ashtanga* yoga. And I thought, "Oh yeah, that sounds good, but I'm going to Ganeshpuri."

They had left Heather with Guruji?
Not with Guruji, but she was living in a house a couple of doors down. They trained an Indian lady to look after her. Anyway, they said to call in on the way through. Six weeks later—it was late March, beginning of April, and it was a hot, dry summer and droughts were on—I arrived

there and found where they were living. The mother and the other daughter had gone off again, to Nepal, and had left Heather there, basically by herself. When I walked in, she was lying there in this cot sweating, with flies around her, and I was like, "Whoa." I explained who I was and I said that I would stay with her until her mum came back.

So I stayed with her and I was just visiting different places in Mysore. Then two Americans came, Gary Lopedota and Stan—I don't remember his surname [Hafner]—from Texas. They encouraged me to come and have a look at the practice. At the time, Gary was Guruji's golden boy. He had been practicing for some time and was doing advanced sequences. So I went along and I watched them practice and it was like, "Whoa, I've got to do this! This is fantastic!" So I was all excited and I said, "I want to start, I want to start tomorrow." And Guruji said, "No, no, no, you wait till Sunday." He said that it was an auspicious day on Sunday, and it was actually Easter Sunday. And so that's how I started. In those days it was very strict, you had to do a month at least, and I said, "How much can I do in a month? Because then I'm going to Ganeshpuri." I did the month and got to the end and I had to stay for another month. I ended up staying for five months. I kept on coming to the end of the month and I felt, oh, I have to stay to learn more. And I only left because Guruji left to go for a tour in America. So I went traveling through India.

Did you get to Ganeshpuri?
No, actually. Swami Muktananda died that year, so I didn't get to go.

I went to Goa first and then Nepal, where I came down with malaria. This was an interesting time, because I was, at that stage, [trying to decide] whether to continue [traveling] or go back to Mysore and do yoga. Was I was meant to go on to Europe and meet other people and travel? It became very clear when I was sick that I should go back to Mysore and continue with the yoga.

There was a month break when Guruji was away. I came back in January, and once he got back I started again. I stayed another five months.

Can you describe your first meeting with Guruji, or your first impression?
I was very green and everything was new, and I was very excited and young, and the whole thing was mystical and magical. He was very stern in a lot of ways. He was very much the authoritarian. As well as being excited, I was intimidated. And that continued for a long time.

Can you describe practicing at the shala *on your first trip?*
I thought I was studying only for one month, so I was eager to learn as much as I could. I was very gung ho, and I was hanging out with Gary, who was also very gung ho and much more experienced, of course, so I would follow him. It was exciting. I was in so much pain but totally in there with it. And it was good because there were very few people there. Mainly I was watching Gary because he was so advanced. It put me in that frame of mind that "I can do." For example, when it came to *navasana*, he was pressing up to handstand between each one, so I thought that was what you had to do, so that's what I did. So learning *navasana* was pressing up into handstand in between each one.

It sounds like Gary was almost more your teacher than Guruji.
He was a huge inspiration. And he had so much energy. He would do the practice in the morning, and in the afternoons he'd walk up Chamundi Hill and back down, do *pranayama*, karate, and circuit training, and then come back and smoke a joint . . . or two.

So initially it sounds like you were intimidated by Guruji and passionate about the practice. How did that change when you came back the second time and the third time?
The first time I was there for five months. Guruji would say, "You do!" so you did. If you had pain, don't even think about getting out of doing anything. It was, "What can I do fast enough to prepare myself?" before he came and adjusted me, because I was being adjusted in almost everything and I was stiff. He used to always say, "Stiff man, strong man but stiff man." So I was too afraid. Basically I was working with a lot of fear but also not knowing how to surrender, how to just submit and give in, not intentionally but in my body. After having malaria, that changed. I got very sick, I lost a lot of weight, and a whole other process was happening in my mind. When I came back it was very different. I could breathe out. I could start to let go. When Guruji was adjusting me, I could actually surrender to it and let go. For example, in *paschimattanasana* after backbends, I could actually [exhales], whereas before I'd be struggling and holding on. I didn't know I could breathe out.

How would you characterize Guruji as a teacher?
He has a lot of energy. He inspired me to go beyond myself. A lot of that

was intimidation, I was too fearful not to, but also he sparked an energy in me that was like a fire to do my best and to work hard. He taught me the attitude of, if you have pain then it's no big deal, you let go of it and you can work with it and you can breathe out and let go of it, as well as not to buy into it and become neurotic about it or to stop because you have pain. Of course, [there are] positive and not so positive aspects to that. It was like having a personal trainer who's making you do your best, making you go beyond what you believe. That was very exciting, that was what I loved.

Did that change over the years, your feeling about him as a teacher?
Not really. I guess I was different than some people in that I didn't take him on as a spiritual guru or see him as being enlightened. He was my yoga teacher. I saw him as a man. And I would take from him the teachings. Of course, as you go on, you realize there is much more involved and it's complex in a more subtle way. But from the beginning, it was like that.

Do you see Guruji as a healer?
He's carrying an energy of a tradition. I believe there is a channeling of energy in teaching yoga, which is a whole healing process in itself. Yes, he's a healer.

How did he convey that healing quality?
There are two aspects. The mind aspect of the letting go, as in surrendering. And also, of course, working with the breath and the relationship with the body, with the pain, of being able to work with that, to not buy into that, and to transform that, to be able to go beyond that. A lot of it, for me, was setting up an attitude.

Do you have a specific memory of a time when you were challenged in a posture and you said, "There's no way I'm going to do that" or "I'm experiencing too much pain," and Guruji took you through that, to the other side?
All the time.

One of the *asanas* that freaked me out in the third series was *viranchyasana*, when you roll over the foot. And as I rolled over my foot my whole knee joint would pop out and stay out, so I'd be in that position and not know how to get back and was freaking out about how to get out of it. He'd just stay there with me all the time and, "You breathe." And finally I could get back out and pop it back in. But each day after that, rather than not doing it, I had to keep on doing it. So it always felt like coming to that one, the feeling I had was that I had to go up to the edge of the cliff and jump off every day. But he sat there with me and made me do it until finally after some time it stopped popping out so much.

I've often heard Guruji say that he teaches real or original ashtanga yoga. What's your experience of Guruji as a teacher of true yoga?
From my perspective, true yoga is yoga what each person can do and continue to do and learn from, so all yoga is true yoga if you're doing it. And because there are different personalities and different bodies, there are different yogas, so that there's something for everybody.

Is there a relationship between what Guruji is teaching and Patanjali yoga?
There wasn't a lot of verbal teaching, from the *Sutras* or whatever. It was actually all in the doing, which I enjoyed because it's more real, it's actual experience. You soon come to realize that what happens in your body, in the way you move and in the classroom, is reflected in life. So rather than reading from scriptures and books, which becomes an intellectual exercise, it becomes experiential. I really enjoyed that and that became my experience and my connection with body, mind, breath, and spirit.

Why do you think he emphasizes the third limb of ashtanga yoga as a starting point?
It's the nuts and bolts of it. It's what we can engage in and work with because we're in a body. It's too easy to get into the head, and the mind is like a slippery white eel. It can trick you very easily, but your body doesn't. So working in the body is very real. I believe we have a body so we can transform, so working in the body is actually a more honest way.

Guruji says 99 percent practice, 1 percent theory. What is your understanding of the theory part?
The simple fact is if you don't do it, then all the theory in the world is useless. That's what the essence is. You can talk about it, you can read about it, and you can study it, but if you don't do it, it's of no value. It's important for us as Westerners to engage in the practice and less in the mind, talking about it or reading about it.

The theory part is learning to really experience the body, to feel the body, to integrate in the body, and to become conscious of what we're doing and of our movement patterns. Then, especially if there are dysfunctional movement patterns that I can correct, this transforms into an emotional benefit, a psychological benefit. Working in the body with consciousness can transform us psychologically, and I believe this is the path to spiritual transformation. The mind is too slippery.

Has his teaching changed over the years?
His teaching has changed because of the numbers. In the old *shala*, we had on some days two or three people maximum, but it used to be eight, then it was I think twelve maximum. The room was very intense and it was very intimate. He was very strong and his eye was always on you. You couldn't miss something. Whereas now there are many more students, and he's become older.

Did you find he's become softer with age?
Of course.

How important is family life and integration of society in this yoga that Guruji teaches?
It's very important that we integrate, that we don't isolate ourselves and feel that we have to go and live in a cave in order to evolve spiritually, that the practice is integrated with family, with working, with daily life, with the stresses of life—with all that life is. It's much easier to isolate yourself and space out than to be in the world with all that involves. So it's actually always a test.

Can you say something about Guruji's work ethic? What would a typical day be? When did he get up?
This was one of the most inspiring aspects: his commitment to teaching, to being there day in, day out, getting up early and being there in the class many, many hours, continually doing it and doing it and doing it, seeing all these people come in and go over the same things all the time. And always the same problems, the same fears one day after another. But he is always there. That was truly amazing, and still is.

Did you ever ask Guruji about the origins of the series?
Yes. [*Laughter*]

Did he give you a satisfying answer?
No. [*Laughter*]

What's your personal opinion about the origins of the system?
Well, I don't believe it came from banana leaves five thousand years ago. I think that's a bit of a cock-and-bull story a lot of people like to believe. It's hard to know, there are so many stories, but I'm sure a lot of it comes from Krishnamacharya, from his teachings and his teachers in north India. I'm sure he was influenced by other activities as well, by the other disciplines in India. Wrestling particularly, the gymnastic tradition, from the training of the English army. But I don't know.

I've heard a number of teachers say that this is a system of yoga Krishna-macharya taught to children. Do you have any idea why it seems so appropriate for Westerners?
It's an intense practice. I believe it was mainly taught to the younger Indian boys who were lean and flexible, who could actually perform most of the *asanas*. For us, it's appropriate if taught and practiced in a way that's suitable for the individual. We have to look at the condition of the person—their age, male or female, their living situation, and any past injuries—and adapt an appropriate practice for them to do. We can still work with the essence of the *ashtanga* system but in a way that is suitable. That's our job as teachers in the West, to work in an intelligent way that everybody can benefit from.

How might you approach different students in different ways?
For example, if a student is only practicing once a week, you're not going to teach them the whole primary series if the rest of the week they don't do anything. If somebody has injuries or certain conditions, we need to look at what to do in order to heal, to strengthen the person, so they can move into the *ashtanga* in a way that is doable for them. There are many factors to look at and we need to modify, to adjust the practice, so that person can feel good about themselves in doing it and get results from it, because the yoga can only work if you do it. So the big thing is keeping people doing it.

What is the value of daily practice, day in, day out, for ten years, twenty years, thirty years? What kind of inner quality is produced by a long-term practice?

If we work intelligently, with daily practice we can start to understand not only what's going on in the body but also the fluctuations of the mind. We can start to see whether we're lazy—if the mind is lazy or if it's really in the body. Something that you do regularly gives us a base to work with and that continuity gives us more experience of it. Which isn't to say that you have to practice every day, because I also believe that somebody can practice once a week. That's better than not practicing at all.

Do you have a sense that one is progressively going deeper as time goes by with repeated practice?

It depends on the practitioner, the intention, and how we practice.

So daily practice without a particular attitude is not going to take you deeper.

No.

What would you say the required attitude would be?

At first it's a letting go, a softening of our attitude. In the beginning we're striving and working toward achieving more *asanas*. But one needs to completely let go of that, let go of this whole goal-oriented practice. Then we need to see our condition as we are, here and now. The next step is to be at peace with that, to actually accept our condition as we are here and now. And from that point, practice with feeling and connection, integrating the whole body and the breath.

Practice with feeling. What do you mean by that?

To actually feel our body, to have a sensation in our body. We can see in each *asana* that there is a connection from the tips of the fingers down to the tips of the toes. We can feel every part of our body and know what it is doing. That means that we are actually integrating and coming into our bodies. Westerners tend to be in their minds. It's important that we transform from being in our heads to being in our bodies in a feeling way.

Presumably, ultimately you want to get back to the mind.
No, you want to get out of your mind.

Completely?
Yeah.

What happens when you've explored the body to its fullest extent? Where does the yoga take you after that?
Oh, there's always more.
    To stay out of the mind, you have to stay in the body. We want to get out of the mind so that we can connect with the feeling in the heart.

How does that happen?
By staying out of the mind.

So by fully experiencing the body, the heart then opens?
We need to give the heart attention to start to then become conscious of the feeling in the heart.

Are there any techniques, or how is that linked in the asana *practice with awareness of the body?*
Letting go of the chitter-chatter [of the mind].

And then just becoming aware of what is actually being experienced in the heart.
Yes, in the body then in the heart.

Once you're experiencing what's in the heart, is that the end, or is it the beginning of another journey?
I don't know, but I feel it's just the beginning. Within the heart, it's a feeling of acceptance, of nonjudgment, of being present and connecting to the joy in the heart.

Do you think it's appropriate for Westerners, and maybe for Indians, too, to move on a path of internal experience rather than having some kind of structured form of teaching, say yama *and* niyama, *or merging oneself with* brahman, *or any of these philosophical ideas that come from Hin-*

duism? Or is it actually more an internal journey into yourself and your own experience?

Yes, depending on what your inclinations are. You have to get away from believing that one way is the right way. It's about the discipline of actually letting go of the mind as we know it, or our external mind. Then we're connecting with [something] more internal, or you can call it consciousness, or the higher Self, or guidance, or God. But in order to do that we have to lose our mind, so to speak.

So you see the absorption in the body as a way of just eliminating the citta-chatter. Then the Self, or whatever you'd like to call it, is revealed in some way, and you can then just pay attention to that. The head is cut off at the neck.

Yes. When you're in the feeling of the body, you're not so much in the head. When you come back into your body, you feel what's going on there, there's not so much external thinking of the past and the future. We can actually be present in the feeling here and now. That's the beginning of *pratyahara*.

How does this carry over into your daily life? What happens after you've finished with practice?

It's always a challenge. It's not that all of sudden you're in the body then the mind becomes quiet. It's always an ongoing awareness—day in, day out, slowly, bringing awareness back in. From being out and getting caught up to bringing it back in and relaxing, relaxing in the body and relaxing in the mind. Our challenge in the West is to continually become conscious: throughout the day becoming conscious that we're breathing, that we're in our bodies, of breathing out, relaxing the body. This is a daily practice.

It seems like a bit of a paradox. When you bring acute attention to something, it's almost as if you're producing tension rather than relaxation. As you relax, you tend to want to fall asleep.

Oftentimes the falling asleep comes from the chitter-chatter. When we're truly connected, there's an alertness, there's clarity, there's a connection with something else, and so there is actually more energy. It's the chitter-chatter, the stress, that puts us to sleep. Unless you're really tired, of course, and lack sleep.

You're suggesting that we should become aware of the body and the sensations in the body, but at the same time relax and totally let go.
In the practice, we can't let go, but with training we become aware of what's working, how much is working, what needs to rest, relax. What's happening with the breath? How's my breath moving? Is it stiff and stressed? Is it soft and relaxed? Or is it deep and smooth? All these qualities are part of being in the body. You can't force yourself to relax, it doesn't work like that. It's actually coming from the opposite direction where, by simply becoming conscious of the feeling in the body, we allow that relaxation process to happen rather than demanding it to happen.

In a sense, you're not trying to relax the body, you're trying to relax the mind.
We can relax the mind by being in the body.

You see the more subtle aspects of the practice as being somehow very much connected with the asana *practice.*
Yes. In the beginning, the *asana* is very concerned about the general movements—you breathe: inhale up, exhale down, etc. With practice, we need to become aware of more of what's happening in the body—how to move the body, what's working, what's not—so that we actually start to connect with and integrate in the body. So that is a continual process with practice of integration and refinement, an ongoing process.

What about the movement from asana *to* pranayama, pratyahara, dharana, dhyana, *and so on—how do you see that progression happening?*
Through practice. If you practice a sequence with intelligence, with being in the body, then we are working with a lot of these aspects already. So that's our foundation, in a way. There are, of course, specific exercises in *pranayama* and meditation that we can do as well. I don't see it so much as you have to do this and this and this. For some people, it's more than enough to be practicing a sequence. For others, they'll be having a *pranayama* practice as well, and others will be practicing meditation as well. They all come together and support each other, but realistically, it's a matter of time and energy.

Guruji implies those internal aspects happen spontaneously or naturally somehow. There isn't a lot of effort required once there's a very strong foundation.

Thinking of it not just as two hours on the mat but twenty-four hours a day as your practice, those special times are there to give us more acutely the awareness and the focus to carry on throughout the day.

So in the early stages, practitioners should be particularly aware of their bodies beyond the asana *practice, throughout the rest of the day?*
Yes. The way that we sit, the way that we walk, our response in stressful situations, sitting at a desk on computers all day, being aware of your body. What's happening? By the end of the day they're using their shoulders as earrings. Are they coming away with headaches?

We need first to look at what we need to do in our daily life to come back into a state of balance and harmony.

What do you think Guruji thinks is the aim of yoga?
I'm not sure if I can answer that question. Ultimately he speaks of God. I guess ultimately being and feeling in connection with God, whatever that is.

He often talks about praying to God. I think that's particularly difficult for Westerners at times.
That's mostly because we've been brought up in Christian traditions and have a certain response to the word "God." For some people, God is somebody up there in the heavens. For others, it's simply consciousness, it's an energy, it's nature. A lot of times we get caught up in the words and lose track of the real essence.

Are you saying that the obstacle for us is language, that when he says "God," we don't really understand what he's saying?
How can we know what God is when it's so huge? We've got no idea. There's no reference for us. So we don't, we can't understand.

How important is it to have a teacher, a yoga teacher? Could you learn yoga by yourself?
It's very important. A teacher becomes a mirror. A teacher can give you feedback on what's going on, what's happening in the body, what's happening with the breath, but also giving you that support and the environment to be in. I think, though, that also we need to not have a teacher so that we are not dependent on having a teacher for us to practice. This is

a big challenge in the West. We become dependent on having a teacher, a space, other people to practice with. So it's important to have a teacher for support, instruction, feedback, and to avoid any unnecessary difficulties along the way. But also it's important to not have a teacher at times.

Do you consider teaching to be a form of practice in itself?
Teaching is first and foremost a service. But also being a teacher, we're being taught. There are two things happening. There's the student learning but also the teacher learning.

There are always new situations arising that teach us by observing how other people move. It helps to get feedback about ourselves. It's a privileged position to be in because it can help our own practice. Ultimately teaching is a practice as well.

What have you've discovered about the bandhas *over the years through your own exploration?*
If you're talking about *uddiyana bandha* and *mula bandha*, in the practice of yoga there is the physical aspect, which I think for us is probably the most important, or the one that we can actually work with, grasp, do something with. The more subtle energetic aspects of it aren't as easy to observe and we don't really know what's going on. So I do believe that physically, if the alignment and the action is there, then energetically it's working and vice versa. The *bandhas* are mostly about the stabilization of the lower back, because it's the lower back that takes most of the stress and the weight of the body, and it's the lower back that's the most vulnerable.

Throughout the practice we need to stay aware of what's happening with the more internal muscles and the alignment of the spine.

What I've found is that as well as the pelvic-floor muscles being activated, and the transversus abdominis from the lower abdomen, we also need to be working a little higher up into the external obliques. We do this by drawing in the rib cage from the front and the side to give maximum stabilization once under load, which is what we're doing with exercises or *asanas* like *uth pluthi*. Here we're putting ourselves in a stressful situation while practicing keeping the navel and the rib cage in and breathing. That position [*uth pluthi*] also gives us a chance to work by dropping the shoulders down and not going into the trapezius while doing it. So there's a lot happening in *uth pluthi* and it's a very important *asana*.

Would you say that lifting up and jumping back is part of that same principle?
Yes.

Do you think the practice has an intelligent design incorporated into it to allow one to develop those bandhas if done correctly?
If the attention is brought to it. One of the difficulties is that, especially if you've come off the street and start doing *surya namaskara*, once you go down to *chatvari* [*chaturanga dandasana*], already you're being placed in a stressful situation that puts us into a dysfunctional movement by drawing the shoulders up to the ears and coming forward. If your attention isn't drawn to it, then you keep doing that and you stay in dysfunction, and by continuing on that way that you actually increase the dysfunction. It's very important from the beginning to learn to do the positions correctly, to learn which muscles to use, and that really means we have to step back a little, isolate, get the awareness of what we need to do, and then work with it progressively, so that when doing a push-up we can do it correctly and safely.

Guruji usually only talks about mula bandha. *What's your feeling about that?*
That depends on what you are calling *mula bandha*. I believe Guruji's teaching is that *mula bandha* is more from the pelvic floor, contracting the anus, the urethra, and the perineum, and that *uddiyana bandha* is more from the lower abdomen drawing in. I believe, but I'm not sure, that Krishnamacharya calls *mula bandha* the pelvic floor plus the lower abdomen.

I know B. N. S. Iyengar, who was a student of Guruji's and Krishnamacharya's, was teaching more uddiyana bandha, *and saying that with* uddiyana bandha, mula bandha *engages naturally.*
Sometimes there's confusion on *uddiyana* and *uddiyana bandha*. We're not doing *uddiyana* when we practice, because you can't. You're holding your breath out when you do *uddiyana*, as opposed to *uddiyana bandha* where you're drawing in, actually sucking right up.

Uddiyana kriya, perhaps, to make a distinction.
Yeah. Doing *uddiyana* helps in being able to relax the rectus abdominis

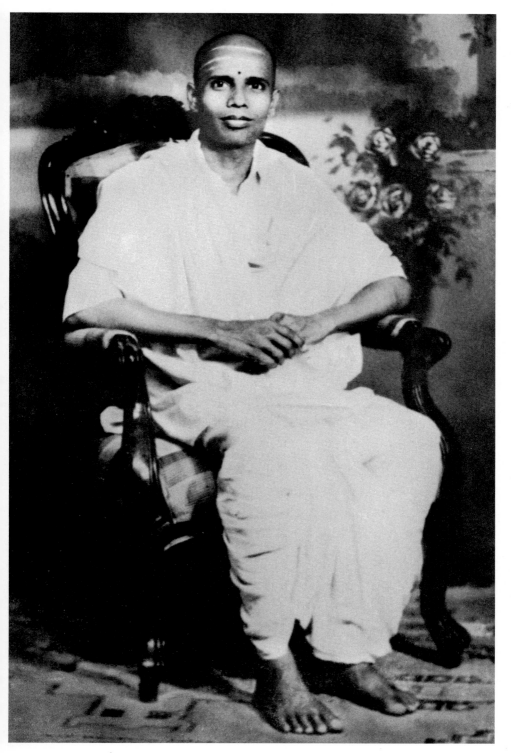

Guruji, Trichy, 1940s

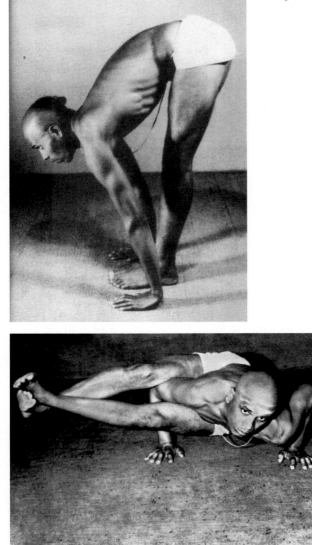

Guruji in trini *position, Kanchipuram, 1940s*

Guruji in astavakrasana, *Kanchipuram, 1943*

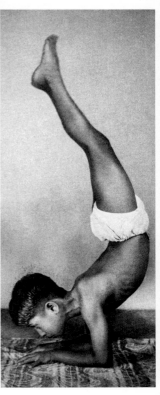

Manju in pincha mayurasana, *1950s*

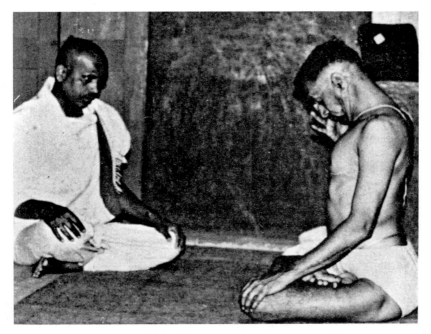

ABOVE: *Guruji and Shankaranarayana Jois, Mysore, early 1960s*
(Photograph by André van Lysebeth)

BELOW: *Saraswathi in* ganda bherundasana *at a UNESCO demo, circa 1960*

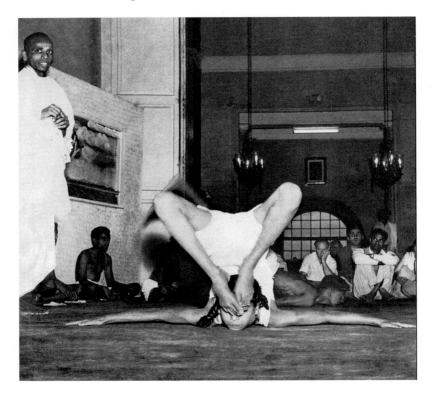

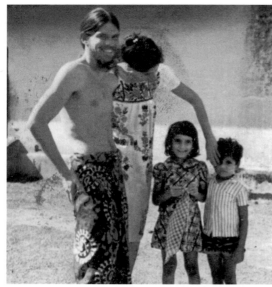

David Williams, Nancy Gilgoff,
and Shammie and Sharath, Mysore, 1973

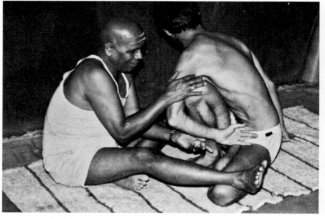

Guruji adjusting Ricky Heiman,
Mysore, 1970s

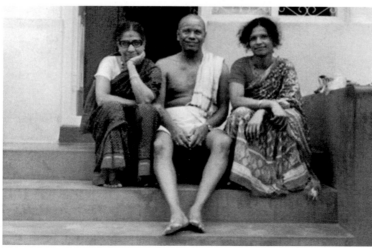

Amma, Guruji,
and Saraswathi,
Lakshmipuram,
1978

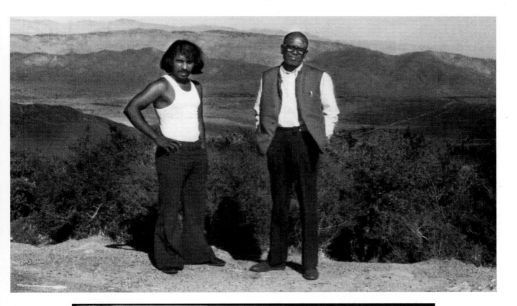

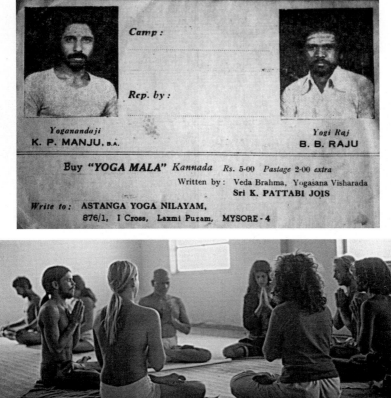

Camp:

Rep. by:

Yoganandaji
K. P. MANJU, B.A.

Yogi Raj
B. B. RAJU

Buy **"YOGA MALA"** *Kannada* *Rs.* 5-00 *Pastage* 2-00 *extra*

Written by : Veda Brahma, Yogasana Visharada
Sri K. PATTABI JOIS

Write to : **ASTANGA YOGA NILAYAM,**
876/1, I Cross, Laxmi Puram, MYSORE - 4

TOP: *Manju and Guruji, California, 1975.* CENTER: *Manju's business card, 1972*
BOTTOM: Pranayama *circle, California, 1970s*

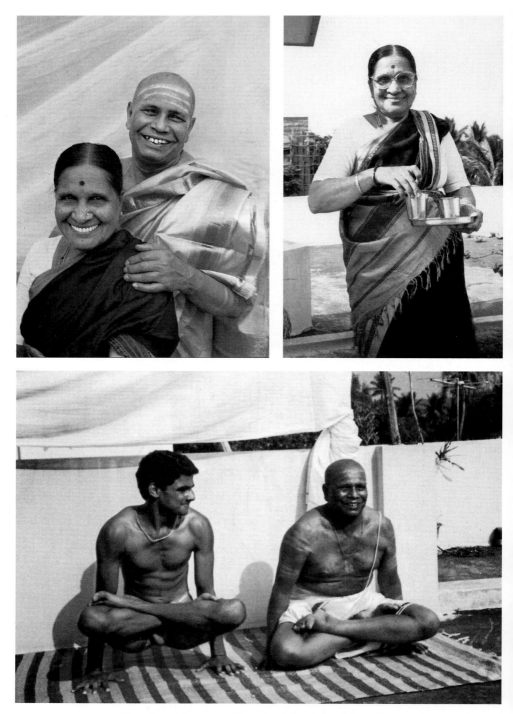

TOP LEFT: *Guruji and Amma on Guruji's eightieth birthday, Mysore, 1995*

TOP RIGHT: *Amma serving coffee, Mysore, 1990s*

BOTTOM: *Guruji and Sharath, Utpluthi, Mysore, 1993*

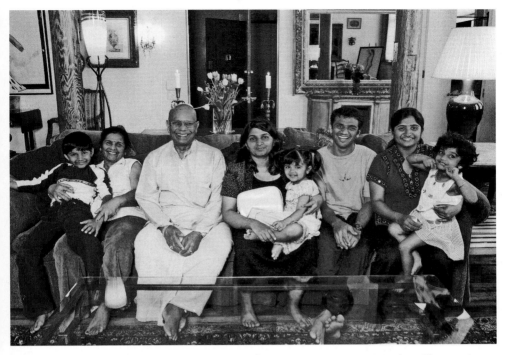

ABOVE: *Guruji surrounded by family, New York City, 2002.* (Left to right) *Prithvi, Shammie's son; Saraswathi; Guruji; Shammie and her daughter, Prakrti; Sharath; his wife, Shruthi; and Sharath and Shruthi's daughter, Shraddha* (Tom Rosenthal)

BELOW: *Guruji teaching at the Puck Building, New York City, 2002* (Tom Rosenthal)

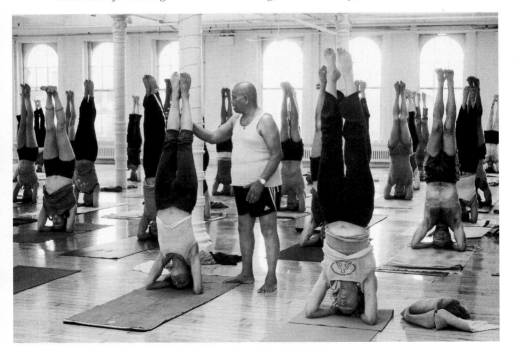

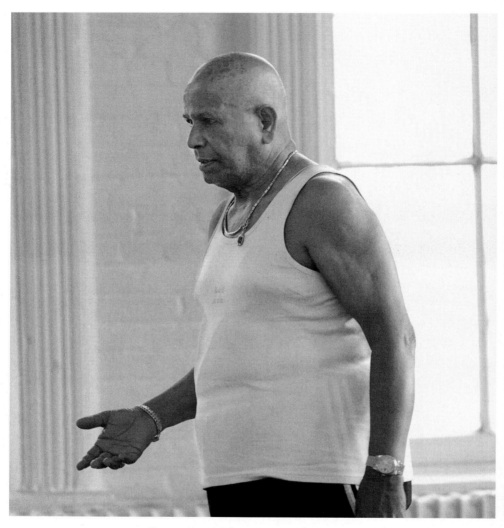

Guruji, New York City, 2002 (Tom Rosenthal)

and drawing in from the abdomen. Mostly, it will bring in the *mula bandha*, but there are times when it doesn't.

Do you think with time and practice the bandhas *start to manifest naturally in practice?*
To some degree, but as I said before, if there's not specific training to bring the awareness there, then we still go into the distressed, dysfunctional pattern.

I think you said that if people were practicing first, second, third series, those who have the opportunity or the ability to go that far find the bandhas *more readily.*
Yes. In the third series we have more arm balances, and you have this contraction of the oblique muscles working, so it makes it more apparent. But for the majority who are just working with the primary series or even less, I believe the extra training is necessary.

Is there something more you'd like to add about the anatomical aspects of the practice?
We also have support systems for the rest of the body. And because *ashtanga* is so strong and we're working the upper body a lot, it's important to learn how to stabilize the shoulders because the shoulder joints are very vulnerable, allowing a large amount of freedom for movement, and a lot of the stability is dependent on muscles. Learning how to correctly align the shoulder while we're doing things is very important. Especially when we get older, we can damage the shoulder. That also goes for the knees, the hips—every joint.

Do you think there's a relationship between progressing in the asanas *and evolution of consciousness for the practitioner?*
Yes, I think that there's a consciousness somehow that's evolving with the awareness of movement patterns and how we work in the body. It's a phenomenon similar to what happens when there is something happening in one part of the world but simultaneously it will start to occur in other parts; different people will tune in to it. We need to pay attention to these new awarenesses in the body and start to use that as a tool for the yoga, to enhance our yoga practice, to make it safer. In that way we can have a more joyful experience in the practice.

By evolution in the asanas *you don't mean doing more advanced postures necessarily, but doing the postures with more awareness.*
Yes.

Some students will never have the opportunity, or the ability, to do the advanced postures. Does that mean that they are limited in their ability to evolve in terms of their spirituality or happiness?
No, it's got nothing to do with it. And in fact, that's a good point, because this is something I strongly believe: that we can bring out the essence, the flavors of more advanced practice into the primary series, or even less than the full primary series.

Can you give an example?
In the third series you learn a lot more about the strength and stabilization aspect of practice. We can take that awareness and place that into the primary series.

It requires an advanced practitioner/teacher to understand those principles and educate a beginning student about them. Is that what you're saying?
That's right. This is something that I'm passionate about. Also, that everybody—regardless of age, disability, if they have injuries—they can still get the full flavor, the full joy, the full benefits of the practice no matter what they're doing. There's too much emphasis on achievement, going through to more advanced *asanas*, and the erroneous belief that you'll become a better person or closer to God by doing that.

Do you think the practice of yoga and moving forward in the asanas *would necessarily bring you to a deeper awareness of yourself, or a revelation of your spirit? Or are there things other than* asanas *to bring you to that stage?*
It's more about awareness, it's not so much about doing more and more and more. It's about what you do and the quality of what you do. The most important thing is awareness. You can work through doing more advanced postures without being aware of what's happening. Somebody who can do *surya namaskara* A with awareness is practicing yoga.

Is surya namaskara, *or one* asana *or position, always taking you to the same place internally, or would you start to uncover deeper layers of yourself, or would you need different* asanas *to access different levels of consciousness?*

It helps to do more *asanas* but it is possible to keep going and exploring by just doing *surya namaskaras* with the right attitude.

Or maybe just the primary series or part of the primary series. That's what most people, if they stick with it, are able to achieve.
For the majority of people, if they can practice the primary series, it's all in there, plus a little more backbending work. It's a lifetime of work to become more aware of what's happening. I often hear people saying they get bored of doing one thing. It's not possible if you're working with awareness, always, every day in your experience, in what's happening in the body, what's happening in the mind, what's happening with your feelings. If you're really tuning in and working in the body, you're in the moment, you're in the present.

Why would it be different each day?
Every day is different in practice. There are some days when we feel good, some days when we don't feel so good, some days we feel more stiff, some days more energetic, some days our minds are more focused, other days it's wandering off all over the place.

So what would be the purpose of doing the same thing day in, day out?
To observe, to become less distracted, to work toward an attitude of indifference, of not judging, day by day, where our practice is. It's a practice of acceptance, day by day, of our condition. With that acceptance, no matter what's happening, if there isn't judgment, we can connect with the joy. As soon as we place judgment or comparison on ourselves, we lose our joy.

Do the fluctuations reduce over the years?
Yes.

Does one come closer to the joy?
Yes. [*Laughter*]

But one will continue to encounter different situations which could potentially cause stress, and you would experience those in your practice. Would you then not be affected?
That's what we're working toward: once you get your foundation, to continually challenge that in order not to stay stagnant.

We are challenged to extend the foundations; a discipline is all about foundations. We're putting ourselves into more difficult *asanas* which challenge us to practice with integrity, to stay aware of the breath, of the body, of what's happening. That's how we progress and evolve in the practice.

So we can establish a foundation with today's awareness, and tomorrow we come back to that foundation and our awareness is different and that foundation is then challenged. Is that what you're saying?
Yes.

Each day we're having a different perspective, so that foundation allows us to really become strong under any circumstances.
Yes.

Do you move from there? What is the next step?
Well, there's fun in challenging the foundations.

Does that go on forever?
Yes, and then life has its way of always being a challenge. I believe the practice and life work hand in hand. Oftentimes life will present itself with experiences and challenges, as does the practice. So we're always being challenged in some way.

So there's an interplay. Life presents you with certain potential emotional disasters, or whatever. You come to your practice and that's in your head. Then you have the opportunity to do your practice with detachment, if that's the right word, working without getting too excited about it. And then your practice plays back into your life also so it's a two-way movement.
Exactly.

Do you think one has to change the way one's practicing from youth to maturity?
When you're younger, you have more energy. You usually have the potential to be more flexible. The ligaments are stronger. As you get older, life usually starts becoming a little bit more stressful—situations with family, with children, with work, with everything that goes on. Then we need to

take more care. We have to become more intelligent in our practice. We have to work in a practice that's appropriate for us, that we can continue to do safely and enjoy and gain the benefits from. We have to keep tuning in to the body and assessing what's appropriate, and not allowing just the mind to take over with what we think or what we're told we should be doing. If we're working from the mind and not connected in the body, we fall down because we're working from the ego, of wanting to do something that maybe we're not really capable of or should not be doing during a particular phase of our life. Joint stabilization and keeping muscle tone becomes more important the older we get for the simple reason that the joints become less stable. As we get older we start to have a leaner muscle mass. So the way that we practice and what we practice can change.

You're not talking about somebody who comes new to the practice at fifty as compared to someone who comes new to the practice at twenty. You're talking about the twenty-year-old continuing to practice to fifty and there's still a requirement to change the way one is practicing to sustain it. Because it seems to me, somehow, that yoga keeps you young, no? It helps you to maintain some of that youthful vitality, strength, flexibility, and so on.
Yes, but we also need to tune in to what's still appropriate, and that's different for different people. So for some they can maintain quite a strong practice as they get older, for others they need to reduce a little bit. It's important that we don't try to make everybody adapt to the one practice. We need to recognize the differences in individuals and adapt a practice that's suitable, safe, and sustainable for that person, because the simple thing is, that if you don't practice, you don't get any of the benefits. It comes down to sustainability, to be able to keep on practicing.

Ashtanga is very confronting and difficult for a lot of people, and a lot of people begin but a lot of people stop because it all becomes too much. The people that stay on it, it's all good, and they enjoy that challenge, but for other people we need to assess their personality and their lifestyle and what's happening and create a practice that they feel good about and can maintain.

There is the perception that ashtanga *is only for a particular kind of person. I mean we often get approached by people saying, "Well, you know, I'm a*

complete beginner. Could I do ashtanga, *or do I need to do something else first?" Or, "I'm very inflexible." In your opinion anybody could—*
Everybody could do it if taught appropriately.

Do you think Westerners have an unrealistic view about the path of yoga?
Perhaps sometimes we place too much on it, or expect too much from it, or become a little grandiose about what we could achieve from it. But we need to come back to a daily perspective, what's happening in the body and in the mind, and working toward moving in the body, getting a little stronger, cleaning out, becoming healthier, and also learning to relax. We need to not get too greedy in our expectations, but to stay with what's real and what's happening in the day-to-day situation.

We discussed Paramahansa Yogananda's book Autobiography of a Yogi. *For me, that was a very inspiring book and it reinforced the idea that enlightenment was possible and that yoga could reveal the truth. What do you think about that?*
Good luck. [*Laughter*] Let me know.

Do you think that's just unrealistic?
I think we have to let go of that idea from the beginning.

So what would motivate us to get involved in the first place?
Usually we're motivated by the prospect of becoming a little healthier, maybe improving our flexibility and strength. Oftentimes people come to learn to relax. Oftentimes it's because their doctors told them they need to do something or that there's been a sickness in the family and they become afraid that they will get that. So we're motivated mostly, in the beginning, by the physical aspect, which is great. The way to continue practice is to become enthused about the journey of becoming more aware. We start by becoming aware of the feeling in the body and moving our bodies, then experiencing the joy in our bodies. We have bodies for a purpose, and we can't discard the body as just a sort of insignificant thing.

What you're really saying is that it's important to become aware of yourself in the present moment, rather than desiring something, perhaps unobtainable or unrealistic, that you're trying to get toward. Be present.

Yes, exactly. That's all we can do: be present with what's happening now. And that's the training in yoga: it is to be in the *asana*, here and now, become aware of when we project into the future, thinking about *asanas* to come, becoming aware when our mind is slipping away to what we did last night or what we'll have for breakfast. Also experiencing and accepting our condition as we are. If you feel some discomfort, then feel that discomfort and experience it as much as possible, and you let it go, then jump back and move on.

Is there one thing that you would say, above all else, that you can be grateful to yoga for?
The journey, the whole journey. I'm very grateful for it. It gives so much purpose and meaning in life, and is a tool to explore, to grow, to evolve, to experience. It's beautiful.

Is there anything that we haven't covered, that you feel passionate about?
Not forgetting all the physical benefits of practice. Sometimes we think that it's about becoming spiritually evolved and all this cosmic stuff, but really, in the here and now, a lot of it is in improving and maintaining our health, of being healthy in the body, of keeping the body functioning well, of keeping ourselves out of hospitals, of learning how to relax and having a tool to alleviate the tensions of life. This is extremely important and this is in the here and now. Yoga has so much potential therapeutically. If more people could practice yoga, there'd be less people in hospital, public health care would be decreased, people would be happier. The whole world would change.

The theory is, as in the body, so in the mind, and the Self is not part of either of those two. So with being content, happy, peaceful, relaxed, joyful, the mind stops the chitter-chatter and the Self just shines, which is all that it does.
Yeah, simple as that. [*Laughter*]. Simple and as complicated as that!

Ibiza, 2008

Heather Troud

At the age of thirteen, Heather Troud suffered a severe spinal injury in a diving accident that left her paralyzed. She met Guruji in 1981 in Maui and then settled in Mysore for a year to work with him. She is in the process of setting up a facility for people with severe disabilities to enable them to experience the benefits of yoga as well as other healing modalities.

How did you meet Guruji?
Through mutual friends, Nancy [Gilgoff], just from his students who knew me and knew him. They said, "You really should meet Guruji and work with him." I was very open to all kinds of alternative and holistic therapies because my parents, my mom was into yoga, Sathya Sai Baba. As I grew up, she was into yoga and Eastern philosophy. And before I had my injury, I felt born to be a yogi and an athlete. I did gymnastics, I was very flexible. I felt that it was from other lifetimes that I had that kind of spirit. When I was growing up, I was always doing headstands and handstands and backflips and walkovers and was just very open.

How old were you when you met Guruji?
I was sixteen.

Were you already into that stuff yourself?
To a certain extent yes, definitely. Holistic, alternative, all kinds of energy therapy, meridian, acupuncture . . . yeah. Then, when he was ready to work with me, I felt it was really a privilege and an opportunity to be able to do that. And after the first two or three times, I started feeling more circulation and tingling through my body, especially my lower body and

my spine. I was feeling a lot more circulation because of the breathing and the *asanas* that he was working on with me. He was basically putting me in a lot of the first-series *asanas*. Slowly I felt more and more comfortable with him.

How did he instruct you what to do?
He worked one-on-one with me. And worked with moving my legs and my spine with the breath, the in-breath and the out-breath, with the different postures and positions. And pretty aggressively, but always to the extent that I would feel comfortable with. I think it was definitely the breath and positioning. I was really flexible from my younger life so I was able to do *padmasana*, and he would then support the lower part of my body and work with my arms and hands to the extent that I had my muscle strength.

So his main instruction to you was really to breathe?
Yes, and to work with the muscle tone that I had. What he did was to increase the circulation and the muscle tone in my legs and my back. And by doing that, I had a lot more feeling return. When I had my spinal cord injury, I was told, "Your spine is completely severed or injured so you won't have any feeling or movement at all." Yet after I did the yoga with Guruji, I had feeling. I was starting to feel and wake up the energy through my whole entire body, my lower body and my spine. He was pretty intimately working with me, and really closely, with my flexibility, my abilities. I'd say he emphasized my abilities rather than my disability, which was really special.

Did you conclude that what you were feeling in your body was not related to the nervous system but was energetic somehow?
Both.

Because you said the nerve was severed.
Right.

You were still getting sensation, or you were again getting sensation, but maybe it was through a different channel.
Yeah, through circulation. And partway through when we were there, Tim [Miller] and Gary [Lopedota] came.

This was in Mysore or here in Maui?
Mysore.

When did you first go to Mysore?
The summer of 1981.

Did you meet Guruji in Maui?
Yes.

Did you work together in Maui before you went to Mysore?
For a month or so. I don't remember exactly how long he was here. And then he said, "You come to Mysore for one year!" And of course my mom was very supportive, and she was wanting to travel and be there and be absorbed in the culture and do the yoga herself as well as be with Sai Baba. And I think it was really powerful for me to be able to experience the culture, spirituality, and that ancient energy by living in India for one year. I had really powerful dreams and out-of-body experiences, experiences of altered states of mind, through my dreams, through the yoga. That is what stayed with me the most even though I haven't done the yoga as consistently since then. I had always been very physical before my injuries, so for me there was no reason to stop being physical, to reach the limits of my strength. Guruji was able to bring that out to the utmost, more than any other guru or teacher I met.

At that time, who came to Maui? This was my home. I grew up here and had a lot of connections. I think our mutual *sangha*, the yoga community, is what really allowed us to be there, and he really wanted to share the work he was doing with me and with other people who were working with me. So Susan came to India, and she worked with him and with me so we could continue what we were doing when I came home. And I continued with her and Stephanie [Nancy Gilgoff's sister].

Over the year that you were there, did Guruji change your practice much? Or was it the same throughout that period?
He included more of the first series, more postures, and it was more powerful. He was focusing on my strengths and changing and supporting my posture so I could stand up. He would stand in front of me and hold my knees and lock my legs and hold me in a standing position. That was really powerful at the time. Then I started feeling pain in my lower back

and spine and hip in different circumstances. So over time, yes, it got more intense.

Do you remember your first meeting with him?
It was in the yoga room. You know, it all kind of ran together, but the first time we worked together, I realized that the therapeutic breath together with the movement was really what everybody needs to stay flexible, and that circulation is the key to health and well-being. So I do remember that, and the tingling. The sensation of oxygenation through my body was like when someone's leg falls asleep or is just waking up, the tingling and pins and needles—that feeling through my body.

You had new sensation right away when working with him? I presume that got you excited.
Definitely.

How did you connect with him as a person?
There was a clear relationship with me, teacher and student, very comfortable. I guess I had experienced and watched other people. I spent time with him teaching other students, and watching other people doing the practice, so I think I could connect with him in a comfortable way. At that time in my life I was just really ready. I was open and ready for something completely different. After my injury I went back to high school for two years, and so I was just sitting and studying, I was really mentally active but not physical enough. So I really, really needed that. I was ready physically and spiritually to have that focus and that meditation and to live in India. It was such a powerful spiritual experience. I can't emphasize how special and intimate it was for me. We connected with a friend of Nancy's, someone who lived on the same street as Guruji, so I lived on the same street as him five houses down. So it was a really personal relationship with him and the family. I fell in love with the culture and the way that the environment was: the same as Maui, Hawaii, in Mysore. I felt that the circle of people who came and went between Maui and Mysore were all ancient beings who came together from different tribes. For me, it enhanced that feeling of how karma brings us together through these different connections, through Sai Baba or Ammaji or all the different gurus and teachers. Guruji made it possible for me to have that experience. Living there felt familiar to me. It was

really so powerful, it was like being home, being comfortable wth the lifestyle. I would like to go back and experience more. Guruji as a person? Yeah, it was definitely intimate and comfortable and powerful.

Did he change your perspective on life in some way?
Definitely. The whole experience did and him being such a powerful teacher. The more Guruji came back to Maui and the more the circle of people in *ashtanga* yoga just spread, kept increasing—it was like this community, family, which was growing. And to see that devotion and focus and discipline—that definitely changed my life, changed my perspective.

What about for you personally? Did he open your mind to another possibility or way of thinking about life?
I think so. I was between high school and college and it wasn't a time where normally—

You would be looking for a spiritual experience?
Yeah. Having the spiritual combined with the physical and the emotional, the combination of the breath and the meditation, the focus, the opportunity to meet him and to focus my life on alternative, holistic, spiritual therapies and studies and teachings.

Did Guruji give you meditation?
Not specifically, just the breath work with the bodywork. The breath was definitely the most powerful tool and I still use it today when I'm getting bodywork or stretching or just breathing exercises or breath control. That changed my life, it enabled me to have that focus when I needed it, when I was going through hard times and pain.

Did you continue to work with Guruji after that year in Mysore?
Just a little in Maui, not very much, maybe once or twice. The classes were so big and there were so many people, so I would come and participate by being there, observing, and being part of the community.

So that year was obviously a special time. Did you go to the yoga shala *to work with him?*

Yes, pretty much five days a week. I went there Monday through Friday and it was focused, one-on-one time.

Did you have fun times as well?
That comes and goes through the whole experience of doing the practice. It's like being on the edge of laughing and crying because of the intensity. I've experienced that since in other types of healing modalities. It's just working through energetic blockages or with certain *asanas*. He would use laughter as a way to lighten the situation and to help me be more comfortable with him. Not so much with words or a lot of communication, it was more like he would lighten up the energy to make it more comfortable to go through the practice.

How did he lighten it?
Just his way of being, just the way he was working with me. The extreme intensity of the *asanas*. He would go "More, more!" like a personal trainer, coachlike: "Come on, let's go for it!" And laugh about it and just really push to the max. Everybody had experiences of being on the threshold of pain and laughter. You have to laugh through some of the intensity to get through.

It seems like your experiences were not so different from everybody else's.
Right, with him.

He wasn't going easy on you.
He was extremely observant, almost psychic: to be able to pick individual people out of a class of a hundred and know exactly what they needed to do to go beyond their comfort zone. That kind of extreme experience people appreciate. We need to be challenged, and it was his job to really challenge our limits and help us breathe and work through them, knowing that on the other side of it is healing and the practice that is with you forever. It's an experience that is unforgettable. I think that's his gift: to make those experiences very memorable and very intense so that people have a lifelong valuable practice through the breath or the body. That was what came to me and it was also through my mom and my sister who did the practice, too, and they really got deeply into it and so it was part of our connection in our family. And the synchronicity happened because

of our connection with Sai Baba who was so close to Mysore, being in Puttaparthi, so I know that is part of the reason that I was able to have that opportunity.

Did you go to see Sai Baba as well?
Yes we did, probably about four or five times, and that contributed to the whole experience. Definitely a valuable part of my life; I'm still working with Faye and getting motivated now to get back into shape and to devote my time to yoga and physical therapy and massage therapy and use the tools that he gave us to continue therapeutically.

Something that I envision is a therapeutic center for peopole with different conditions or different disabilities, where people could come and do yoga and we could have different modalities of physical therapies, like a gym therapy and having different machines. So that's really what I wanted, and I've considered leaving Maui but I think it's not an option—leaving Maui. I think it's going to have to happen here. So part of my vision is to bring that yoga therapy to more people who are open and willing and needing it.

If you went back to India what would you enjoy most? What would be the thing that would take you back?
Probably a healing center with meditation and yoga—the combination of the spirituality and the therapy. I just really enjoyed the temples, the day-to-day energy of the chanting and the rituals. That stayed with me for a long time.

Did you feel the spirituality in the yoga?
Yeah.

How did you feel that was transmitted?
Through the breath and the discipline and the focus; Guruji's joy in sharing his being, for opening his heart and his soul to so many people.

Do you have a sense that he had access to something, some experience that he wanted to share?
His generosity, really, of sharing, like he knew that this discpline and this practice would be effective and carry through generations and generations and really spread, that was his purpose: to really share his intensity

and his joy with as many people and yoga teachers as possible. Powerful, really powerful.

He had that vision already that it would spread so far.
Yeah, I think so. Because of the students. When I was there for a whole year, seeing the students come from all different countries and different places to study, just seeing that, knowing that he had that intensity, that his special gift would be able to be transmitted through the other teachers, the yoga teachers, and of course his family: his son Manju and to Sharath and Saraswathi. They were like a liberal kind of alternative Brahmin family because of their experience with the combination of the Western and Eastern cultures. They wanted to have that autonomy, that freedom. To have the liberal philosophy combined with the traditional Hindu caste system and the Vedic teaching and all of that. That was really the most interesting thing about the family: they were open-minded and outgoing, interested to experience Western ways and integrate that into their home life, their community. I have studied psychology, sociology, and peace studies, and the larger perspective of the United Nations. I specifically spent time studying the culture and sociology of India and learned a lot. And the value of the spirituality through yoga has really changed Western and Eastern relations forever, so that's one of his gifts.

Do you think the movement of yoga from East to West has helped to change our global perspective?
Definitely, because when I was growing up my mom was already doing yoga and she was studying Eastern philosophies and practicing, really building regular practices.

It's true these things weren't available before.
Right. And going from the sexual and drug culture and all that *revolution*, bringing it into the discipline, to getting the alternative, the healthy high, as opposed to all the other drug-related and other experiences [people were pursuing]. In the West it's just hard and sad that all the other pleasures take precedence over, in general, the holistic approaches. But now it's changed and it's getting more and more popular and it is definitely because of Guruji and all of the Eastern influences, definitely. He has touched hundreds or thousands of people.

Maybe tens of thousands.
Yeah. So that's what I love about having had that opportunity for that connection.

Did Guruji help you to re-relate to your body or to see yourself or experience yourself without attaching to something completely physical?
Well, both. It helped me have more awareness and consciousness of my body and at the same time have the detachment of being able to be comfortable in my body. And a lot of people see me in my wheelchair and they are just looking at me and are thinking that I'm a normal balanced person without knowing the day-to-day challenges of just keeping a healthy consistent living. So I think the whole experience helped me to just have the love and joy, and keeping that in my heart. So, yeah, not so attached to the physical, it comes and goes—the physical.

Did Guruji help you re-relate to your body as an athlete?
Definitely, because I hadn't therapeutically taken the time or had the motivation to process or to actually mourn the loss of my physicality. It was like "Okay, keep going!" and keeping up with life. It was more "Well now I can be a mental but not a physical being"—that was how I was treated and how I felt after my injury. But then when I got to do the yoga I felt I could definitely embrace my physical body as a gift. After that I had more strength and courage to do a number of things I wouldn't have done otherwise: piggyback for miles and swim many miles, snorkel and kayak and do a lot of, to me, just essential therapeutic activities. To have the strength and courage to do that, to keep going, to keep motivated and inspired about being part of the joy of my physical body. And there was, along the way, a lot of other support for me to be that way, to have partners who would be able to help me have a lot of physical therapy, swimming, hot tubs, and so on.

You were cut off from your physical life but you were able to come back to it.
Totally. Just kept me motivated, inspired by having that experience and having that accomplishment.

Is that what you needed? Inspiration?
Definitely, because otherwise, I think, the sadness or the mourning of

that much loss, of going from being intensely, extremely physical to not having that available to me . . . I've known other people and seen how that could be all-consuming in terms of depression or addictions or just escaping, just using anything and everything to escape from the loss and the pain from such a severe and traumatic injury. So to be able to be at that young age with Guruji and for him to really embrace me in my condition was really meaningful, valuable—invaluable.

I guess it emphasized to me how our bodies and our relationships go through many, many lifetimes of growth—evolution and growth. I was so blessed, I felt so blessed that I had that opportunity. It was so really incredible to have it and for it to be part of this lifetime's experience. And then I've written about it and so that might be something to cherish as well, kind of a memoir/autobiography of my life before, during, and after my injury. That's one of my goals to be able to write. That's really my vision, too: to be able to write about my experiences and to share, to help other people with their experiences. The spinal cord is the core of our bodies and our beings, so that's something that's been such a powerful lifelong challenge and lesson. This is the thirtieth year of my injury, so I think that's brought it even more into the light for me and helped me to just focus and to let go of all that is not working and to embrace what is healthy for me.

Probably everybody has said how Guruji was so young and energetic, and at my age it was just wow! He was really devoted to his practice and spreading *ashtanga* yoga. It was really cool.

Maui, 2009

Brigitte Deroses

Brigitte Deroses was among a large contingent of French students who traveled to Mysore every year from 1983 until 2000. She would regularly take her daughter, Annabelle, who is mentally challenged, and Guruji would work with her in her practice. Brigitte teaches in Calais, France, and continues to be a shining guide for her students as a teacher who deeply senses the spiritual aspects of *ashtanga* yoga.

Why did you start to explore yoga?
I was always interested in a certain research of relaxation, of sophrology—that kind of thing—but I could not find anything that pleased me. At a certain moment I met Philippe Mons, who was doing *ashtanga* yoga with a physical therapist in Lille. It immediately moved me because when I took an *asana* I thought of nothing else, while with everything I had done before, I continued to be stuck in my head. And the departure point for this research, after all, was because [my daughter] Annabelle had been sick and I myself was really not well in my head. So I absolutely had to find a way that would allow me to accept my life. I got hooked on this path, which instantly brought a lot of things, and I understood quickly that it could in fact help me like psychoanalysis. So that was it.

When did you start the practice?
In April 1983 with Philippe Mons, and I think he spoke to me immediately about a trip to India. He was leaving in November and I decided to go with him, but I didn't know anything about Pattabhi Jois. It was the practice that interested me. We left with Jean-Claude Garnier and a few of his students and that was our first trip. Meeting Pattabhi Jois was for

me a revelation. I said to myself there is something here, and I immediately felt a desire to practice by myself and to continue. I felt it was something that would carry me my whole life.

Describe your arrival in Mysore and your first meeting with Guruji. What was your first impression? Can you say something about Guruji's character or personality?

I didn't expect anything. I had no movie playing in my head and when we arrived, immediately after landing, we didn't even stop at the hotel but immediately went to say hi, and it was so warm, there was Amma, Guruji was reading his newspaper. He offered us coffee and said, "You start tomorrow." The next day we practiced. There were some impressive American students, somebody called Dennis, and we saw them practice and at that moment we realized how immense it was. They were already in second series and we were allowed to sit and watch. We didn't know anything. Guruji took us in the afternoons. He asked the Americans to come and help because we were total neophytes. We didn't know how to do anything, not even a sun salutation. I found Guruji well-meaning, welcoming, with sparkly eyes, and I did not speak any English but felt that Guruji didn't need to talk to me. We understood each other through the gaze, because he touched us and we understood everything, and yet I didn't understand his means of expression, and he especially didn't understand mine, yet he didn't need to talk. We communicated through touch and gaze.

Can you say something about Guruji's energy, how that influenced his teaching?

At the time I was very impressed by his energy because he was always attentive to everyone. As soon as you tried to skip a posture, he would say, "You there, you haven't done that posture!"—like that. I was very amazed that he was so attentive to reading everybody. And everybody had the impression they were his favorite and he did that for everybody. It was afterward that I understood that when he made us take the postures he paid us special attention, so you got the impression that he liked you a lot. We realized that we were each his favorite, his unique student. And that was his manner of making us advance. I understood that much later. But in the beginning I thought, "Oh, he likes me." But he loved everybody.

Do you see Guruji as a healer?
A healer of the soul, not of the body, of the soul, because when he came here the first year in 1991 [to Château Renaud, and then Lille], I took my family, and he looked a little at Annabelle, and he said to come to India with her. I never told him that Annabelle was sick, but he felt it, and indeed after that I took Annabelle every year and she worked with him.

Would you say that Guruji teaches a standardized practice or does he adapt it to the individual?
I think he adapts it to the individual. I did not understand that immediately, because in the beginning you have the impression that he asks the same thing of everyone. But the more advanced you get, the more he becomes different with his demands.

Often students have a blockage at a certain moment in their practice, but it is not only in the body it is also the mind very often. What is Guruji's role in the process of psychological transformation?
I believe he makes us think, he places us in front of our own difficulties. Sometimes he is intransigent about the hour we arrive. I remember at a given moment I lived very far from the *shala*. I had to go with a rickshaw and I arrived late and in my head I said he will not say anything to me because he knows I come from far and he told me, "Do you see what time it is? You're late. Tomorrow come half an hour early." And in fact, at that moment I didn't understand that you have to be there without preferences or attitude. You're not there to be pampered but to advance.

When you experience limits in practice, how does Guruji help to go beyond?
On the level of the body? I didn't experience that really, because I really didn't have many difficulties until the year 2000. It was difficult in terms of stamina but I didn't experience too many difficulties in my body. Starting in 2000 I had a back problem, and there I felt blocked on the level of my body, so I needed time. But I understood immediately that my mental life changed, evolved, from the moment that I was blocked in my body.

According to you, what is the relationship between ashtanga *yoga as taught by Pattabhi Jois and the* ashtanga *yoga of Patanjali in* The Yoga Sutras?

I think, in fact, it is the same. They are both as demanding in the same way, they totally are one into the other. They are the same.

Why does Guruji place the emphasis on the third limb of ashtanga *as a departure point?*
Asana? I think it is because he wants us to understand the physical effort which gives us tenacity, willpower, in order to be able to develop discipline. He inculcates discipline so that we understand that we should be attentive to other people and practice the first two limbs. But you have to go through the physical to understand the two limbs which come before. You have to be peaceful in your head, you can not go immediately to the first two limbs. That's why he makes us start with *asanas*.

Did he speak about the other aspects?
I think he must have spoken about it on Saturday afternoons, but I didn't understand. [*Laughter*].

Guruji suggests prayer and devotion to God. Westerners often find this difficult. Why do you think he considers this to be so important?
When you recite your prayer, you have to put yourself in a certain state that allows you to detach from all the rest. It is true that it is important, but it also took me time to integrate that because it is not our culture. Now it is indispensable. I could not start a session without starting with a prayer. But in the beginning, even in my practice room I had a hard time, because I thought the students would say, "What is this?"

Guruji always says 99 percent practice, 1 percent theory. What is your understanding of the theory?
What does the 1 percent represent? I think as soon as you practice, everything comes by itself. Of course, you have the desire to go further and to be interested in theory, but practice is by far the most important: the discipline of getting up in the morning and doing it. From there, theory becomes easy as you evolve progressively, but you definitely cannot start with theory.

What do you think his definition of yoga is?
I think he says that if you do yoga correctly, everything will come to you. You level out all difficulties, you accept everything that happens to you,

you accept what cannot be changed, and you change what can be changed, I believe.

Where is it going? What is the destination we are going toward?
Toward *samadhi*, toward enlightenment.

What is the importance of the householder in this lineage?
Family life is very important for Guruji. I think it is essential that you have to integrate yoga with your family life and, above all, not isolate yourself and not do yoga only for yourself. It has to be spread out to your whole family and everybody, your students, but it is not a personal affair at all. Moreover, he shows it with his own attitude. When we saw him with his wife and his daughter, his grandchildren, he was always surrounded with his family. And he speaks about them and asks news about how are your children, and how is Annabelle. He is very attentive to all of that.

Can you say something about Amma, her relationship with Guruji and the students?
She was really an exceptional person, and especially with Guruji. She was completely in his service and he placed a lot of importance on her, too. When you asked him a question he would turn toward Amma and he would say, "Maybe you should ask Amma." So we had the impression that he was the teacher, she was serving him, but they were actually mutually serving each other. And with the students, it was the same with us, the French, she was very, very kind. In the morning, she offered us coffee. Very attentive. They were fantastic, truly.

How would you see the way he lived his life as a moral, ethical person?
He is an example because he has always been very simple and welcoming, warm, and he worked long and hard. Because he was a teacher he gave a lot to other people, and little by little he progressed on the level of wealth. He does a lot for his village, he gives a lot to foundations, so maybe now he looks like he is a very rich person. But I think it is something that is practically normal, because he paid a lot with his person, he worked very hard, and he helped and still helps a lot of foundations.

Can you say something abut the special quality of life in Mysore as you experienced it?

Guruji is such an important person in Mysore, so we are respected through him because of the image that Guruji has given. It doesn't come from us.

Did you ask Guruji about the origin of the ashtanga *system? Do you think it originated in the* Yoga Korunta, *or with Rama Mohan Brahmachari, or with Krishnamacharya? Or do you think that Guruji developed it by himself?*
No, I think that it comes from *Yoga Korunta*, of course, and perhaps Krishnamacharya has maybe improved it, but in the beginning it is very ancient and it was already fixed. It is not something that was invented by them, it was researched.

What is the value of daily practice, day after day, over the years? What is the inner quality developed from long-term practice?
It is to oblige us to a discipline, and to not be satisfied with any posture. You never win, you have to keep going for another posture, the one you do today, you might not be able to do tomorrow, and in the long term it gives you mental power because it carries you.

How does he teach the subtle aspects of the practice? Do you have the impression that they are integrated in the asana *practice?*
For me it is in the *asana*, for it is by practicing certain *asanas* that you unblock certain mental attitudes, especially *kurmasana*. That is an important posture, I think. It is indispensable, essential, it is a key. Once you pass to *kurmasana* you are already a little evolved. I think it is in the *asanas*.

What about yama *and* niyama?
It is the totality of the *asanas*, it is not in one posture. It is the daily practice that makes you more attentive or well-meaning, or ethical or moral. The daily practice brings that with it.

How important is it to have a teacher?
A guru? It is very important, I think, to have one single guru because he becomes your reference point and you do not lose your way. When you start by trusting somebody from the beginning and this person does not disappoint you, there is absolutely no reason to not follow them or to go looking for anyone else. I never had the desire to change even when in

my body it was not going that well. Even, for example, when I studied with other teachers, I never considered them guru. My guru is Pattabhi Jois, the first that I have known and with whom I had the desire to work.

Guruji does not do his asanas *anymore. Do you see him as a practitioner of yoga still?*
Yes. I do not know if this is true, I've never known the reasons. I heard that he stopped at fifty when his son died. But I never have had a problem with that because I think he reached a stage where he could let go of the *asanas* because he was beyond that. He had the prayers, and his attitude toward us suffices. That was his practice. It was to help us and make us advance. That's how I felt it.

Can you say a few words on the important role of breathing?
I had a few classes on breathing when I arrived at the third series because that was his attitude back then. I was completely lost. I think I was not ready yet, so I didn't understand what was happening. It is only now I realize how important the breath is, and I try to speak as early as possible about it to my students. I think if I had better understood back then, I would have progressed quicker.

What is the importance of food in the practice of yoga?
I think healthy, light food is important because of the purity that one wants to experience. What you swallow has to be good and fine and respecting of your body like a temple, a shelter for the soul. So don't eat just anything. It has to be related to the level of the effort you have to make. You have to eat things which bring you energy, but not just anything, otherwise you don't feel correct and well.

What is the relationship between the body and the spirit in your view?
You have to come to the point where it is a union. That is very difficult. That is what yoga is, it is coming to a point where you do not make a difference between the body and the spirit. And you never attain it, you always have to continue to make effort because, for the moment, it is not that yet.

Do you see ashtanga *yoga as a spiritual practice?*
Yes, totally.

What are the aspects of the practice that are not material?
It helps to be without judgment, to accept others without judging them. For example, if you see someone who eats and drinks a lot, when you do yoga you manage not to criticize any longer. You say, "I do differently," and that is how it is. He is allowed to do what he wants to do. You can advise but not criticize anything, and I think it appeases judgment, you are not riding judgment, you don't judge anymore.

What is the relationship between the practice of yoga and the teaching of yoga?
You cannot do one without the other. You have to practice your own practice to be able to teach it, otherwise it is not yoga. You have to go through difficulties to be able to understand—you become a better teacher when you have difficulties. For example, in the first series I didn't have any difficulties at all, and I kept pushing people saying, "Oh come on, it is easy, you just have to make the effort, have some willpower." But when you get older and you have difficulties, you know that it can be painful to get into certain postures. And you are more indulgent in terms of caring, or more attentive.

What is the most important factor for a healthy practice of yoga?
Desire, to be in the mood to practice and to know that it is part of you, and to know it, the desire to practice, to be enlivened by it.

Certain students will never be able to achieve the most advanced postures. Does that mean that they have less hope of spiritual evolution?
I thought that for a long time. In the beginning you think, "I have one more posture to do, I have one more posture to do," and you want to go further and further, and at a certain moment, even if the body refuses to go further, still you continue anyway to practice what you can, but your mind continues to advance.

What do you think is the relationship between evolution in the asanas *and the evolution of consciousness?*
The more you advance in the *asanas*, the more difficult it gets, and the more you have difficulties, the more you have to concentrate and to be detached from everything that has a parasitic effect on the spirit. So of course there is a relationship between the evolution of consciousness

and the difficulty of the *asanas*. Something you can do easily can let your mind act in a parasitic way, but when it is more difficult and requires more concentration, yes, there is a relationship to the evolution of consciousness.

Do you need to change practice for a younger or an older person?
Yes, because as you age it gets more difficult. There are problems with the joints, of arthritis or other difficulties such as reduced energy. So you have to adapt, you cannot be as demanding of older people as of younger people. Younger people need it to be playful a little but you cannot expect the same of older people. You have to adapt, of course.

Would you like to say anything about Guruji or his teaching which I did not ask?
I would like to say that Guruji completely changed my life. He brought peace into my life when, at the time I met him, it was total chaos because I had a sick child and I thought life was just not possible. Now nothing has changed, my daughter is still sick and there are many difficulties and I bear it not without difficulty, but not as a burden. He took away the burden from me, he took away something that was heavy, that was weighing on me, and he made me light again. I thank him every day. I go in to teach my class and I thank Guruji.

Since the year 2000, since the new *shala*, I don't work with him anymore because I didn't manage to move from Lakshmipuram. But I could not go to Mysore without going to see him. And there is not one day when I do not think about him. His pictures are everywhere in my *shala*, he is like my father, somebody very important who transformed my life, who truly helped me a lot. And I experience always the same emotion when I see him, even if I don't work with him anymore, I always have a lot of emotion. I will never be able to thank him enough for having transformed my life.

Calais, 2008

Tomas Zorzo

Tomas Zorzo first learned yoga at the age of fourteen from his brother. The desire to meet Guruji took root after seeing his photo in André van Lysebeth's book *Pranayama*. In 1985, Tomas fulfilled that desire and traveled to Mysore, arriving there sick with dysentery that he had contracted in Mumbai. Guruji helped to heal him, and Tomas has been a student ever since.

How did you become interested in yoga in the first place?
I was on a spiritual quest. When I was fourteen years old, my brother bought a book called *Yoga, Youth, and Reincarnation*. He was one of the top climbers in Spain and this was one of the first books like this which appeared in Spain. He was just interested in gaining flexibility for climbing. When I saw the photographs in the book and read a little of the philosophy, I started to practice. Copying my brother a little bit, who was five years older than me, I practiced by myself in the morning and I felt fantastic.

When I was eighteen, I entered a personal or spiritual crisis. What should I do with my life? I was a student and a revolutionary. I started going to political rallies because it was the time of Franco, the end of the dictatorship in Spain. I went to jail for one month because of these revolutionary things.

When I came out I was depressed, but I was reminded of this beautiful feeling I had when I was fourteen years old.

Do you see a relationship between your political and your spiritual inclination?
Yes. You have an aspiration to become a better person and change the

world. But what I found was that [change] was not possible with the political system. That same aspiration brought me to yoga. The political way does not achieve anything. There has to be a transformation from inside.

My sister came back from Japan with new ideas of a macrobiotic diet, Zen, and so on. She gave me a book by Swami Vishnu-devananda, and I used that book like a bible. It helped me come out of that depression. I started to practice yoga again.

I spent one year practicing and then I went to Barcelona to find a Sivananda teacher. There was one American lady whose name was Radha. She was a talented teacher and she encouraged me to go to Canada for the Sivananda teacher training. And then the search started. I was not satisfied with that. I wanted to keep practicing and go to India.

How did you become interested in Pattabhi Jois and ashtanga *yoga?*
When I was young I was very interested in what was physical. You get seduced by the *asanas,* the difficult *asanas.* You want to keep improving your *asana* practice. I got *Light on Yoga* and said, "Wow, this is much better than Sivananda yoga." I started to read *Light on Yoga* and practice from the book. Then I came across a copy of André van Lysebeth's book and saw a photo of Guruji doing *pranayama.* I felt it looked very authentic, which was something I was looking for, and I thought I would like to meet this man. On my first trip to India I was at the Sivananda ashram in Rishikesh taking Vedanta philosophy training for three months. There I met a man from Holland who was hitchhiking around India and he gave me a beautiful impression of Guruji and Mysore. He gave me the address and told me Guruji was a very good teacher and had been a co-disciple with B. K. S. Iyengar. So on the next trip to India, in 1985, I went straight to see him.

You had not been exposed to Guruji's teaching?
I didn't know anything. *Surya namaskara* A. Nothing.

Do you remember arriving in Mysore and meeting Guruji?
The first time I went to India I got very sick with amoebic hepatitis. A doctor told me I had to leave the country, so I had a lot of fear. I had been close to death. On my second trip I was afraid to fall sick again. No mineral water, toilet paper, etc.—it was difficult to travel in India. First,

I went to do *vipassana* [meditation] in Bombay and then on to Mysore. But on the way to the *vipassana* course I got dysentery, so I could not sit the course. I was very sick with a high fever and I was thinking it was amoebic hepatitis again. Thanks to God, a Spanish Christian priest helped me and I spent a few days recovering there. Then I went to Mysore, but I was still very sick. I met Guruji and told him how sick I was. He said, "Oh, you remove all these medicines." I had all these medicines which the hospital had given to me, about fifty tablets of different colors. "You just throw these out and just practice, practice, practice. This will clean the liver and other internal organs and you will be just fine." So I went to practice and I remember the first class was tough because I was very weak. He took me as far as *janu shirshasana* the first class and I came out with more energy than I entered with. That started to hook me. It was very powerful and I could feel the therapeutic effect immediately. Each week I got better. It took me one month to recover completely from the sickness.

Did you have any doubts when you met Guruji, or did he give you confidence immediately?
I remember writing in my diary, sitting on the bench in front of the Lakshmipuram police station waiting for class. He had told me to come at 6 a.m. I wrote, "This man, he is going to kill me, he is adjusting me so strongly." I was afraid I was going to be broken from his strong adjustments. He was on top of me in every *asana* and I was feeling, "Oh my God, he's going to kill me," but instead of that he was healing me. His adjustments were very good. He treated me with such love and care on that first trip. It was superb.

When I went to India, I had fear of getting sick again. India felt very big and I felt very small. I had fear of food, fear of touching anything, everything was dirty, India was just huge. And when I came out after those first two months with Guruji, I had the feeling that I was huge and India was small. I had the feeling that the *prana* was huge and I was not afraid of getting sick again.

How would you describe what Guruji was teaching you?
On my first trip, I couldn't take him as a guru. He was just a good teacher and he healed me. But it hooked me. I don't know what—the practice, the *asanas*, the energy in the *shala*, his power? The next year, I

wanted to show him that I was strong, that I had been practicing. I was in an ego situation. He was so tough that I was coming out after each practice crying. He was treating me very badly. I remember talking with Peter [Greve] from Germany, who was my friend, and he was telling me, "Yes, it sometimes happens. He can be tough with egos." I didn't want to see that. I remember after the backbends, and I was young and quite flexible at the time, he would never say, "Good," but he would growl and say, "You! Bad breathing!" And I had such a reaction against that, that when he was adjusting me in *paschimattanasana* I didn't allow him to bend me. I was pushing backward. He was making these noises, grunting with effort to push me, and I remember leaving in tears. The next day, I thought, "It's over, this is not my guru." I decided to go to practice but I was not going to look at him, just forget him. And then he came to adjust me, and he was saying in some adjustments, "Better, better." I started going through a big transformation. He was making me humble and I was starting to feel he was my guru and it was the beginning of my surrender to him. So his teaching was very much on the psychological level.

So your relationship with him was established on your second trip, and you took him on as your teacher. What do you think he was teaching you in terms of a philosophical/spiritual system?
Guruji is very practical, you know. I was coming from all these gurus talking philosophically, not practically. It brought me down, it brought down the spirituality to a human level. It's not like God is something in the sky. Humility, courage, surrender, trust: all these things were in his practice, in his teaching. It felt very earthy. The spirituality was very earthy. I was a little in the clouds. Looking upward toward God, but you have to look down and deal with the practical. I knew that. He never gave me any *asana* unless I asked for it. I knew that. I was very shy and had a fear of rejection at this time in my life. So he never refused me when I asked for a new *asana*. He never asked, but always was waiting for me to ask.

Many people experienced the opposite. People asked and he would say, "No, no, you are not ready." So his teaching is very psychological.
Yes. But very physical as well.

Can you say something about his personality, his character?
I saw him in different stages of his life. I saw him on early trips when he was just like a wild man. On one of his first trips to France I spent a lot of time with him and saw him differently. I had the opportunity to assist him in his teaching. I learned the way he was adjusting, I was copying him. I saw how he was relating to different French people, adjusting to how they eat and smoke. He never judged. He was just laughing. He was looking through the person to the heart of the person, not how they were appearing. I could see how he was relating to different people in different ways. I realized that when he seemed to be treating me harshly, it was the result of something not clean inside of me. He was reading my state of mind.

Do you think he had some kind of siddhi *[magical power]? Or perhaps he was very observant.*
He was very empathetic. He was teaching through empathy and he was looking into your Self.

Do you see him as a healer?
I remember him touching and adjusting me with very healing hands. If healing is putting you in your place, in your center, yes. I saw situations where he was bringing people to their center.

Do you think that was through his sensitivity?
He was connected with the source. He was quite spontaneous. I remember he was crying a lot when his wife passed away. He was adjusting me in *paschimattanasana* and he was crying at the same time. I loved that he was so natural, a real human being, not pretending to be a guru. But probably attached to the money. [*Laughter*]

How did Guruji react to different students in different ways?
We have different natures. He was looking into the individual nature. One time, when he was having all his teeth removed, he was very grumpy. He didn't give any *asanas* to anyone. No one received any new *asanas* the entire month or two months I spent there. Only my son Ananda, who was eleven years old. He was the only one who was having any new *asanas*.

How many times have you brought Ananda?
He started when he was ten years old. He would go with me or with Camina, my ex-wife, every year until he was sixteen. Then he distanced himself a little from the practice, then he started to come back to it by himself at around nineteen, I think. Now he goes to Mysore by himself. Our intention was to put the seed in him. The best gift we could give to our son was what we love most: the practice. This is my heritage. And he is now an authorized teacher.

Can you say something about how Guruji taught him?
Nicely. Gentle. He was always very gentle. He took him quite quickly through the primary series. The first time Ananda spent a month there he got to *baddha konasana*. The second time, he finished primary. He was practicing at home as well. Guruji taught him the same method, but he understood that he was a boy, though he had very nice concentration.

Have you seen Guruji adapt the practice for different students?
I saw him adapt to different situations, teaching people with severe back pain differently, for instance, a few *asanas* from the intermediate series. People who were not flexible at all and not able to do primary could do some *asanas* from intermediate. He would adjust if someone was sick—not much, he was quite strict with the series—but sometimes, depending on the person.

Often students get stuck in practice not just physically but psychologically. Can you talk about how Guruji helps people move through difficulties?
He frustrated people. Students would come with a lot of desires. Some desire to conquer new *asanas*. He was always cutting that. You need to confront these frustrations to grow as a person.

How do you think he helped people?
You have desire. You are craving. And then you want it more. And then Guruji says, "No, tomorrow." I saw some people have tantrums wanting a new *asana*. And Guruji said, "No!" I saw people get upset and run away. People who are very well-known yoga teachers in America, but they couldn't cope. [*Laughter*]

What about the opposite? Sometimes there is fear or maybe weakness.
Yes. When you are breathing deeply and doing all the movements and *asanas*, it increases your *prana*. When you have more *prana*, you have more of a sense of being grounded, you feel stronger, and then you can feel stronger in all areas of your life. My sister came with me one time. It was just after a [relationship] separation. She was feeling depressed. She spent only three weeks there, but she always felt very grateful for those three weeks because she could cope with the rejection of her partner and find a new job. This practice in India gave her a lot of inner strength.

What about fear in an asana?
He says, "Don't fear. You bad lady!" [*Laughter*] He's there in front of you, ready to give you an adjustment, and he just says, "Don't fear. Why you fear? Just trust." Sometimes he was pushing you to the limit. Sometimes he wasn't pushing you; you were pushing yourself. But he was there with you, to help you to trust. The practice, the intensity of the practice, depended on his presence in the yoga *shala*. When you were practicing and you saw him, everything was vibrating in that yoga *shala*.

So just really through encouragement. And if you were stuck or at a limit, he would push you.
Not pushing; encouraging you. He helped you to be patient. Practice, practice, practice. You need time. That is something some students knew. They would spend a lot of time there. You need time to make any progress at the physical and psychological level. As Westerners, our relationship with time is that we want everything fast. He was saying, "Tomorrow. No, tomorrow. You need time." He was removing this anxiety. He was making you confront this anxiety. This is part of the inner change. "I want to start third series!" This was my case. I came many times but didn't stay longer than one or two months. Each time I came back, I had to start at the beginning. It took a long time to learn one *asana*, and another *asana*. They didn't come quickly and then I had to go home. Then the next year, the same thing, maybe one more *asana*. But in the end, you just want to practice, you don't care anymore. You just practice.

What do you see as the relationship between Guruji's teaching and Patanjali's Yoga Sutras?

I asked Guruji, "Why don't you to teach meditation?" This was in France, and he said, "Western people are only interested in the physical practice." But I remember, especially on that trip, because not many people were able to speak English and I had the opportunity to be quite close to him, I asked him spiritual questions about meditation and psychological questions. He was keen to talk about that. Unless you were really sincere in your questions, he wouldn't talk about spiritual things. I remember him telling me, "You ask whenever you like." He was available at a personal level. He taught Patanjali yoga, but in a very traditional way. Unless the students are ready, he will not teach, unless your motivation was very ready. But I saw him teaching people concentration and meditation and giving mantras.

Why do you think he thought it was important for people to have such a strong asana *practice? Because this is what people were interested in?*
This was what he learned. It came from his tradition. He came from a strong practice, like Iyengar. He thought this was the method, as well as seeing the limbs of yoga as a step-by-step process, especially *asana* and *pranayama*. He always used to say, "*Asana* and *pranayama* are difficult. Meditation is easy." If you do *asana* and *pranayama*, your body/mind will be clean and you will then be ready for meditation, and meditation is a state of consciousness which you will fall into. When you have this strong *asana* and *pranayama* practice, at a deep, deep level, *yamas* and *niyamas* will come as well. You will have the mind to reflect on your *yamas* and *niyamas*. Practice has to be *asana* and *pranayama* because meditation is more a state of consciousness you fall into. Concentration you do during the *asanas* and *pranayamas*, meditation is a state of divine revelation: you see the Atman, or God, everywhere. You can't say, "I'm going to look and see God now." You see or you don't see; it depends if you are pure and clean. He was working at the ego level on the *asana* practice—this was his method.

Can you explain a little more about the yamas *and* niyamas—*why he isn't teaching them first and how one develops those thoughts?*
How can you teach nonviolence? You are either violent or not. You have ego, and you have desires, and you want things, then maybe you want to take things in a violent way. You don't need to touch anything to be violent. You can be violent in a cunning way: psychological violence, spiri-

tual violence. You can be violent in many different ways. If you just are peaceful, then you practice nonviolence. If your ego has been reduced, you can practice *yamas* and *niyamas*.

How can the ego be reduced?
In my case, it has been reduced. But unless it is destroyed, the ego starts again. [*Laughter*]

How?
There is no technique. I think you need aspiration. When I went to Mysore, I had this aspiration of an opening. You open to the guru and you allow the guru to work on you. In my case, especially on the second trip, he was very tough and that helped me to become humble. Guruji was working with me at this level: developing good qualities and releasing negativity.

Do you think the guru is necessary for developing yama *and* niyama? *Or do you think* asana *and* pranayama *practice is enough by itself?*
It's the attitude with which you do the *asanas*. What makes the practice a spiritual one is your attitude, your listening to and trusting the teacher. That makes it a spiritual practice. Without the right attitude, it is only physical exercise.

Do you not think that asana *practice can change your attitude?*
It can help, but you need to change some deep patterns. That is where you need the help of the guru, the teacher, to help change the psychological and physical patterns. With *asanas*, you change the patterns of your body; but with the guru, if you have that resonance, you can change patterns of the mind, too.

You seem to be saying the teacher is important for taking the next step.
The teacher is important, but what makes the teacher is the student. There is no teacher without a student. So the most important thing is the student's capacity to learn. And then you recognize the teacher.

What sort of attitude does the student need toward the guru?
Humility and trust and opening to him, to receive from him—the capacity to learn.

Mostly, people don't have that. They come with ego and ambition.
The teacher has to see that and go down to the level of the student. A
real teacher will see that this person is not ready to learn in this way. In
Guruji, I saw a lot of this. He did not spend any of his energy with people who did not want to learn. He made it so hard for them that they had
the choice either to surrender or to go away. He was a master of not
wasting a single bit of energy with students. This is why he was so happy
teaching.

What is the essence of what Guruji is teaching?
To connect with the source of life through the *prana*. When you start to
practice, you feel the *prana*. And then comes the question: From where
did this *prana* come? We didn't create it. It was created by the breathing,
the *asana*, and the movement. The question is: What makes this practice
spiritual? "I created this energy!" [says the ego]. From what is it coming,
this *prana*? At this moment [of questioning], it becomes spiritual, but
through the body.

*So you think rather than teaching a system of knowledge or philosophy, he's
teaching you to observe the process that is happening within you. Then you
start to question for yourself.*
At least it happened this way for me.

*He always talks about praying to God. Why do you think he finds that so
important?*
God is the source of everything. In the end, peace and tranquillity is
coming when we can surrender to the source. So we pray to the source
because everything is coming from there and everything is returning to
there. I remember asking him about the *drishtis*. One day he said to me,
"There is only one *drishti*, that is God." I sometimes felt that very strongly
after practice. I remember coming down the stairs and he would look at
me and recognize that I was having this strong feeling internally and I
felt we had some kind of resonance, and we just laughed together and
didn't say anything. I just bowed down and said, "Bye, Guruji. Thank
you."

*Guruji says 99 percent practice, 1 percent theory. Why do you think he
takes that approach, and what do you think that 1 percent is?*

We don't have to take it so literally. [*Laughter*] Who knows? If you want to know the taste of the food, you have to taste the food. You cannot talk about the taste of the food. Practice is bringing you a good taste of the food. And you need some theory, too. He is a practical person. Too much theory takes you away from the goal.

How does it take you away from the goal? Doesn't it point you toward the goal?
Too much theory without practice is like building castles in the air. You can talk about compassion and love and God, but if you don't practice or feel it inside, it is just theory.

It's strange that these physical exercises are in any way connected to compassion, or love, or God. It seems like quite a big jump.
It's the attitude. And then the connection to the guru.

So the teaching is not the asana, *it's the challenge in performing the* asana, *how that psychologically affects you, and then how your relationship with the guru helps you to overcome those challenges and evolve.*
Yes. But the *asana* is real as well. They have been practiced for centuries. *Asanas* create a transformed body—the postures and the breathing have a purifying effect. It's a scientific method. But you are not going to become enlightened or a Buddha from sitting in the lotus, you need an appropriate attitude in the pose.

How important is family life for Guruji? We have an idea that yogis remove themselves from society rather than integrating. Why do you think family is important?
He is a practical person, just like Krishnamacharya, and wants to bring spirituality into real life. No escaping from the world. Maybe in the traditional yoga they renounced everything and lived in caves, but Krishnamacharya and all his important disciples had families. And it is important in the sense that you don't have to renounce life to be a yogi.

But it's almost as though you shouldn't renounce. Guruji would say, "You get married, you have children!" What positive value does that have on the path of yoga?
Well, it puts you in touch with the difficulties of life. According to *The*

Yoga Sutras, to reach the state of yoga, you must have detachment, nonattachment. It's a paradox, because attachment is psychological. How powerful an experience it is to have a child, to love the child as much as you like but without attachment. If you don't have a child, you won't confront that situation. You can love romantically, but you can remain protected. When you have a child, you have to love the child without attachment.

Can you explain? Because many people are confused by the idea of love without attachment. Detachment is something to be afraid of because you may lose everything you are connected with. How is it possible to be loving without attachment?
The purpose of our spiritual life as human beings is to pass through the difficulties that life brings us, and to allow these things to pass through us without getting hooked—to become more like a witness to the events without craving, just to be aware of them. That is the difficulty. Life is just change, and maybe your wife passes away. To see Guruji's wife pass away was very interesting. He felt attachment toward his wife. And I remember him telling me something in Sanskrit like, "Time is being eaten by a rat, you have to accept that, everything has its expiration date."

You have to accept that everything is changing, everything is passing away. I remember Guruji crying and telling me that. "Yesterday Amma was here. Today, is gone. Yesterday here . . ." And he was crying so strongly. He was not pretending. He was in the middle of suffering this attachment to his wife. He was not going to see her anymore, and he was suffering. And at the same time, he surrendered himself completely to this suffering and it was interesting to see how he recovered. He was smiling again one month later. He was so happy. And he was not happy because his wife was gone. He could express his love toward her but he could accept that things were changing. *That* is detachment. You have to say goodbye to things that are living. You cannot control that. Life is bringing you so much, especially if you have a family. All the time things you want are not coming, and things that you don't want are coming. You see the attachment and the aversion and desire and everything right there.

What is interesting to me is that people usually think of love and desire almost as one thing. When there is love, there is desire, natural desire—it is impossible to love without attachment. It gives such pleasure so you want more and more. I think of love as being more about the way you act, it is a way to serve. Rather than you receiving something, you are giving. Most people think, "I love this relationship. If I don't have this relationship, I will feel empty." Rather than "I love this person and I want to serve this person and give them the best." I think that is perhaps one of the most challenging ideas for most people on the spiritual yogic path.

This is why Guruji says, "You see God everywhere." They say it also in the *Upanishads*. The only way to reduce suffering and attachment is to see the divine in everything, in every person, in every situation. When we have that *drishti*, we accept the situations of life better because we are relating to something which is infinite, something which is beyond ourselves. That should be the purpose of life. When we are just caught up in the conflict of existence, we are in a very low level of consciousness and are caught up in the dualistic mind. All spiritual traditions suggest the same solution. The Hindu tradition talks about seeing the one in the many. In Christianity, you see Jesus Christ in the heart of everybody. It's the same. You don't have to go far to find the same truth.

Can you say something about Amma?
She was very important to all the students. I remember Manju telling me, after she passed away, that she was the only person who could change Guruji's state of mind. When he was upset, Amma would make him laugh. So she was very important. But they had fights. Maybe not too strong. I remember in France his telling me, "Tomas, you come to our home and bring the students. If not, Amma and me, we fight." [*Laughter*] So we would gather in the evening at his house.

Can you say something about the energy he had for teaching?
Sometimes when I had a night off, I would pass by the school and his light was on at one or two in the morning. He would get up very early. He would take a bath. Prepare the fire to heat the water. And probably in that time he was doing his *puja* and meditation. He would start to teach us at four and would sometimes continue until twelve thirty as the *shala* became busy. Then he would teach Indians in the evening. He loved teaching and was never tired of it and was always enthusiastic.

Can you say something about Mysore and its support of the practice?
It is changing now, but before, it was a beautiful small city with a lot of

color and very Indian. You had to use simple rooms and simple hotels. Now progress has come and you can find *everything*. But at that time, the rooms had nothing. And it was very good for the mind of the students, because we took on a simple life.

India and its simplicity has a healing touch. We came to Mysore and we dropped all the problems we were dealing with in our Western lives. We came to Mysore empty. And you see the pumping of water, and people with very little, and happy. Families with nothing and super-happy, welcoming you and inviting you to have lunch when they have nothing to eat. So on the unconscious level, everything made us more relaxed.

This is why I think it was very bad when the students started to have motorbikes and luxury rooms. This is too easy. Then you are—

Bringing your life from the West rather than immersing yourself in the local way.
Yes. In the past, it was simplicity. We had nothing.

What is the value of daily practice? Year after year?
First, you keep your body strong. Life demands that you have to be strong and healthy. Also, when the person starts to practice, they change their habits in a healthy direction. At the psychological level, you start to develop willpower, which is also necessary in life. When you practice every day, you develop willpower. When you relax in the *asanas*, you are developing the quality of relaxation in life. So the *asana* practice is giving you strength and relaxation and also the possibility of reflection. You can see, according to your state of mind, how the practice will be affected by what you are eating. So the practice is a mirror. You can see many things. When life is falling apart, you still have your practice: it brings you balance.

What about the subtle aspects of the practice? Do you feel that just by practicing asanas *that states of meditation will naturally evolve?*
You have to put something into it from this side. I remember one time Guruji said, "There are some people who never learn. They always repeat the same mistakes." It's very easy to fall into some kind of a mechanical practice.

Guruji was no longer practicing asanas *when he became your teacher. Did you still see him as a yoga practitioner?*

Yeah, because I always thought that yoga was not only *asanas*. This was my approach from the beginning. In India, you have yoga for different stages of life. When you are young, you have *asanas*. As you grow older you change the practice. Toward the end of his life, his practice was in mantras, meditations, and in teaching.

How do you incorporate Guruji's philosophy in how you teach?
I want to transmit to students what I felt when I was practicing with him. I try to transmit his presence into the *asanas* and to the students. I try to be how he is: honest. I teach the way he taught me and try to be as authentic and sincere as possible.

What do you see as the relationship between teaching yoga and practicing yoga?
Teaching is practicing. We have to define what is yoga for us. Is it *asana* and *pranayama* only? Jumping? [*Laughter*] What is yoga? Yoga for me is getting in touch with something which is very real, which is the life in us, the source, through the *asana* practice. We call it *prana*. It is the life force, something which is beyond us, something impersonal. I try to experience that through my practice and to make my students feel it. This is not related to whether or not you are an advanced student. Some people are advanced because they are flexible. Some will find difficult *asanas* impossible because of age or for other reasons. But everyone can feel the same. It does not matter how advanced you are, if your practice is correct, if your the breathing is correct, you can be an old man or a cripple and you can still be in touch with this *prana*.

Are you saying that you don't see a connection between an advanced practice and being an advanced yogi? If you just apply the correct technique, no matter your physical condition, you can reach the same psychological and spiritual state?
And health, because this has nothing to do with flexibility or whether you can twist your bones 30 percent or 90 percent. Two brothers, one can sit in *padmasana*, one can't, they are almost the same age. Two different genes, two different natures. You have to understand that. If not, we are competing against ourselves, pushing ourselves to do things we should not do. Hurting ourselves.

You said teaching is a practice. Can you explain?
To be in touch with something that is beyond ourselves, the source, that is the purpose of my life, and the purpose of everybody's whether they know it or not. Then everything in life should become yoga. But we make the *asana* practice, the teaching, concentrated. We focus. It's like a prayer. When you pray, you are thinking of God. Ideally, you think about God all the time. We choose the moment for our practice, and we treat it as something sacred. In that moment, life has deep meaning. And we can find this strong meaning in just two hours of practice.

So it's similar in that it's a concentration of your yoga awareness in your practice and in your teaching. You have to transmit something similar.
Yes, similar.

We hear a lot about mula bandha *and* uddiyana bandha. *Can you talk about your own understanding and how that's evolved over the years?*
Guruji was never very specific about that. He was practical, physical. He would put my hands where I had to contract when I was doing the breathing. He would test if I was having anus control, especially the first few times. But to me, *mula bandha* is an action that is created when you exhale into the lower abdomen to protect, massage, and help purify the internal organs, and to stabilize the lumbar curve in the lower back. When we exhale, we pull the lower abdomen in, and to increase the effect of that action, we contract the anus, which is *ashwini mudra*. So we do *mula bandha*, which is the action of moving the lower abdomen toward the spine, squeezing the anus, and that creates, at the physical level, an effect on the lower back, stabilizing and protecting the lower spine. On the physical level, it has this purpose.

You said contracting the lower abdomen. Did you mean uddiyana bandha *or* mula bandha?
That is *mula bandha*—the action of contracting in the lower abdomen on exhalation. *Uddiyana* is like the extension of *mula bandha*, where you suck in the whole abdomen on an exhale retention. I understand [this is] the way Krishnamacharya taught it—that *mula bandha* is the contraction of the abdomen below the navel.

Because Guruji was not so specific.
He would say contract, but I observed some people who practiced wrongly because the breathing technique was transmitted wrongly. They kept the whole abdomen too tight and breathed very shallowly, only in the upper lungs, because they [held] their whole lower abdomen very tightly toward the spine and this created a lot of anxiety. You can do a bad practice with bad breathing and get crazy! And then, if you are also doing a lot of jumping *vinyasas* with that bad breathing? You get very excited. And this is called anxiety. You can go crazy if you don't breathe correctly.

Can you say more about the importance of breathing?
Sometimes you do the practice and it becomes mechanical. You don't end with tranquillity and peace. When you have a good practice, you end with peace and tranquillity. You had a good practice? You are not peaceful, but you put your feet behind your head? No, you are just agitated. So it depends on the effect. *Asanas* have an effect, and the breathing has an effect. How we relate the breathing to the *asanas* is very important. The breathing has a stronger effect than the *asanas* on the nervous system. You can do *paschimattasana* because you are flexible, but with agitated breath you end up agitated. *Paschimattasana* should give tranquillity, but it can end up causing agitation if the breathing is very fast. The breathing has to be always equal—Guruji always used to say that. There are three types of breath: short, medium, and long. For *asana* practice it should be medium for keeping the heat. The heat that is created is good heat. If the *asana* practice has fast breathing, it creates the wrong heat. Krishnamacharya used to teach very, very long breathing. This created a very tranquil state of mind. Very fast? The effect is agitation. To avoid making the practice mechanical, you have to be aware of the connection between breath and movement, and if possible make the breath a little longer than the movement. If you do that, it is impossible for the practice to be mechanical. Make the breath a little longer than the movement, and it is like a new practice all the time.

What is the importance of food in practice?
Diet has to be properly balanced. We have to find out what is good for us. That depends on the type of person, the type of work you do. Some people like more fruits, some more cereals. Everyone is different. For me, the macrobiotic style suits me best. But for others, not. [*Laughter*]

What you eat, and how you eat, are important. And how you cook the food. And how much you chew. I was in a macrobiotic place in France and was impressed that people who were chewing fifty, one hundred, two hundred times, just by chewing, they were healing themselves, bringing tranquillity.

What effect can a poor diet have on yoga practice?
Ayurveda says that sickness comes from food that was not digested properly, not absorbed or assimilated. If we don't chew, if we eat with agitation, we won't absorb that food properly.

And if we eat the wrong substances.
Yes.

But why is it important for us in the practice?
We reduce *tamas*, heaviness. The positive effect, the healing, is by reducing *tamas*. *Tamas* creates sickness. We reduce *tamas* by avoiding *tamasic* foods. It brings a positive effect to our health and in our practice.

Should practice change as you get older?
We have to adjust. In his book, *Yoga Mala*, Guruji talks about adjusting. When you are young, you do many *asanas*. When you get older, you focus on a few main *asanas*. It's part of life. When you are young, you can climb trees. When you get old, it's hard even to walk.

But it seems like people who practice ashtanga *yoga stay young.*
Not forever.

But it seems he's teaching people in their fifties, sixties, as if they were young. He's always encouraging you to have more energy and strength.
He helps you to go beyond yourself all the time. But as you get older, there are things you cannot do. You have to adjust the practice to a different stage of life. Krishnamacharya said this beautiful thing: Life is like a river. At the beginning, there are waterfalls and the river is full of energy—this is youth. Then the river becomes more focused, calm. At the end it loses its strength, it gets wider, and it disappears in the ocean. Our practice has to adjust to these three stages of life. When you are young, you practice *asanas*, jumping—you develop everything in youth. Later,

you have to sustain, you are more focused and calm, but you get more energy from the practice. And then the river disappears and we need to adjust the practice again. In the end, Guruji was just meditating and praying. But that is yoga as well.

Guruji talks about purification. It seems quite easy to understand how the internal organs and muscles can be purified and become more healthy, but he also talks about the nervous system and sense organs becoming purified. Do you have any ideas or understanding about that? Is this physiological, psychological, or on a pranic level?
A purified nervous system means it is tranquil, strong, and stable. This is expressed in relaxation and concentration. When we don't breathe well while doing the intermediate practice, because of all the backbends they can increase stimulation and make us crazy. Backbends work the nervous system in an intense way. When you can do all these backbends and not feel agitated, it's a sign that the nervous system is calm, purified, tranquil. You have to do backbends as if you were doing *shavasana*—that means perfection.

Perhaps it's the combination of physical foundation and appropriate attitude.
And breathing. Breathing has an immediate effect on the nervous system.

How does that happen?
Forward bending results in relaxation. Backbending is stimulation. Upside-down poses create stability and balance. These are the most valued postures. This is why shoulder stand and headstand are called the queen and king of *asanas*. Inhalation results in stimulation, exhalation in relaxation. If we breathe fast, it creates stimulation; if we breathe slow, relaxation. If you do forward bends with a slow and proper breath, it is going to create a tranquil effect. If you do backbends with proper breathing as well, it creates proper stimulation to achieve balance. *Hatha* yoga, the sun and the moon, the strength with the tranquillity. But if we breathe crazy doing backbends, we hyperventilate and create a state of anxiety. The combination of breathing and *asanas* has a powerful effect on our nervous system on a therapeutic level. For instance, if you suffer from anxiety, doing a lot of backbends and breathing fast, you aren't going to sleep well.

What is the physical effect of the breath on the nervous system?
When you inhale, it works on the sympathetic nervous system. When you exhale, it works on the parasympathetic nervous system. This is why we have to bring it into balance all the time. All effort is initiated by the sympathetic nervous system, while sleep or relaxation is more the parasympathetic nervous system. *Pranayama* is how we control the nervous system. When we inhale, you have to make an effort. Exhale is just happening, you don't need any effort. But to inhale deeply you need to make an effort. When you make an effort everything becomes tense. If you say "Inhale," a person may screw up his eyes, raise the shoulders, move the head up—it creates that action. In *pranayama* when we inhale, we move the head down and look into the heart. You don't raise the shoulders. You just inhale peacefully. So you are breaking the pattern. When you exhale you don't fall into *tamas*, you keep the back straight. Otherwise, you would naturally collapse the back on exhalation. When you exhale, you engage *mula bandha*, you support the spine and avoid falling into this heaviness [*tamas*]. In this way, you change the nervous system, you gain mastery over it. And this is probably how Krishnamacharya was able to stop his heart from beating.

How do you view both your internal experience and your way of being effective in life as a result of your thirty years of yoga practice?
I started practicing *ashtanga* yoga when I was twenty-four, and now I am over fifty. The practice has given me support in passing through difficult moments in my life. Sometimes you feel like life is just shaking you from one point to the other and it's easy to lose control. The practice gives you support. I am thankful for that, because we don't control life. Life can be difficult. The practice brings you balance and you don't become depressed. When things are positive, you enjoy them more because you are more awake. In the negative moments, you have the support.

It seems that your perspective is that yoga is a support for you to do the things you have to do, rather than something that transforms and changes you.
First it is the support, and then it is there to transform life. You need the support first; then, how to transform the life? That is the big challenge, the superior yoga, but how? This is called "transformation." First is realization. You need to realize some strength, some power within you. Then

the most difficult thing is to take these realizations that you have into your daily life, to bring light, and to transform the life. This is why I like Aurobindo's teaching—bringing the realization into life makes life divine. Life is intense, we need support and balance. Then to transform life, that is the superior yoga.

Is there something important that you would like to add?
Asana practice should not be our goal. Having *asana* as the goal is often the reason we injure ourselves. If we don't respect our nature, our body, our physical nature, and we want to do *asanas* that are difficult because we compare ourselves with others, because we want to do *marichyasana* D in order to reach *navasana* and our hip doesn't open and we try to force ourselves into poses. This also applies to teachers. We think it is important to put the student in an *asana*, and then we hurt the person. To me, the *asanas* are just the expression of the flexibility of the person. The goal is not *asana*, we use *asana* as a tool to attain flexibility and strength. But we have to respect the body. If that tool doesn't work, we maybe need to adjust the *asana* a little bit, or maybe wait until the student is ready. We have to realize that we will not reach enlightenment by being able to sit in *padmasana*. Maybe we achieve *padmasana* and also end up in the hospital with broken knees! [*Laughter*] We achieve enlightenment with broken knees! We need protection. Guruji used to say, "You take slowly." This "You take slowly" is very important.

Is there one thing above anything else that you are most grateful for which you received from Guruji?
Many things. From him, I have a profession. I'm helping people, and they are grateful for that. The practice and his teaching have helped me. The contact with him has helped me. His presence and strength and the connection with his force, the *prana*, whatever you like to call it. I feel grateful for the sense of health and happiness I have received.

New York City, 2009

Richard Freeman

Richard Freeman met Guruji after an extensive period of spiritual undertakings which began in 1967 and included living as a monk in India, becoming an avid yoga practitioner, and devoting himself to philosophical studies. He has been instrumental in spreading *ashtanga* yoga in the West.

How did you first find out about ashtanga *yoga, and how did you find your way to Mysore?*
I don't remember when I first heard about it, but I knew of its existence for a number of years. First, through the work of Desikachar—the concept of *vinyasa*, that things occur in sequences and that you can practice yoga *asana* in sequences. And then I learned that Pattabhi Jois was going to come to the United States and lead a workshop at the Feathered Pipe Ranch in Montana, and so I signed up right away. When I met him I was enthralled by his radiance and his kindness. We almost had an instant connection. And fortunately, we were in a place that was isolated. There were two classes every day and hours of time in between to talk, and it was an exciting experience. I was swept off my feet by Guruji when I met him.

What was your first impression of him?
I was impressed by his smile, his radiance, his overall sweetness. I found him extremely accessible. He was willing to tell me anything I wanted to know, and that was actually rare in teachers. I was swept off my feet.

I've often heard Guruji say he teaches real or original Patanjali yoga. What was your experience of him as a teacher of true yoga?
When someone says they teach Patanjali yoga, the eight limbs of yoga,

they are implying that not only do they teach *asana* and *pranayama* but also *samadhi* and all of the stages of meditation and then the release, or the self-realization through *samadhi*. My experience of Guruji is that this is what his interest is. Practically his only interest in life is to fulfill the whole yoga system. His emphasis is, of course, on intense *asana* practice at first, but through that *asana* practice with the *vinyasa* methodology he is also teaching the fundamentals of *pranayama* and meditation. And much later on in his system, these particular parts are separated out and refined. But in a sense he is teaching the eight limbs initially through *asana* practice, and when one picks up the thread inside, we find that the other limbs are very easy to practice. And so he is saying the first four limbs of yoga—*yama*, *niyama*, *asana*, and *pranayama*—are very difficult, but if you are grounded in them, the internal limbs are easy and occur spontaneously, naturally.

Does he actually teach them by themselves or are they just incorporated in the asana *practice?*
He teaches them on a one-to-one basis when he wants to. If someone is really interested, dying for it, he teaches the internal limbs. Practically, you have to be experiencing them already so that it's easy to teach. If someone is burning with desire, then they are so close that the teacher doesn't have much to do except say yes, that's it.

Is samadhi *far off for us?*
Samadhi is very close, according to my understanding. Practicing yoga, you gradually develop the ability to observe what is happening in the present moment, and when you observe very closely what is actually occurring, then that is *samadhi*. And what is occurring is very close to us. Usually we are looking at some other place rather than at what is actually happening. So yoga *asana* and *pranayama* allow the attention to focus on what is actually happening. Present feelings, present sensations, and the present pattern of the mind become sacred, they become the object of meditation. So many people try to practice meditation but are trying to practice by observing what isn't present. They are trying to look behind this, they are trying to look anyplace, let me see anything but this. But when you practice *asanas* enough, when you practice *pranayama*, the very sensation that you are having presently is what is sacred. You stop looking elsewhere and *samadhi* starts to occur.

So how does Guruji's system bring you face-to-face with that experience? Or does it? Is it specific to this type of yoga, or is it part of any yoga teaching?
It would be part of any yoga teaching. The question is: Does the system work, or does the collection of systems and methodology work? And in many cases, in many schools of yoga, not a lot is happening. Yoga traditionally has been passed down from teacher to student over thousands of years, and often the lineages are broken, so it is like a wire that is broken and no current flows through it, so the actual internal teaching doesn't get transmitted.

Do you know how far back this lineage goes beyond Krishnamacharya's teacher? Do we know anything about Rama Mohan Brahmachari's teacher?
No, we don't. Of course, Guruji has a family lineage which is the lineage of Shankaracharya. And he is constantly making reference to Shankaracharya, to teachers in the Shankaracharya lineage, and he has much involvement in that, and his yoga guru, Sri Krishnamacharya, also has his yoga guru and his family lineage. It's a complex thing to study.

How important is a guru when practicing yoga, and how does Guruji perform that function of separating the light from the darkness?
The guru is practically the key to the whole system. I suppose in theory, if one were extremely intelligent and extremely lucky and extremely kind, you could learn yoga from a book and you could do very well and get very far. But with a teacher, you develop a relationship, and something right at the heart of that relationship carries the essence of the practice, and so the various techniques that you might learn, even the various philosophies you might learn, are placed in an immediate context by the guru. That context is simply one of complete, open relationship, complete presence. It's a great thing. So if there's a great teacher around, take advantage of it! If there's no teacher around, practice anyway.

How would you characterize Guruji's teaching method?
When I first met Guruji, he reminded me very much of a Zen Buddhist teacher in that he used very few words in his classes. The words he would use were like koans, they were puzzling, at least to most of the students. And often, he was just trying to wake you up with what he was doing. It wasn't so much the content of what he was saying. He would sometimes try to distract you or to place you in a kind of double bind

where you might just laugh and let your breath flow and all of a sudden find yourself doing a posture that you had feared two minutes before.

I remember doing backbends in Mysore with Guruji. We were just standing and arching back and grabbing our knees which is, if you think about it, very scary at times. I was all set to do it with my arms crossed and he looked at my shorts which were soaking wet and cotton and he said, "Oh, nice material!" just as I was starting to drop back and made me completely forget my preconceptions. And the backbend was no problem at all.

When there is fear going into a pose, does he have a technique to take you deeper, beyond your body's apparent natural capacity?
I think what he does is he makes you drop your presuppositions, your preconceptions about your body and therefore about your limitations. Oftentimes you'll approach him and say, "Oh Guruji, this muscle is hurting" or "This bone has this problem." And he'll just look at you and say, "What muscle?" In other words, he is inviting you again to look with a completely fresh mind to see if there is anything really there. And by dropping the concept you have around a sensation or feeling, you release them. Many times the concept is the limiting factor. He's a master at that: seeing if there is some fear or some attachment. And usually, in a very kind, sometimes gentle, sometimes abrupt way, he'll get you to reframe a situation.

Is he imparting that skill to Sharath?
I think naturally he is. That's just the way he relates to people, and so Sharath is bound to pick it up I think.

It's interesting because Sharath is still involved with practicing with Guruji immediately present, which is an intense way to practice. So Sharath experiences sometimes a lot of pain, sometimes his own fear, and so he is very sympathetic with the students, very compassionate, because he has learned to be compassionate with himself when he practices. Guruji is also that way, but he doesn't do *asana* practice anymore and so he just takes you right into it.

Can you say something more about the way Guruji teaches, his method?
I found him to be something of a trickster in his teaching methods. He'll emphasize a particular aspect of what he'll call the *vinyasa* methodol-

ogy—that certain poses have to follow other poses. Then, if he sees that you've taken him too literally or that you've become too attached to that, he'll completely drop that. I remember once in Mysore, I finished a series with him and we then went to watch the *Ramayana* on his television. About an hour later he looked at me and he said, "Oh backbending!" [*Laughter*] And I said, "Oh Guruji, very cold now." My conceptualization was, there is no way I'm going to do backbends, especially with him. I was completely cooled down, completely ready to go back to my room and take a nap. He just smiled and said, "Oh, no problem!" So we went back to the practice room and he wanted me to stand there and drop into the deepest possible backbends. Again he just laughed, and I did it. And so the rules about *vinyasa* and things are context-dependent. In other words, in certain other contexts they don't apply.

So he taught me to develop a flexible mind in relationship to the methodology of practice. He is also very strict in how he follows those methods, but then he also wants you to see them from a deeper context so you can actually experience yoga and also be free of the methods, too.

It seems this strict methodology breeds dependency and you can get attached to it, too.
He sometimes encourages that kind of attachment, and then one day he'll pull the rug right out from under you and say, "Oh, I never said that." [*Laughter*]

Or you are just dying to get another pose and he'll hold off—
For months and months and months, and then a new person will come and he'll give him the pose you wanted, right next to you, and then he laughs. So much of the practice is the mind, the breath.

Do you have words to describe the essence of what he's imparting?
I don't think what he's imparting can be said. But I think there's nothing else really worth talking about, because he is teaching a kind of openness of the mind and the heart which is so stunning that, at least at times, you don't know what to say, you are awestruck and can't put it into words. That's why there is such an art, I think, to teaching. Krishnamacharya once made a comment to a friend of mine: yoga is not mechanical. I think Guruji is always teaching that through a very formal system. You have to follow the form very carefully, in fact you have to pour your being

into it with intensity to create *tapas*, internal heat. But then you have to be completely not attached to it. And somewhere in that changeover, where you are able to follow form precisely but then not identify with it, the real yoga comes out.

Is it a spiritual practice he's teaching?
Yeah, I think it's spiritual in the way most people use that word. You could also say it's beyond spiritual. If someone has a concept of spirituality, this is much more interesting than anything they could imagine. But it's definitely a totally spiritual practice. However, if someone comes to it and has no interest in what they believe spirituality to be, if they just take up the practice for improving their health or fixing some biomechanical problem in the body, it'll prove effective but it will also put them in touch with their core feelings. And just by touching those core feelings they will start inquiring into what is real. They'll start to ask: "Why am I suffering all the time?" "What is true?" And so they've come to the right place. And so yoga in a sense is like a fountain. People will go to it, for many different reasons but because they've gone to the source they start to get a taste for it, and they might not really understand why they like it but they'll keep coming back to the source and eventually they'll just jump right back in.

It is spiritual in the sense that the Atman, the soul, is revealed, but at the same time there is a methodology as well, so is it somehow a fusion of those two things?
Exactly. If we say that what is of most interest to the open mind, to the open heart, is beyond expression, beyond words, also therefore beyond technique, our first reaction is "I won't do anything." But the fascinating thing about practice is that what is manifesting as the body and the mind is composed of strings and strings of techniques, and so yoga is actually the art of using techniques with incredible skill and through that one naturally arrives at a place where there is no technique anymore but freedom. This is one of the major themes of the *Bhagavad Gita*, one of the extremely illusive themes, that the truth is ultimately formless because it generates all forms. How can it be approached? How can you realize it? It's actually through seeing forms with an open mind and allowing the body and the mind to complete their natural tendencies to complete their forms, and in that you release form.

So you have to see all the forms that your mind wants to manifest to actually see behind them, and that goes for all the different asanas as well.
Yes, each one is sacred, each one is like a mandala, or in the Hindu tradition they use the word "yantra," which is a sacred diagram. Yantras have very distinct forms, so a yoga *asana* has a very distinct outer form and a very distinct internal form, and if you are able to go into it, in sometimes excruciating detail and intensity, and you see it as sacred, if you are simply able to observe it without reducing it to some concept or theory, then you are free from that form. The very heart of the yantra or mandala is you. Then another form comes which happens to be the next pose in the series, and eventually you are able to see all of these as an expression of the same internal principle. It's just that at certain points we get confused and we're not able to see it as sacred, as spiritual.

Has Guruji described to you different mental forms that relate to the different asanas?
No, he hasn't, just practice. What he has done is he's given me a lot of things to study, books to read, hoping that I will be fascinated and extract information from them.

Why is there such a strong emphasis on asana practice in this system? What is the function of going back to the same place daily?
The practice is like a mirror. We go to the mirror every morning to tidy ourselves up before going out into the world, and the practice is like a mirror for what's in your heart and what's in your mind. If you are able to approach the practice from an internal space, it's always new. The same old pose is always fascinating because you are using it as an object of meditation rather than as a means to get something. And that way you are able to practice and practice and practice—perhaps forever.

What is the attitude one needs to get that experience?
I think the key to *ashtanga* practice is *bhakti*, which is devotion or love. The eight limbs are accessories to that heart. *Bhakti* is probably the closest thing to what yoga is. And so guru *bhakti*, which is a direct relationship or love for the teacher, is one aspect of *bhakti* that is extremely helpful.

You are saying the essence of yoga is bhakti, *devotion. Is yoga at the heart of every religion?*
Yoga is the direct experience of your original nature. You could call it God or you could call it Allah, Vishnu, Shiva, but oftentimes we don't really understand what those terms mean, or those terms don't have a meaning in relation to other ideas in our mind, so it has to be experienced. But many, many religious forms and traditions are practiced to give you this experience, and in that experience you find freedom. So I would think yoga is something that is more essential than religion.

What is it like having Guruji as your guest?
Having Guruji as your guest is very much like going to your first yoga class with him. It's a combination of a lot of work, because he has so many particular needs that are primarily cultural, and we also love him so much that we really want to make it nice for him—setting up his kitchen correctly and finding a place where he can sleep, finding where he can rest and feel at home. So it's a mixture of anxiety—of doing something that is nearly impossible—and then he's like your grandfather, someone you are really glad to see, so sweet. He's also so easy to please as well as hard to please. If anyone gets the chance, I recommend that they invite him to their home. [*Laughter*] And you can study your own mental states just before he arrives, and after he arrives the incredible relief. It's part of the teaching. Doing the actual practice is much easier!

In many ways Guruji seems to be down-to-earth, a man of this world. How does this yoga penetrate into his everyday life?
Part of his charm is that he's so down-to-earth and appreciative of simple things that are immediately around him, and I think this is because of the nature of the yoga practice. As he would say, you start to see God everywhere or in everything. I think one of the main thrusts of his teaching is that this, this is it. Many people look at yoga *asanas* as "Well, we are temporarily going to work the body to get away from this," and all the time keeping the preconception that the body is not a good thing, rather than really penetrating the body, and as well as the body, our immediate environment, our immediate lives, penetrating them with our intelligence and then our compassion. That's what he's done to his own body and to his own environment and so he's totally present with what is really happening. It's such a relief to be around him for that reason.

This is a lineage of householders, not renunciants. How significant is that?
It's a lineage that recently has many householders in it. I'm sure it had renunciants in it. One of the nice things I've found is that it's the nature of
the yoga practice to make you wake up to what is really happening in
your body, in your mind, in your environment right now. You start to see
them, just as we are seeing the postures, as sacred. We see everything in
the world, all the forms, as sacred. Seeing them that way, we are able to
engage with them, work with them completely, and that's really the way
to be free. If you see them as a threat, like many renunciants will see the
world as a threat—"I have to go off to the forest or cave so that I can
make my mind quiet"—then their quietness depends on the absence of
stimulation, the absence of form. But in a deep yoga practice, the peace
and tranquillity are not dependent on anything. So anything that comes
to the mind, whether it be a sensation, a feeling, a family crisis, or a catastrophe, is the object of meditation, it's sacred energy. Through householder life, through married life, through participating in the world, the
yoga really blossoms. Guruji is a fine example of that. He often jokes that
the householder life is seventh series, it's the really hard one.

Can you talk about Amma, the role she played in Guruji's teaching?
What's that saying? Behind every successful man there's a woman?
Amma was so wise, so down-to-earth, so aware of the immediacy of the
divine, that she was the perfect complement to Guruji. And they would
always talk about everything together, especially after classes. She was
also a walking encyclopedia of Sanskrit texts and Indian philosophies.
He would often be quoting things and he couldn't remember a line. He
would just turn to her and she would be able to repeat verse after verse
verbatim. And she was also able to laugh it all off—so she didn't hold on
to it or take it too seriously.

*You had just mentioned Sanskrit texts, and that Guruji had given you books
to read. Were you reading in Sanskrit? Were you working on the 1 percent
theory?*
Yes, I worked on the 1 percent. [*Laughter*] Actually, the study part of
the yoga practice is *svadhyaya*, according to *The Yoga Sutras*, which is the
study of the Self, initially through the study of the tradition and the
scriptures. It's a concentration of the same information you will get from
Guruji. And really 1 percent of Indian philosophy is theory and the other

99 percent is freeing your mind from it. The text is designed to make your intelligence fluid so that no theory is going to trip you up. It is so remarkably consistent with the type of practice *ashtanga* yoga is, the way that the scriptures flow from one point of view to another point of view, just as eventually your intelligence has to flow in your practice from one pose to another without getting stuck in any particular philosophy or theory. I look at yoga as freedom from philosophy, freedom from theory, freedom from religion.

How has Guruji helped you with an understanding of theory?
He has given me things to read, things to chant, and told me to practice meditation on certain forms or deities as well as *pranayama* practice and of course *asana* practice. I think mostly through his smile he's kind of let on that there is something light, almost humorous lying in the heart of this dense philosophical system. There is, of course, some language barrier when talking philosophy with Guruji. But he talks like a Zen teacher, speaking metaphorically or to put you in a bind where you start to find out for yourself what really counts.

Did Guruji teach you Sanskrit, or had you already studied it before you went to Mysore?
I studied Sanskrit before I met Guruji, but he has taught me Vedic chanting. He's very much concerned that you pronounce correctly, that you get the right intonation and the right meter, because traditionally that's what really gives the power to the chants. It's a respect for detail and form that makes you concentrate your mind, that makes you use your palate as you chant in such a way that you create internal resonance. He's very excited about chanting, chants a lot himself.

Do you feel that Guruji is a self-realized being?
I feel he is, but I don't know for sure. You don't really know, but he certainly touches that chord in me. When I'm around him, just his presence makes me start to wake up and to look more closely at everything. I don't know if he's self-realized or not. How would I know?

Boulder, 2000

Dena Kingsberg

Dena Kingsberg began practicing yoga in Australia with Graeme North-field, eventually leaving her studies as an art student to pursue yoga full time. Along with Annie Pace, she became one of Guruji's most advanced women practitioners. She lives in Byron Bay, Australia, with her husband and two children.

How did you first become interested in yoga?
I came from a family of two different religious beliefs so I was never completely clear in which direction I should focus my own faith. My father traveled to India every year of my life. He collected religious artifacts and wandered the Himalayas. Perhaps I inherited his natural curiosity, for when I first came upon the word "yoga," I was fascinated by what I had understood it to mean and felt that it was a definite direction for exploration.

How did you first come across it?
A girlfriend took me to a yoga class, it was Satchidananda style and we did a lot of interesting *asanas*. What really held my attention was the way the teacher sat in *padmasana* for an extended period of time and remained remarkably still. I was studying sculpture at art school and working as a life-drawing model to support myself, so I understood how difficult it was to stay still like that. I found her serenity in this complex pose was strangely moving.

How did that lead you toward an ashtanga *practice?*
The class sparked my curiosity but it was an isolated experience. Later

that year, when my father passed away, I made my first trip to India. I had my eyes open for a yogic opportunity but not really knowing where to go, who to go to, or how to begin. The road eventually led me to Bodh-gaya where I met a community of Tibetan Buddhists, who just melted my heart with their warm and welcoming smiles. And that was where my spiritual spark ignited, practicing in the lineage of Mahayana Buddhism. Strangely, it was not in India but on my return to Australia that I chanced upon Graeme Northfield and first encountered *ashtanga* yoga.

He had recently returned from Mysore and was really passionate about Guruji's teachings. I started practicing with him casually, but slowly it became my priority and I would miss art-school classes so that I would not miss yoga practice. After a year, Graeme moved on, leaving a small group of us to practice by ourselves. I felt a surprising amount of anger and disappointment at his decision to leave. I was more attached to the practice than I had realized.

Some time after that I drove my car across a causeway and was swept into a rising river. The car and I were fully submerged before I could get out. On the surface I was fine, but in the months that followed I began to lose confidence and become more and more introverted. I felt like I was losing my way, shrinking. I thought of the most terrifying thing I could, and that was to go and seek out Guruji in Mysore.

So you wrote a letter?
I don't recall the protocol, but I had directions! I had met up with a girl-friend in Madras and we traveled to Mysore together. "Go to the police station in Lakshmipuram and turn left," or something like that. When the rickshaw pulled up outside the house, both Amma and Guruji were sitting on the front porch and I had the feeling that they were waiting for us. I was hardly breathing, I was so nervous. We got out, he smiled, and she laughed. They asked who our teacher was and when we said Graeme, they were incredibly welcoming. They served us coffee and we sat down in their little entry room feeling delightfully at home.

Do you remember going in for your first day of practice with Guruji?
When I arrived the first day there was a class of Indian students finishing up. I watched through a little window from the staircase. It was fascinat-ing, primal, such an intense energy coming out of the room.

Do you remember how Guruji started teaching you?
Graeme had told me, "Stand up straight, begin, and don't stop." I had a relatively clear primary series, and that was my practice on that first day. Guruji may have adjusted me in a few poses but I remember the back-bends, as he took me higher in *chakra bandhasana* than I had ever been before. It was quite the introduction.

How long did you stay on that first trip?
Three months, and I remember having a calendar on the wall and mark-ing off the days as they passed. The intense yoga and the rawness of India made it quite challenging. If I could survive these three months then, theoretically, I would be in the next phase of my existence. That was the plan. I was very clear at the time that it was going to be a one-off experience.

Can you describe how the teaching unfolded with Guruji during that first period, and how things changed over the years in your relationship with him?
Guruji moved me relatively quickly into the second series, which I found quite intense. But once I was back in Australia, I realized that I had a certain longing to stay on that edge of intensity. There wasn't any other place I could imagine that was possible other than the room in Lakshmi-puram. So I did all I could to collect enough funds to get myself back there. It was an ongoing theme for at least the next ten years. It was all about being with Guruji and facilitating that education. I had once had other dreams for myself, other plans, but yoga simply outshone them.

Guruji's smile was the beginning of the relationship, and every other possible expression of human communication followed, from him being sweet and encouraging, to him being inquisitive, to him being what ap-peared to be angry, to myself feeling extremely unworthy. He would say, "Why you so stiff?" and I would be thinking, "Am I really so stiff?" And he'd be yelling, "Why don't you practice?" and I'm thinking, "But I do practice, I always practice." He was pushing me to the edge. For many years I was holding it together with my will, trying to seek his approval, to be good enough, to be worthy enough, and to be accepted by him. I would do whatever it took. One time, he pushed and he pushed and he pushed both physically and emotionally until the bubble burst and I started to cry and he asked, "Why are you crying?" I replied, "Isn't this what you wanted?" Then he just laughed, and I laughed, too. And then began another phase.

Did your relationship with him change after the tears came?
It changed my relationship with myself and I was then able to see more clearly that his intention was simply based on love and his approach was to use whatever tools were required to move us through the practice.

So prior to that point in time, it was a little confusing as to why you were drawn to him. And after that you were more clear.
I was clear that it was right. Exactly why it was right is not so clear. The pull to it was as subtle and as real as gravity. Perhaps subconsciously I was looking for a father figure. He has certainly played or fulfilled that role, as well as others, over the years. A parent can be both harsh and soft in their intention to bring out the best in their children. I trusted in the method and felt blessed to sit at the guru's feet. I just belonged there.

What is it that Guruji teaches?
He helps us to understand that our insecurities are not necessary and that we are each of us essentially okay. Guruji teaches that knowledge of the true Self is possible if we continue to practice. That eventually the veil that obscures us from self-realization will fall away, illuminating our true nature. That if God is in all things, then God is also in you. And if you can get out of your own way long enough, then perhaps you'll feel it. Sometimes I feel it.

How did his methods bring you to that realization?
Repetition of the same practice daily brings some insight into behavioral patterns, our personalities, and the workings of the mind. Same practice, different experience. It's an honest and often uncomfortable look at one's Self. Guruji's commitment to the method inspires trust that allows one to let go of self-set limitations. Under his touch, the body and mind find a new relationship beyond fear, both present and detached.

As the physical body transforms to accommodate the unfolding series, the emotional body unravels with it. I had unwavering trust in Guruji that I would always land in a safe place. Because of that trust, my physical body and all that was dragged along with it has made remarkable changes.

It sounds very much like a personal journey rather than there being an agenda on Guruji's part to impart a certain type of knowledge. Is he facilitating your own personal exploration?

Both. Guruji wants you to be well and whole and to understand. It was always clear to me that the process wasn't going to happen quickly. When I first arrived in Mysore, I got the impression that all the female students were named Mary—because Guruji called them all Mary—and it wasn't until you repeated your visit, that you showed some dedication, some sincerity, that you were even worthy of a name. And then as you came again and again, affection became associated with that and with the mutual commitment to the journey.

His agenda was simply to impart the "correct method," the one he learned from his guru. When Guruji appreciated your sincerity and dedication to the path, he took extra care to be sure that what he was presenting was understood with precision and clarity, as it was likely that those people who were ongoing in their studies would then be sharing the practice with the greater community.

How does Guruji's personality come out in his teaching?

He would not tolerate disrespect or ambition. He would be truthful when it wasn't always comfortable. He was endlessly patient and kind to beginners, compassionate if you had pain, sweet, affectionate, and loving. It was difficult not to adore him. He holds up the mirror, metaphorically, and he holds that mirror at the right angle to collect the light so that it reflects back on you.

Do you see Guruji as a healer?

Guruji embodies the practice. He carries great light and wisdom. His vibration is finely tuned and his hands are filled with *shakti*. Perhaps the practice is the medicine and Guruji is the doctor who knows just what and how much to prescribe. I'm sure many of us have never felt so well as when we are in his hands or in his presence.

What is Guruji's role in the process of helping people go through changes?

Guruji pushes you right to the edge of your limitation. Because he has walked this path before us and shared the process with so many, he is familiar with the landscape. His confidence and experience inspires a trust that allows a student to let go. He will hold you gently as you pass through or catch you if you fall.

Do you have some examples of how he worked with you in those intense moments?
There was one particular posture that caused me a lot of grief. Each day when I got to the pose before it, Guruji would say, "Tomorrow: *buddhasana*—some difficult!" *Buddhasana* is an intense foot-behind-the-head position in the fourth series. I would get up very early in the morning, at two o'clock, and start warming up my hips in the hope that I would be able to move smoothly into the pose. When I'd get to that pose the following day he would say, "Oh! No. *Buddhasana* some difficult, tomorrow you take it." So the next day I would get up very early in the morning and start warming up in the hope that I would get comfortably into this next pose and then he would repeat the cycle. We would get to the same place and he would say, "Oh, no, *buddhasana*, difficult posture, tomorrow you do it." This went on for some time. I was lacking sleep and my anxiety was building and I was getting frustrated and exhausted, not because I didn't have the pose but because of the pressure of the waiting, the building pressure. And then it was almost as if I gave up. On the one morning I didn't get up early to warm up, I was given the pose. I slipped into it effortlessly and I could feel the rest of the students in the room opening their hearts with support and relief because the tension had finally been broken. But I couldn't move after that day for quite some time. It was a structural renovation of my body on a deep level. I was left confined to my room and my head. The internal process was as uncomfortable as the physical. I guess Guruji knew it was coming. The other practitioners who had been past this point enjoyed a laugh of empathy as I tried to walk and regain the use of my body. But time passes and the body adjusts and facilitates this new liberation. Qualities of humility and patience accompany it. You change, you open, energy shifts, and you move on to the next challenge.

How important is family life and integration into society in the system of yoga that Guruji teaches?
Guruji teaches that yoga is not just for *brahmacharis* and *sannyasis*. It is a path to knowledge for all people. As the years passed, I started spending

more time in Mysore than at home. I thought that if I had no other distractions I would be able to focus and go deeper with the practice. So I packed up my things in Australia, intimate relationship included, and planned to settle in India for an indefinite period. When I communicated this to Guruji, he just laughed and said, "No, that is too easy for you. You have to go back. You have to teach. You take one husband, you make two children." So how important is family life to him? Well, at the time it seemed a lot more important than it was to me. But Guruji is always all about family. Amma was the twinkle in his eye. His life companion for more than sixty years. When she passed away, Guruji said to me, "Nonattachment is easy only in theory." Family was and is everything to Guruji, and I mean both bloodline family and the family of students that he has given and devoted his life to. He said it is important for practitioners to have children. They would be special children. My feeling was that it was a way, a small way, to heal the world. You start with family.

Can you explain a little how relationships support yoga practice?
I imagine my experience with support in a relationship is likely to be very different than many. I was fortunate enough to choose the right partner—I had a little help from Guruji with that. Relationships are an essential adjunct and support to yoga practice. The world is our playing field, a stage for transformation in life. The people we share it with, the relationships we have, are the greatest of teachers. We learn so much about our conditioned mind and our patterns of behavior as we interact with others and our expectations, fears, and attachments rise to the surface. If you are clear enough about your path and you walk it with determination and commitment but with enough compromise to accommodate those around you, then there is nothing more amazing than having companionship on that journey. However, when there are distractions caused by other people, then you are forced to be clear how sincere you are about the practice. Finding the balance is challenging and sometimes difficult, yet this is often where the true yoga lies. Guruji and Amma performed a marriage ceremony for Jack and me in 1997. The one line he repeated in English over and over was "one thousand years don't change it" (your partner, that is). It was also suggested that as Australia is a spacious country we should have ten children. We managed two. Our daughter, Zoli, arrived in the year 2000, and Guruji gave her the name Lakshmi. Our son, Izac, followed in 2003, and Guruji gave him the name

Ishvara. He gave them chocolate each morning at 6 a.m. in the yoga *shala*.

Can you say something about the energy Guruji put into his teaching?
Guruji was and is a remarkable man. If someone new would come to the *shala*, he would sit down with them and give them his undivided attention while talking them through the beginning motions of the practice. He would do it over and over and over again, never tiring of the repetition. He saw to each person in the room personally. We were all like seeds of a crop that would fruit, whether we are at the initial phases or further down the path. Each time a new student came to him it was as if he was unwrapping a present. As the class size grew from a handful to hundreds, he still saw to each one in turn with personalized, focused devotion. It was remarkable how he held such unwavering joy with every new face. What an inspiration!

Do you see ashtanga *yoga as a spiritual practice?*
Essentially, it is the quest for truth. It is a path for those with longing to know the silent whisper of God's voice. Each day, we breathe, we bend, we extend, we fold and unfold [through practice]. The next day again we breathe, we move, we move a little further, we unfold again. Again and again in the same place, penetrating deeper and deeper, peeling away the layers. Letting go. The practices strip us back. Through the struggle of it, we disentangle from the bondage of conditioned existence. We shed the layers of cultivated Self. You are neither your job nor your position in society. You are not your education or your image. You are not the people you attach yourself to. You are not simply body or mind. Stripped back of everything that separates us, blinds us, our awareness directed inward instead of outward, a spiritual awakening seems inevitable.

Why do you think Guruji starts with emphasizing asana *practice, the third limb?*
The first two limbs, *yamas* and *niyamas*, are the individual's responsibility. They will evolve as awareness deepens. Our practice begins by removing impurities and blockages from the body. For this we need to move and create heat, we need to light the internal fire and produce sweat to begin the cleansing and eliminating of accumulated toxins. The unfolding *asana* practice cultivates strength, flexibility, and balance of body and

mind and prepares us for the more subtle internal practices that follow. Breath, sensory withdrawal, and concentration are entwined and interconnected, not separate. Guruji starts with the work of unraveling the past so we can come into the present. Meditation is the doorway to liberation of the spirit. *Asana* practice and all that it encompasses is the path to that door. You've got to get to the door before you can pass through it.

How do you think the asana *practice purifies the mind and body to be ready for meditation?*
The practice is a purification process, a therapy to make us well. From this state of being well other things can unfold. We turn our attention inward, reducing distractions by withdrawing the senses. *Drishtis* direct the gaze to a soft focus and we listen to the even sound of the breath. This rhythmic repetition of movement becomes familiar and soothing and the mind slips away into the space between thought. Then the practice becomes a moving meditation, an invitation to stillness.

I think of it like this: Perception is a window. This window has been marked with the passing of time. Impressions are left upon it by our conditioning. It is colored by life's experiences, our upbringing, relationships, and culture. It is damaged by disappointment, trauma, and loss, clouded by uncertainty and confusion. I see the practice as the process of cleaning the window. Each day we dip the sponge into the bucket and wipe it across the surface. After some time, the change is apparent. A clear opening arises where it was clouded before and this unclouded vision brings more light and clarity. It's enough to keep you dipping. Sometimes there are marks on the glass that are difficult to remove and sometimes there are areas in the practice that are difficult and it seems that we will never be able to pass beyond them.

Repetition is the key. We go back to the same place over and over without expectation or judgment again and again in both the practice and in the cleansing until eventually catharsis, either subtle or dramatic, occurs as some stubborn or trapped part of us breaks free. A grief, a fear, a trauma, a secret, a sadness. Once it settles, there is clarity or lightness, a freedom of movement or a breakthrough in the practice that was not there before. That illumination and transformation inspires faith in the wisdom of the method. Days, weeks, months, years pass, and slowly the mind settles and the window of perception clears.

Guruji always says 99 percent practice, 1 percent theory. What's your understanding of the theory part?

As I appreciate the theory largely in theory and not in realization, perhaps we should start with the practice part. That window is not going to get clean just by looking at it. Another metaphor if I may. It's a little bit like playing the piano. In order to be a pianist, in order to create music on the piano, you have to go the piano. Having a piano is not enough. You have to touch the keys, make contact. Anyone can play, touch one and then another. From single notes to scales. From scales to a melody. With practice and effort an effortless grace arises, and with it the magic of music. At some point in the process it would be really helpful to have some understanding of written music. But that understanding alone will not produce the same outcome. It is the sound that has the ability to soothe the soul. It is the same with yoga. You can read endlessly, and though the words may be insightful, without practice it is the author's insight and not yours. Make your own music, discover your own discoveries through practice. Then the intricacies of the theory will hold valuable meaning for you.

I have a memory related to this. One particular student asked Guruji to describe the nature of the kundalini rising. Guruji proceeded to give a lecture in a mixture of Kannada and Sanskrit. After about forty-five minutes, with the whole class sitting perfectly still and looking on in awe with their mouths wide open, the student who asked the question said, "But Guruji, I don't understand your answer because I don't speak Sanskrit." And Guruji said, "It wouldn't matter what language I gave the answer in. You are not able to have the understanding until the work is done."

My understanding of the theory part is that by stilling the mind and purifying the nervous system through the practice of the eight limbs of yoga, discrimination between *prakriti* and *purusha* is realized, thus removing the veil that obscures the light of our true nature. That all things are God. That with faith, devotion, and practice pure consciousness will be realized. Guruji says to me, "You are still thinking the wall is a wall. The wall is not a wall." Somewhere in there is the 1 percent that moves me.

Why do you think Guruji considers prayer and devotion to be so important?

Guruji says we think too much. And when we think, it is with a limited capacity to understand. "Do not think of here, do not think of there, just sing songs to God, that's all." He is trying to guide us to see that understanding doesn't just happen with the mind, that the deeper understanding happens with the heart, so he encourages prayer and devotion. Those who are devoted to God offer the fruits of their work to God, see God in all people and all things, are close to God, not separate, and will reside in peace. Surrender and devotion will open our hearts and bring us closer to this truth.

The practice of yoga requires not only *tapas* but also *svadhyaya* and *ishvara-pranidhana*. It is a devotional practice and it's about finding the heart of the Self and unifying that vibration with all those things we don't yet understand. How can you express the experience of the heart in words? Perhaps best through prayer.

You were an artist. I don't know if you are still involved in art, but I have always felt that art and spirituality are very closely connected. Do you have any insight into the relationships between the two?
As an artist, when you are involved in the moment of creativity, when you are totally present in the now, there is a sense that something moves through you. This at it's most potent seems to bypass the mind and speak of the soul. Time stops. I am still an artist, only now "I" am the work in progress.

Would you say that Guruji teaches a standardized form of practice, or is his teaching tailored to the individual?
Both. The initial elements of the practice are suitable for everyone, but how the practice unfolds—at what pace, how intensely, to what level—is tailored to the individual, and that's the beauty of the Mysore style.

People think of this practice as being made up of primary, intermediate, and advanced series, and they get obsessed about it being a particular way. But what I've experienced in talking especially to the older students, who had a more individual relationship with Guruji because there were so many fewer in the room, is that they were being taught different sequences depending on their needs.
My personal experience was the first option of the two that you described. Primary followed by intermediate and then advanced series. However, I am aware of variations in Guruji's approach over the years. These earlier students you mentioned shared the room. Guruji's experi-

ence teaching the practice has evolved with his understanding of the students and perhaps his need to accommodate the ever growing numbers. I've seen Guruji working individually with people with illness or physical structural limitations in a very personal, healing way. He modifies the practice so it will work as a therapeutic tool for each situation. He fits the practice to the student. There have certainly been variations on the theme of standard practice in both Mysore-style and conducted classes, and many different approaches over the years to the *vinyasa*, from simple to elaborate. There has certainly been a noticeable change in method and type of student from Lakshmipuram to Gokulam in recent years. I think it's best not to be obsessed with anything. Particularly believing that you have it right. Everything changes a little with time.

Ultimately, whichever way we have learned, we are essentially all heading in the same direction. The method is like a box of tools. How those tools are used individually will depend upon the need, the understanding, the temperament and capacity of student and teacher. Perhaps the idea that it should be "this way," this standard way, is emphasized to protect the purity and integrity of the practice so it will not be diluted or lost in translation.

What is the value of daily practice, day in, day out, over the years, and what is the inner quality produced by a long-term practice?
When the commitment to a daily practice is made, then there is no longer a battle of will I or won't I. The resistance no longer wins. Once the practice is a constant, then the thing that changes, the variable in the equation, is the practitioner. You get to see yourself, have a relationship with the Self. It is through this repetition, through the observation of the variable, through self-inquiry, that we see the fruit of the practice. It's like any relationship with a person. In the beginning it's superficial, even though it might be very sweet. There are qualities that can only be found and developed over time and with commitment.

What are the inner qualities which are cultivated?
Those who practice for a long time with a positive attitude and without interruption following the correct method have a quiet knowing, a sense of well-being, a tangible spark. There is a precious acceptance and there is a possibility of union.

With consistency and commitment, the practice can penetrate from the superficial to the profound. Over the years, the qualities of the practice change. What starts as a predominantly physical practice becomes delicate and subtle. And though the movement continues, there is an internal stillness as the poses unfold. Mental dialogue that once held center stage falls way as the body and breath surrender to the familiar comfort of repetition. Where once great effort was required to tame an awkward body and persistent mind, time inspires a steady grace.

What about the subtle aspects of the practice? Do you feel they are somehow integrated into the asana *practice? Does one naturally evolve from* asana *practice to the more subtle*—pratyahara, dharana, dhyana, *and* samadhi?
It appears so. Guruji says, "Practice and all is coming." Time will guide the senses inward as concentration is refined and will still the mind to a single point. Then meditation is its consequence. There will always be those collecting *asanas*, they are still traveling outward. Soon they will stumble on something that slows them down and turns their focus inward. It's all part of the journey.

How do you try to incorporate Guruji's spiritual philosophy in the way that you teach?
I have practiced this method to the best of my understanding religiously for more than two decades. I believe this work itself has left a mark upon me as a person and therefore as a teacher, I hope to be a natural representation of the teachings.

What do you see as the relationship between practicing yoga and teaching yoga?
Teaching yoga is an amazing yoga within itself. One's life, one's process, one's practice is a visible example to others. Once you involve other people, then there is a challenge to maintain equanimity. I feel that teaching is an extension of practice and the whole path of yoga happens from the minute you wake up to the minute you wake up the following day. It doesn't ever really end. Teaching is a very challenging form of practice. To maintain equilibrium while interacting, to be without judgment and stay objective, to teach with compassion and sensitivity while holding firm to the integrity of the lineage takes considerable diligence.

Ideally everything you do somehow embraces the eight limbs as described by Patanjali. Every breath you take is conscious, every interaction and choice you make is conscious and with pure motivation. Teaching yoga not only provides an incredible forum for personal growth; it is both a responsibility and a privilege. The more I practice and explore the path, the more I appreciate how little knowledge I hold. When I teach, I try keeping this in mind.

How do you find teaching affects your own personal practice? And how do you find the practice affects your teaching?
When my practice is undisturbed and spacious, when I am able to find focused stillness, a connectedness arises. From within this space, teaching is natural, effortless, and harmonious. I have had a great love affair with this practice. I love teaching it, sharing it, and being a part of the journey for others. It fills me with balance and joy and light. As a teacher I strive to bring the best of myself to the students, to guide them by example. My practice stays as focused and religious as life's events permit.

Practice provides a stable foundation to teach from. Sometimes teaching makes me tired and sometimes when I am tired it fills me with energy. I think becoming older and becoming a mother also takes its toll. Having said that, the gifts from teaching and the gifts from parenting are so precious that one appreciates the wisdom of a path for householders.

Someone once said to me that the second most difficult thing you could do in a lifetime is to become enlightened and the most difficult thing that you can do is have a successful relationship. I'd like to try both. I try to have a successful relationship with every person that crosses my path. As a representative of the path of yoga, as a yoga practitioner, a yogin, and especially as a yoga teacher, I believe it is essential that my lifestyle demonstrate unwavering ethical integrity.

Do you think women and men practice differently? I know that some women are concerned about doing the more advanced practices. They feel like their bodies are becoming more masculine.
I don't buy into it at all. I do not feel that the more advanced series steal femininity. There is nothing more beautiful than a strong woman. I do not think that as a female I have struggled any more or less with either strength or flexibility. There are delicate male practitioners who demonstrate grace and elegance. There are powerful female practitioners who defy gravity. They are all beautiful to me.

Why not be a strong woman? Why not be an old, strong woman? The choice is ours. This practice is difficult for everybody. Male, female, young, old—we all find our obstacles. It's a difficult but rewarding path. The changes to the female body are only more masculine if you identify strength with the male. If something was lost on the way, it was probably nothing I needed. I love my yoga body. Whether it is attractive to another is not a major concern. Femininity comes from within. My female peers are women of dignity and beauty.

However, each woman needs to be true to herself regarding how appropriate, relevant, necessary the ongoing practices are. I don't believe that the number of *asanas* is a measure of how potent the practice is. I have not concerned myself with the differences between male and female, whether it is harder or easier. The comparison is not helpful. We must make this journey with the gender we have.

As somebody who has been practicing for a long time, can you say something about your understanding of the bandhas?
Bandhas are the essence of the *asana* practice. With them one can build, regulate, and maintain the flow of *prana*. Without them, there is no spark generated, no energy cultivated, no lift, flight, or potency. They are the key to an internal understanding. Gaining them, maintaining them, igniting them takes time and focus.

Do you consider that these things evolve and develop naturally with correct practice over the years, or are there some techniques that one should apply?
Some long-term practitioners seem to be devoid of understanding of *bandhas*. Perhaps they spontaneously arrive in some students and not in others. I believe that a little focused attention from the offset is helpful. It's not something you really want to try and tack on later. If the *bandha* is introduced, at least in concept, from the first breath, then it's a seed that has been planted.

Can you say something about the role of breathing in practice?
If someone asked me what constituted a fine yoga practitioner, I would say it's someone who can keep their mind focused on the breath. If someone asked me what constituted a fine *ashtanga* yoga practitioner, I would say it was someone who could keep their mind focused on the breath while activating *uddiyana* and *mula bandha* and cultivating *ujjayi* breath. You'll notice that that definition in both cases showed no measure

of where someone was in an *asana* practice. The breath is the beginning, it's the first step and every step that follows.

Why is the breath so important?
The breath is our most powerful tool. Without it, life ends; with it, life begins. If we develop it, enhance it, empower it, invigorate it, extend it, the quality of life will mirror those things. In practice it's the fuel, it's the focus, it's the mantra, it's the strength, it's the surrender, it's the connection to the spirit, and it's your best friend.

How do we come into a relationship with it?
Inhale consciously. Spend time with it intimately.

Do you see it as a tool also, something you can use for effect?
It's the master tool, especially in the form of *ujjayi* breath, and even when it is most natural and relaxed. The breath is the spirit running through you. How it moves through you will mold each moment of you.

It seems to me it has a natural inclination to flow through you, but then when we get into a difficult asana, we restrict its natural flow if the mind is not attentive.
Guruji uses the term "free breathing," and some of the *asanas* bind us so tightly that it makes free breathing difficult. And so we attempt to cultivate free breathing in a difficult situation. This practice is just a metaphor for an uncomfortable or difficult situation out in the world. When we find ourselves in difficult situations and we feel restricted emotionally and in the breath, then we use the tool of free breathing to try to be open and as present and relaxed and full in the breath as possible. And that in turn will make the difficult situation in life more comfortable.

What do you think are the most important considerations for a healthy, life-long yoga practice?
A healthy, lifelong practice is really the aim, as it's going to take a while for the fruits of our labor to ripen. In the beginning of *asana* practice, we are concerned with trying to do the best we can with what we have, our movements limited to the freedom and flexibility that is already available. Once limitations prevent progress, caution is then required. If one

adopts an attitude of attaining an *asana* at all costs, then damage, discomfort, or pain often result in a reluctance to continue.

Once one establishes an intention to practice for a long time, or a lifetime, then it needs to be done with patience and an anatomical awareness so as to awaken parts of the body, particularly of the spine, that are blocked, stiff, or compromised in order to spread the load of the *asana* practice more evenly throughout the entire body and reduce the pressure in fragile areas.

I guess what I'm trying to say is, it's not what you do but how you do it that will affect the longevity of the practice. I believe that flexibility is the gift of an even breath. We need patience to mature in the practice, patience to remove blockages both physical and emotional, time to integrate practice and change into daily life, and a holistic approach for safe personal evolution. Eight limbs not one. This is really important.

That sounds like it would be almost impossible to achieve without the help of a teacher. How important do you think a teacher is on the path of yoga?
If you have a teacher, then you are blessed. If you have a teacher who practices, then you are twice blessed. If you have a teacher who practices and cares about you, then you are triply blessed. It's a gift. How important is it? Sometimes it's difficult to have a clear picture of where you are and of how you are proceeding. Having delusion about where we sit within the process is very natural, so it's helpful, especially if the teacher has no agenda beyond taking care of your ongoing practice. Obviously it's the ideal situation: guidance, reference, correction, alignment, support, an objective view are very helpful.

What do you see as the relationship between achieving asanas *and psychological evolution?*
The scope of *asanas* is never-ending, and they become more contortionist, complex, and bizarre as they unfold. Some of us need to drag our bodies a long way in order to facilitate the cleansing process. Those of us with stubborn, egotistical natures feel the need to drag ourselves even further, twist ourselves harder, and bend ourselves deeper in order to appreciate that at the end of the day, we simply need to focus our attention, open our hearts, and head back to a place of stillness. There are undoubtedly insights that present themselves along the *asana* journey— precious victories, awakenings, and unveilings. Still, I believe that psy-

chological evolution is related to the continuation of practice as much as to *asanas* achieved.

Is there anything that you would like to add?
I reside in gratitude. What an amazing practice this is. The way it shines a light, that it inspires people to get out of bed in the darkness and to work so hard at what seems almost intangible gain. And at a time when there is so much potential for despair on our planet, so many, because of Guruji and this path of *ashtanga* yoga, so many people who may well have been lost have illuminated direction. Guruji is older now, he struggles with his health and he may not be with us physically for much longer. I only hope that we can do him proud.

Goa, 2009

Peter Greve

While biking through India, Peter Greve found himself at Guruji's doorstep. One of the few students who learned to speak and write in Kannada, Guruji's mother tongue, Peter formed a rare relationship with Guruji. He currently resides in Berlin, where he is a physiotherapist and runs an *ashtanga* yoga school.

Tell me how you became interested in yoga and how you started to explore it.

It started with Buddhism. I read a book about the Buddha and Buddhism when I was twenty-one. At that time I was smoking and drinking and this book by a German Indologist was very clear and it was like a shock to me because the philosophy of the Buddha was striking. It was like, wow, that is so, so complete. And it's not just intellectual, it's true to life. The rational aspect is strong in India, but [Indian] philosophy covers all aspects of life, unlike a lot of the European philosophy.

And at that time I was living with a woman who did yoga, but I was completely uninterested. I was working as a taxi driver and I had the opportunity and the money to leave and go to Asia. At that time I was also studying philosophy at the university, but not really seriously. So I went to Burma and Thailand. It was such a different world, I couldn't believe it, so much more traditional and without Western influence. I was in Mandalay, the second biggest city in Burma, in the north, and they had no electricity. And all the traffic was bicycles. And at night all you heard were these bells ringing, people were giving signs like *ring ring ring*, and you could hardly see anything. I spent three or four months in Asia, and began to long for change in my life. I kept on reading about Buddhism, and if you read about Buddha, you come to read about India because the Buddha was Indian, and you get to know that Buddhism grew out of and is very much influenced by yoga. I went back to Germany and decided to start yoga and also decided to do a second trip, to India. So I worked again, drove a taxi, earned money, and bought a book called *Light on Yoga* by B. K. S. Iyengar. My first yoga practice was learning from this book. I tore the meniscus in both knees almost right away. I tore one side and showed the doctor the next day what I had done with the other leg, and the same happened again.

You tore your meniscus in the doctor's office?
Yes. I didn't do anything crazy. I just put one foot on my other thigh. At the time I was still smoking. Smoking means that the metabolism of the body is very bad. Then I have little bony legs, my hips were not open, and the knee really takes on all that stress.

How long were you working with Iyengar's book practicing by yourself before you were put out of action?
One hour! I opened the book and tried it and then it happened. And that was shortly before leaving for India. I already had my ticket. I went to the hospital for eight or ten days. They said, "You need to have this part of the meniscus taken out." Two or three weeks later I traveled to India. My knees were fine again.

When you went to India, were you looking for a teacher?
I didn't know about any teacher. My idea was to go to India with a bicycle because I had taken a bicycle to Malaysia and Thailand. I started to cycle from Bombay toward Goa and I thought, "Well, let's see what happens. Who am I going to meet?"

I was in Pune on my way to Goa on the bicycle. There were many Westerners, and I wondered what all the Westerners were doing there. They were mostly there because of Osho, but some because of Iyengar. I met a French guy who had spent two years in Mysore and was on his way back to Europe. We became friends. He had three days left in Bombay, so he showed me a little about India. He had studied at the Mysore university for two years, not doing yoga, but he knew about Pattabhi Jois. He showed me an article about Pattabhi Jois from *Yoga Journal*. And I saw this picture of Guruji standing in *samasthiti* and read about *ashtanga* yoga and thought, "Well, that's it! It's powerful and dynamic and seems not to be esoteric." So I traveled down by bicycle and bus to Mysore.

I came to Mysore and I got sick—stomach and diarrhea. I went to a hotel and I was there for two or three days lying in bed. And I didn't know how to find him, so when I recovered, I asked some Indians. They looked into the telephone book and picked out the telephone number. One of them called Pattabhi Jois and said, "There is a Westerner who wants to meet you." He gave me the directions. It was in the morning. I went there, I rang the bell, and he opened [the door]. I said, "Here I am. I want to learn yoga." He asked me to come in, we sat down, and in just two or three minutes he said, "Yeah, no problem you can start yoga. To-morrow you can come, six o'clock." Very simple, very friendly, very open. And not many questions. Just a nice talk. When I left, the last thing he told me was, "Don't forget, every month, two hundred-fifty dollar." [*Laughter*] That was my first meeting with Guruji.

The next morning at that time there were six or eight people. I saw people doing amazing things in the room. At that time Brian Kest was there and he was lifting up from *navasana* to handstand, and he did it five times. "Wow, this I want to learn." And so I did. Guruji showed me how to do *surya namaskara* A five times, *surya namaskara* B three times. And I was going on to do *surya namaskara* B a fourth time, and he said, "No, no. Lay down. You take rest." And I was like, "Oh, what a pity." I was very eager.

He didn't ask you to take lotus? Normally, he gets people to go into lotus the first day.
No. The first time, I did only ten minutes' practice and he told me to go home and come the next day.

Did you tell him about your knees and your surgery?
Yes, I told him.

That's probably why. How long was it before he had you doing padmasana?
After about one month in Mysore and halfway through the primary series.

How about the rest of your trip?
My plan was to travel with the bicycle for six months. I left some of my

money at the German embassy in Bombay. After I decided to stay in Mysore, I needed the money, so I took the train to Bangalore and the bus to Bombay, which is another twenty or twenty-two hours. There was some trouble in Bangalore. The bus didn't come and people were very angry and went to the police station at one or two o'clock at night. There was lots of shouting. All the people who had tickets for the bus got hotel rooms. We walked through the dark night of Bangalore with a policeman in front guiding us to the hotel. Very early in the morning I got a bus but had no seat, so I was sitting in the middle. After a few hours, it was very comfortable to sit upright like that. A chair makes you become tired. I went to the embassy, got the money, and then I again traveled back with the bus. Again, twenty-two or twenty-four hours. And then Bangalore back to Mysore. I arrived at one at night, two at night, went to sleep for two or three hours. And at four or five in the morning I was back on the yoga mat. It was like a trip on drugs. With very little sleep, you're flexible and energetic and that was a very wonderful experience.

How did the practice unfold for you and how did Guruji work with you on the first trip?
First of all, it made me feel very good. After practice, I felt in my power, I had good energy. This was a new experience. I quit smoking a few months later. I struggled really hard. For one year, every day I said, "This is my last day." Finally I gave it up. This was the first time for many years I'd done something for my body. To breathe and to bend and to twist was an incredible feeling. I remember lying in *shavasana*. It was very intense and I was like, "Wow! Now the day can start." It felt very clear and fresh, and that was a new experience for me. It took me three months to learn the primary series. We were very few people at that time, six to eight. And then in December/January we were maybe twelve or fifteen people. Guruji was always behind me because in the primary series there are a lot of sitting forward bends. He was always pushing, pushing, pushing, and I was pulling, pulling, pulling.

Were you resisting or helping him?
He was helping me and I was helping him. I was very stiff. I was pulling on my feet and I couldn't forward bend. With straight legs, my fingers were by my knees. He was working very hard with me. This is what I wanted.

People complained to me, "He's always with you and we get no attention." This changed once I had learned the first series. We had a very good time. He never shouted, never bad words. We liked each other a lot.

What does Guruji teach and how does he transmit that?
He teaches you to do your practice. That is what matters. He's giving you a lesson. Basically, he taught me *asanas*. But what he transmitted was concentrated energy. In the room you could feel his presence, and that he was very serious about doing the practice. It's fun also but it is not, it's not just playing around. He transmitted his teaching by his energy, his presence and by few words. And by his touch, of course, his physical presence and his adjustments. You could always feel, when you got an adjustment, that he knew what he wanted. Very present. One of the typical things he would say throughout the years was, "Don't delay." That was something I heard again and again when people yawned or started to fiddle with their toenails.

Procrastination. When people talk instead of act.
He didn't let people even think about talking. It was a concentrated emphasis on doing your practice. So he could get really . . . not angry but demanding. The teaching was very much about doing. Do your practice, do this experience of practicing. And, as I understand it, bring your practice up to a certain level. You are being confronted by your body, your emotions, your feelings, your breath, your thoughts.

Then it becomes a personal exploration from that point on. It brings you into contact with those things and then it is for you to deal with them.
Yes. He never asked me, "How does it feel?" And he gave me no precise adjustments by words. About the breathing, "free breathing" is, I think, the only thing he ever said in the years I was there. "You do *asanas* many years and then comes *pranayama*, in the tradition of Krishnamacharya," he said. "You do *asanas* many years," when people asked about *pranayama*.

You never heard him say, "Breathe with sound."
No, I didn't. I did it because everybody did it.

There's a certain amount of learning you get from the students around you also.
That's so important. He also never said anything about *mula bandha* and toning your abdomen. He said the length of the breath should be equal and nothing else. It's important because this lets you experience free breathing. You can do whatever you think right if it is free, if there are no obstacles for the breath, for free movement of what's connected with the breath and the diaphragm. What I have experienced in my own practice, and I believe many other people will have had similar experiences, is that I superimposed some kind of technique on the practice. If you force the breath into a pattern, this is not good. For me it was not good, definitely. My brain would say, "Breathe this way." It was not good for my body. I think that it had prevented me from feeling and prevented me from making the connection between breath, mind, and body.

Do you mean physically feeling your body or emotionally feeling?
Both. Definitely both. Learning to breathe freely and well has a lot to do with a sense of physicality. And to relate to sense, to feel where there is pressure—in the abdominal region, the breast region, the throat region, and so on—and how that is linked to emotions. Breath is deeply related to how we grew up, our anxieties. Breath patterns are intimately linked with our *samskaras*, our past experiences, wishes, etc. Pressure can be a good feeling but it can also be a bad feeling, and that's something everybody needs to experience on his own. No teacher can tell you. A teacher can only look from outside. He cannot see how it is deeply connected with your emotions and feelings. That's why the physical practice is not just a physical practice. The physical practice throws you into contact with your whole being, with your past especially, with your karma, your *samskaras*, and makes you face it and listen. When you start yoga, you listen to your present moment. The present moment is the accumulation of your past.

The present moment is the past?
Yes, in a way. *Samasthiti* is standing equal. But you cannot stand equal because of your conditioning. When you try to stand equal, you are connecting with your history, your karma, your *samskaras*. That's why I don't understand when people say it's just a physical practice. Yoga is so much more. You can find it in a nutshell, you can find it in the whole pose. And

I didn't learn that in Mysore. I had to go through bitter and bad experiences until my body stopped me and told me, "Listen to your body, listen to it work, work more sensitively." When Guruji said, "Free breathing," in a way that's what I'm now doing.

It took you fifteen or twenty years to really understand what he was saying because the conditioning was so strong?
Yes, the conditioning was so strong. And the other students influenced me. All the experienced people were doing this *ujjayi*, forceful breathing, and I think everybody is doing it differently. Richard Freeman does it completely differently than how I did it because he had integrated it in a different way. At the time I didn't understand that, and I didn't ask anybody. I thought it was like law: in *ashtanga* practice, you do this kind of breathing.

Imitation or comparison with other people in the room is limiting.
Now, when I look as a teacher, it's so simple. How is somebody standing? How is the moment when you finish one *surya namaskara* and before you start the next *surya namaskara*? This is a kind of a break. What are people doing at that moment? What is their presence at that moment? How are they standing at that moment? Many people finish a *surya namaskara* and they're like this . . .

Their shoulders sag and their posture is—?
Yeah. The quality of the yoga practice is what counts because you take the quality of the yoga practice into your daily life. The quality of the yoga practice depends on the breath, and the breath depends on how mindful and concentrated you are, especially how mindful. And that means you need to come in contact with your whole being, with your physical, emotional, mental being. And then you can have such a wonderful awareness. It shows you the way. Otherwise, you're pushing, imposing something on yourself which will stop you altogether one day. You will give up, your body will stop you with injuries, or you'll lose interest.

You said earlier how the breathing was an indication or an expression of your samskaras, your history. You'd probably agree that the breathing is also a vehicle to transform that. How does that actually happen?

What does free breathing actually mean? That's the question. I think it means that you're really listening to the present moment and letting something breathe that's not the ego, not the "I." Breath is something that is so, so old, and the director of the breath is in the vegetative nervous system. We can change the breath, but only in cooperation with the body. Free breathing is like really listening to the present moment. That means, according to my experience, that one breath can be slow, one breath can be faster, one breath can be long, one breath can be shorter. And especially about the breaks—after exhalation or after inhalation. When you look at a child, the breath sometimes stops. Or during sleep, sometimes it stops and then suddenly there's a very deep inhalation. When this happens, there's a letting go of tension, a letting go of movement patterns. It has a lot to do with accepting, with acceptance of who you are, where you are at this moment. Free breathing is "Here I am and I am fine how I am" not "Oh, I have to achieve this." If you accept how you are in the present moment, and the present moment is the accumulation of karma, then something changes on its own.

So if you can release the breathing, then the mind also releases, and the samskaras *can also then transform.*
Releasing the breathing sounds so simple, but it means to accept the feelings, thoughts, and everything that is happening in the moment. You live the moment you practice. That means to accept the positive as well as the negative. That comes with yoga and Buddhist philosophy, to step back and say, "Okay, there are good feelings and there are bad feelings." Just let go and accept how it is, and suddenly you feel you are not clinging to them. That makes you free.

We want to control everything, but the breath is an example of something we cannot control, at least we can't without being loving toward our body. What am I doing that my body cannot breathe freely? It's not that I can will myself to breathe freely; I have to put aside tension in order that it can happen. I work in such a way that this old brain stem, where the breath is controlled, can take over. The brain stem is the conductor. The orchestra plays the music.

Good breathing unites breath and body and mind. Where is the tension? How is it linked with my emotions? Are they really so bad, my emotions? What if I build up more tension *here* and release some tension *there*? Suddenly the diaphragm can move freely!

What you're saying is that the breath is an autonomic process controlled by an ancient part of the brain, the brain stem. When we engage in yoga and we have an agenda, we superimpose another pattern on top of that which creates rigidity.
This is exactly why old yoga texts say *pranayama* can destroy you. If you're just struggling against resistance, you can do very bad harm.

Can you say something about Guruji as a person?
He's very down-to-earth and very direct. Always looking for a smile, for a joke. A lot of humor.

He has a direct and strong personality and can get people to do things. Sometimes he would get agitated, but mostly he's easygoing, nice. He can—especially in the teaching—have bursts of anger sometimes. I experienced him as a very caring man. Without many words. Just a simple question: "How are you?" And that would be it. I felt that he was deeply caring.

Have you had experiences with Guruji taking you to what you think is your mental and physical limit and beyond in the asanas?
Yes, definitely. [*Laughter*]

Can you describe experiences you had where he radically changed your understanding about what you could do?
From the first moment you practice with Guruji, he gives you this energy to do your practice absolutely to your limit. I was so stiff and he was my first teacher. The first yoga class I ever had was with Guruji. So my first experience was, go to your limits. And not only that, but he would give you strong adjustments. From the very first day it was totally to my physical limits.

Did you experience pain?
When I got to Mysore, I had a few injuries. It's never a pleasure to work with an injury. Then there is pain when one pushes beyond limits. Or because one has not found the connection between mind and body. I think if one is not connecting mind and body, then you are working against resistance and this does not feel pleasant. Yoga practice was really a workout. And the reward was afterward, lying in *shavasana* and coming out of the resting with just a feeling of having achieved something.

How did you feel when you came out?
More connected with my energy, like I was walking more easily, more erect, feeling freer with the body and in contact with my power and energy. But I remember also that this didn't last long. I hadn't found this connection yet. I had this up and down of energy between the days. So the next day you need it again and you need it again. Practice became something I needed to get this experience of feeling energetic. I think now that practice should always feel pleasant. Always.

What about sweet pain? You know, when a joint opens and there is a release, sometimes there is pain in the muscles and then when you come to shavasana *there is no pain anymore. There's pain in the moment, you meet a certain resistance, and you release it.*
This will happen only when you are in your body, when you are breathing well. Really sweet pain is not connected with bad emotions, that's the difference. There is pain that is emotionally not good, and there is sweet pain that you feel is in a way good for you. Pain that is associated with bad emotions is never good. It is a false gain. You gain more flexibility, more strength, but the body takes it back later. A month later, a year later you have an injury, you have a breakdown, you get sick—the body takes it back. So the release or opening of a joint, muscle, or connective tissue is always in connection with some little sweet pain. The person senses it is good for them, that a good change is happening. And it is, again, about being in contact with oneself.

Should we be using a part of the brain which is not active in thinking? When one then experiences an unacceptable level of emotional pain, it's simply a question of not being ready to let go. But if your breathing was correct, if you allowed yourself to release the breathing, the emotion could become sweet pain and release itself.
Definitely.

Why does Guruji consider prayer so important?
He never mentioned it to me. In the first years, we didn't do the *ashtanga* prayer. That started in 1991. It seemed to me that he never wanted to impose it on us.

A lot of his teaching seems to come out of the questions of the students. There's no pressure from his side. The practice itself somehow is sufficient as a foundation, and then afterward more will come.

Yes. For instance, when students started touching his feet, and I didn't do it, he never gave me the impression that this was obligatory. Also with the prayer, I think his students asked him, "Can we do something?" I'm not sure, but as far as I remember we didn't have this, then suddenly it started, and I think it started because a student asked him to do it.

It seems that Guruji is giving technique and then leaving you to do the work. If you want to ask questions, he will answer, but otherwise he expects you to just practice, practice, practice, and this will change your mind.

Yes, and this is in a way his character, his personality. He is very intuitive. He senses where somebody is. Otherwise, you can't explain how he teaches everyone differently. Some people he stops when they want to do more; with me, he always wanted me to do more. With some people he's nice, and with some people you feel he's very tough. Guruji's way of teaching is really nonverbal. He senses where the student is and leaves it to the individual to practice.

If I hadn't met Guruji, I don't know if or when I would have started yoga. Guruji would say, "All is coming," and I stayed with the practice and I had to go through the transformation that came, but that was after my time in Mysore. For me, the main points came after Mysore, but it would not have taken place without Guruji.

This system of yoga has been passed down through a lineage of householder yogis. Krishnamacharya was told by his guru, who was also a family man, that he should have a family and teach yoga in society. What do you think about that?

Yoga is wonderful for almost everybody. And the majority cannot live in a cave. Family life teaches one so much about relationships and responsibilities. And also to step back from the idea that "I'm the most important person in the family." You have to learn that you are not the only one in the world. For many people in the yoga world, practicing can be something selfish—indulging in "I" and "my." This changes with a family.

We have yamas *and* niyamas *but we understand, and Guruji often says, that they are very difficult so that's why you do* asana *first. But obviously they are critical. Do you think that if you were just to continue the asanas, all the other angas of ashtanga yoga would naturally unfold? Or would you need to make some moral progress independently of that?*

Not moral progress, but I think for the inner steps—*dharana, dhyana,* and *samadhi*—that you need to be ready and also have a guru. The moral and the physical aspects naturally, but not automatically, go together, because if you decide to do yoga, you're ready to change something. It's very simple. It means that you think about the world and that you take care of yourself. And if you can share that with others so that they can also have the opportunity to take care of themselves, you are in moral aspects already. If you just do yoga for fitness, you need not think much about the moral. However, usually, after a while, if you stay with the yoga, changes start to happen. People start yoga for fitness but those who stay with it will eventually come to the deeper aspects.

When I say moral, I don't mean being a good person or a bad person in the Christian sense. What I mean is cleaning up your act, acting in a sattvic *way, in such a way that you're true to your Self. And it seems to me really the only way to be true to your Self, capital S, means also not taking from others, not harming others. That those kinds of acts or behavior result from limited access to the Self, and from anxiety, fear, and so on. So you almost have no choice but to evolve morally. Otherwise, you cannot breathe freely.*

That's really a keystone in the yoga practice. Krishnamacharya said that if you can breathe, then you can do yoga. And this is really the number-one sentence of all yoga: Can you breathe, and how can you breathe? If you can work with that, you can come to the point not to judge but to accept the good and the bad and to be open to that.

If you accept good and bad, you don't feel like you're a victim of circumstances. You are responsible; you're above it somehow.

If you are a victim you think, "I can take, it's my right, others have not suffered like me!" One can detach from that. When you look at the present moment, one is open for the future and for anything to happen. That allows one to take responsibility, to find the dharma. That's an important aspect of yoga, not to do it for the little ego but to find out also about the work we have to do in our life, the dharma we have in our life. It's not just "I become a doctor or I become a painter." It's something one has to struggle for to find out, and this dharma that one finds out for oneself is not on a scale—"This is the highest dharma and this is the lowest"—but without judgment: this way is more work, this way is less work.

It's like your personal combination code, which unlocks your karma and samskaras *to bring those things to fruition.*
Yes.

How important was Amma?
She was like an anchor. She helped him live a normal life, to find his place in a family. She was doing the work in the background that gave him the opportunity to unfold as a father. He was like a father and grandfather to me at the same time. He had this stellar combination to me. I think this quality of householder and father for his children would have been different without Amma.

When they cooked for us it was always so wonderful, and this is something that they really loved to do more than anything—feeding the students. Guruji was always happy when the theory talks were over. But to serve and to cook for his students, and to put out the carpets [for seating], and this game he liked to play while feeding us: "More, you eat more!"

How about Guruji's attitude toward his work?
He was energetic and took his work very seriously, [with] the strong belief that what we are doing is not just play. It has a very important place in life and in society. I think more and more this is true, that yoga has so much to offer mankind and human beings, and this was his work ethic.

Any final thoughts?
Over the past twenty years, I had the opportunity, the luck to learn something that has changed my own practice so much and shown me how important it is to be really open, open for new explorations and not to take things as dogma. I see yoga as such a wonderful contribution, especially the tradition of Krishnamacharya. He was so ahead of his time in so many things, like teaching women. So there's a tradition. But this is the time, *now.* Let's see what adjustments we can make, proper adjustments.

Is there one aspect of this journey that is most important for you?
The most important thing for me is to share, the opportunity to take part

in sharing with others. To live in a country that gave me the opportunity to learn, to study—I don't take that for granted, I am very thankful for that. I came from yoga to this [physiotherapy] and found such a good combination. But behind it, the main thing is that people share knowledge, they share experience with each other. Guruji shared with us, and other teachers shared with us, and at the university or the school or in the family we share experiences, and I see that as the main way for evolution to take place: that we are open to share. I'm really, really thankful for that. Having these opportunities is not something we should take for granted.

Berlin, 2008

Annie Pace

Annie Pace has been a devoted student of Guruji's since 1986. She upholds his exacting methods of teaching at her temple, Shakti Sharanam, in Colorado, where she combines yoga teaching with the other healing and consciousness-oriented disciplines that she learned over many years of study in India.

How did you become interested in yoga, and how did you start to explore and find your way to Guruji?
Back in the '70s, I read *Autobiography of a Yogi*. It took me years to make it to a yoga class. Then I went to one at the recreation center in Denver, Colorado, in 1979, and the class taught a little of this and a little of that, a couple of *asanas*, and I went to six classes and that was it—four poses. Did those four poses every single morning, every day before I went off to work at the corporation in my panty hose and suit and pumps, and discovered that ten, fifteen minutes every day was making a huge impact on my life. So I started taking yoga classes and dabbled here and there and got into the Iyengar world for a while because that was what was available in Denver. And then I met Richard Freeman, who turned me on to *ashtanga* shortly after Guruji came to Colorado. Then I went to Mysore and the rest is what it is.

So you started off by reading philosophy.
A little bit, one book. Started off by doing some poses, so what happened was that I was experiencing *abhyasa* [spiritual practice]. I didn't know what *abhyasa* was, I knew nothing about practice, but what I knew was that doing something, even a little bit consistently over a period of time with good intention, was helping me a lot.

Can you describe meeting Guruji?
The first meeting with Guruji was in Boulder. I believe it was '88. I was nervous. Richard had made a very big deal about preparing everyone for the guru and all the protocol, and dos and don'ts and blah blah blah. We all got sufficiently nervous and after meeting Guruji and doing class with him it was this huge relief—what a loving and endearing man. How could I ever have been nervous? At the same time he commanded a lot of respect, so I can say it was a very pleasant surprise. I appreciated even then the guru's humanity.

And how was it you came to Mysore?
Guruji said at that first meeting, "You come!" And I said, "When, Guruji?" And he said, "You come October." And I said, "Okay," and that was that.

Can you describe arriving in Mysore and how you got settled into the practice there?
Arriving in Mysore was a beautiful experience and again, a relief, because I had spent a few days in Madras and there had been conventions going on, prime ministers and rallies and it was absolutely insane. I asked myself, "What have I gotten myself into?" I had just signed up for three months of this and after coming to Mysore and landing at the Hotel Metropole and being treated like a princess I felt much more at ease about India. But the moment before going into class at the old *shala* I waited, standing outside the curtain. There were only six people in the room and a total of twelve people here practicing—that was 1989. I just stood outside the curtain and I heard the room breathing like a living being. It was Tim Miller, Chuck Miller, and a lot of the first-generation practitioners inside on the other side of the curtain. I just felt the room breathing and its heart beating and I was a little nervous but mostly intrigued. Of course I moved the curtain, stepped in the room, and felt like I was in the womb.

Can you describe what Guruji teaches and how he transmits his knowledge?
Guruji is a man of few words. His energy teaches more than anything. From the beginning, I appreciated his compassion and his unconditional acceptance of any level of student. I came in with some background before I showed up, but a few weeks later someone walked in off the street

having never done any yoga before and I watched Guruji next to these seasoned practitioners—how he was with them, how he was working with me, and how he gave his unconditional love and attention to this first-time student, teaching her *surya namskara* A. I will never forget that.

Can you say something about what it is that he teaches?
Guruji teaches us how to live. He teaches us poses, but he teaches us life. He teaches us householder yoga, he teaches us respect, he teaches us how to look our demons in the eye and he questions us on that. No one had done that with me before. When he looks you in the eye and says, "Why fearing?" No one had ever said that to me before.

Can you say something about his character?
He is a very loving, sweet, endearing human and I appreciated his humanity, his householder life, his humility and accessibility. On some of the first trips, in the '80s and early '90s, he and Amma would serve us food. They would set up the floor with banana leaves [as plates] and he would serve us meals at festival time. That's not what most people think of a guru as doing. So he teaches us all of it.

Do you see him as a healer?
Yes.

Why? What do you think makes him an effective healer?
I think anyone is an effective healer, teacher, helper, or guide who has the capacity to reach *any* individual. This could take on different forms, so his way of knowing just what the right medicine is for every different person is truly amazing.

When you say "medicine," what kind of different remedies does he have for different people?
Medicine for me might be beating me up and hollering at me and getting me troubled and working me until I was a noodle, and medicine for the next person just might be a smile and a pat on the shoulder. That's what I mean by adaptability with appropriateness. The teacher who has the experience can provide the right medicine for the right student.

What kind of attitude toward him and the practice did you find was helpful in establishing your own practice?
Trust. [*Laughter*]

Would you say Guruji teaches a standardized form of practice, or is his teaching tailored to the individual?
A lot is up about that question these days: Why is the system changing? Why is someone doing it one way and someone else is doing it the other way? And Guruji is telling one person one thing and another person another thing. The answer is adaptability. Different students, different medicine, but we are all going through the same place. Bottom line is, there is a system, the system doesn't change. Appropriateness can appear within the system in adapting to the individual, and it doesn't mean changing the system, it means appropriateness. Appropriate use of individuals' energies, appropriate teaching styles, communication styles for different people and different times in people's lives, even different days of the week or hours in the practice.

Often students are stuck at certain points in the practice. What do you see as Guruji's role in the process of breaking through those obstacles and helping students progress?
Often his role is pushing the right button, and he has a knack for finding the right button to push. And that might be verbally, it might be physically, it might be harshly, it might be by his sweetness and his laughter. You may be seeing a trend here to my answers—adaptability, flexibility within the form, he has the knack for that. We are all so different. There's no script in *ashtanga* yoga. There is a system but there is not a script.

Have you had experiences of Guruji taking you to what you think is your mental and physical limit and perhaps beyond? And how did he do that?
Yes, many, many times. I've been coming to Mysore now for twenty years and that provides a lot of opportunities for that to happen. It's taken a lot of forms with myself over the years. In the beginning it was, "Why fearing?"—just asking a simple question for getting me to look at my mind. And sometimes it was physical, sometimes it was humor. Continuously changing forms but always breaking through my self-imposed limitations.

When learning advanced B section back in the day, trying to get into *buddhasana*—this is the one where the leg goes behind the back and the arm goes over the ankle—learning the pose every single day, I would get to that point and Guruji or Sharath would come and help me get into the pose. So we had this little thing going on where at *buddhasana* I would wait for them to help. I didn't think I could do it by myself. One day I waited for them to help. There were only six people in the room. And I said, "Guruji," and he ignored me, and I tried some more and I grunted and I groaned and then, "Sharath," and he looked the other way and so they had this wonderful little game going on, totally ignoring me. You couldn't hide in that room, it's not that they didn't see me or hear me, they were just not going to help me. And I sat there and I breathed and I fumed and I was frustrated until I got actually pretty angry. I was feeling very neglected, very abandoned. Where were my teachers? I can't get this done by myself. Whah whah whah went my mind until out of this frustration, "Well then, fine then!" and my mind said, "I'll just do it myself!" I put my arm over my ankle and let out this enormous grunt. It was "Ugh!" It sounded like I was giving birth and Dena, who was in front of me, turned around and said to me, "So Annie, was it a boy or a girl?" And the whole room laughed, it was just too much. But I won't forget that one. And then I realized, okay, I could do it myself. They knew the time.

What do you think is the relationship between ashtanga *yoga as Guruji teaches it, and the* ashtanga *yoga of Patanjali in* The Yoga Sutras?
The practice that Guruji teaches is the vehicle for the Patanjali yoga in the same way that the breath is the vehicle for the *prana*. It's very convenient, because we use our body and our bodies are always available to us, we don't go out without it. So same, same.

Why does Guruji emphasize the third limb as a starting point?
Because of what I just said. There is *asana*, there is our body, it's something that every human being can relate to. Everything else is not as tangible.

Does he talk about the other limbs?
Yes, he does, in lots of different contexts over the years. It's hard to encapsulate that because it's always being referred to—*yamas* and *niyamas* are always referred to whether it's in conference, in class, in a posture, or

over coffee. In posture maybe, not in words, but in Guruji's way of communicating—nonviolence, not being greedy, being honest, all the basic things are right there when you are practicing in relationship with the guru.

What do you consider to be the essence of Guruji's teaching?
The essence of the teaching is that God is everywhere and if we practice we will realize that.

Guruji always says, 99 percent practice, 1 percent theory. What is your understanding of the theory part?
It's good to have some understanding of the method of the eight limbs. What is the point ultimately? We will find that through practice. I could go on a long time about theory, but what is the point? The point is how to realize God. The practice is the vehicle.

What do you think Guruji's definition of yoga is?
Yoga is knowing God.

How important is family life and integration in society in the system of yoga that Guruji teaches?
It's very important, and of course Guruji exemplifies that as does his entire family. Especially now. Watching four generations practicing householder life together under one roof is pretty amazing. Even back in the day, householder yoga was very important. Often, when we come back from India and we go back to America or wherever we came from, people who aren't familiar with Guruji's family or how the *ashtanga* yoga is taught often have the assumption that we have gone off to an ashram for many months. And they will ask, "So what's it like at the ashram? What ashram? Is it in Mysore?" And I usually need to explain that it's not really an ashram, no one tells us when to get up and when to poop and when to pee and when to eat. Certainly some recommendations are there, but we are not on a program where we don't have to think for ourselves. So in addition to Guruji and his family exemplifying householder yoga, I think it's very powerful and certainly more impactful to integrate the teachings when we aren't in a place where somebody is ringing a bell telling us when to do what. We show up for practice in the morning, you have however long your practice is—one hour, two hours, three hours, four

hours in the day—and the rest of the day you're out on the street making your own decisions. What will I have for breakfast? Who will I hang out with? Where will I go? How will I spend the day? Should I be a vegetable by the pool today or do shop-*asana*? Do I want to be a hermit? There are so many options. Someone said to me earlier, "Too much opportunity!" Many, many, many decisions to be made each day. In this way, I see that we can much more immediately integrate the practice, the teachings, into our life when somebody isn't telling us what to do. And we have the opportunity to make many more mistakes. And we have the opportunity to learn more things.

How important was Amma in supporting Guruji in his teaching?
Very important. Amma was always very stable, always supportive; there was much *shakti*. How important? Very important, would be the answer.

Could you describe Guruji's attitude toward his work?
His work is his life, so I can't separate that and say this is how Guruji works or this is how Guruji lives. His work is his life, and that's probably the answer to the question right there: there is total integration, it's all one. There is no difference.

Could you describe the context from which Guruji comes? His cultural, ethnic background and how that impacts him as a person and what he teaches? And do you think that, by virtue of his connection with Westerners, he's moved away from it to an extent?
Guruji had a hard life. He wasn't rich when he was young. He didn't have an easy life. I won't go into the historical data about Krishnamacharya. Most of us know that story. It wasn't easy for him and he always knew what it was to work hard. And he had respect for his guru. He lived a good, not necessarily easy life. How did he come away from that? You can't come away from your roots. I don't think any of us can erase our heredity, our past, our past karma, but we can certainly integrate it into the present. And Guruji has a knack for relating to Westerners. Not all Brahmins his age can communicate with the Western mind the way that he can. Little did he know way back when that he was going to be having so much connection with Westerners, but on the whole he is able to do it and do a good job.

I'm sure you asked Guruji about the origin of the ashtanga system. Has he given you a satisfying answer? Did it come from Rama Mohan Brahmachari? Krishnamacharya? Or did Guruji create it? What's your understanding?

Guruji did not create it. And Guruji has never implied that he created it. People who don't know Guruji and don't know the system have made assumptions and publicized information that may not be so accurate. As for Guruji creating the system, Guruji making it up, he has never, to my knowledge, implied that. It comes from the *Yoga Korunta*, it comes from his guru, his guru's guru—back, back in time.

So you think the basic system, the basic series of asanas, he received that from his teachers. That's your impression?

It's my impression and I don't question it.

Do you think he put his own personal stamp on it?

No.

I've heard many yoga teachers say that this system is something Krishnamacharya taught to the young Brahmin boys, to children. Why do you think that we Westerners are so attracted to it?

Well, we have young minds and the body is something that the Western mind can relate to. The Western mind cannot so easily relate to God and enlightenment and the subtler aspects of yoga. The body is a pretty gross thing. We can all relate to that—you don't go out without it. It's always there. It's a good access point.

What is the value of daily practice, day in, day out, over the years? And what is the inner quality that is cultivated through long-term practice?

Abhyasa is consistent practice over a long period of time with clear intentions. Whatever our practice, if we are doing it consistently, even if it's a small practice, we benefit a lot. There comes a point where certain aspects of the practice do become integrated and Guruji told me this point is twelve years. After twelve years, okay, we start to become established in a practice. These phases start at three months, six months, nine months, one year, three years, six years, twelve years, and so on—these chunks of time. When we have been practicing for a long time, we can

then actually step away from the practice for our family duties or whatever might be calling us away and step right back into the practice and
be right on the boat. With a short-term practice it's a little harder to get
back on the boat. Whatever practice it is, it becomes established over
years, over decades, over lifetimes. The inner quality is a steadiness that
comes from that integration.

*What about the subtle aspects of practice? Do you feel they are somehow in-
tegrated into the* asana *practice? Does one naturally evolve from the* asana
practice to the more subtle aspects of yoga?
If one is truly practicing the practice with all of its ingredients—the
vinyasa accompanied by *ujjayi* breathing, the *bandhas*, and the *drishti*—
it can't help but integrate and expand on subtle levels. If someone is
practicing *asana* as exercise without *bandhas*, breath, and *drishti*, I think
it could remain limited to the physical level. But having said that, the
body and the mind are always linked, so even one who exercises every
day is going to benefit and their mind is going to benefit. But the fruit of
this practice is multiplied again and again and again by all of those ingredients, by practicing consistently over a long period of time with
devotion.

*What kind of obstacles do we have as Westerners to attaining the goals of
yoga?*
Well, a stiff mind, stiff body, television, computers, cars, cell phones—
there are many obstacles in our material world. *Yogas chitta vritti nirodhaha.* If yoga is the stilling of fluctuations in the mind, and the mind has
too much opportunity, too many choices . . . I think that's a big handicap
for Westerners or people brought up in cultures like ours. There are too
many bloody choices out there and therefore more and more *vrittis*. The
less choices there are, the less *vrittis* there are, the process becomes simplified or more streamlined through the course of practice. Even though
there are still 816 brands of toothpaste on the shelf, we don't necessarily
look at all of them. So our choices in our mind become less.

How important is it to have a teacher?
It's very important. It can be dangerous without a teacher. Benefits can
happen, someone can read a book, learn a few poses, and learn something and do a practice and there will be some benefit. But there are

more dangers without someone watching us, without someone whom we can place faith in, and that's a big part of the practice: trust and faith in a teacher and having a relationship like that. Many of us as Westerners have not had that in our life, so it adds a whole other aspect to the practice.

Can you say something about the important role of breathing?
The breath is the vehicle for the *prana*, so the breath is important. The breath is the driver, and the beauty of that is as long as there is breath in our body we have the opportunity to experience the fruits of the practice, no matter how broken our body might be. It's the breath that will take us to the *bandhas*. It's the breath that links the body and the mind. Through the breath we can still the mind.

Can you say something about bandhas?
Bandhas are very elusive. I think very few of us have experienced the real deal. But if we have an idea what it is we are looking for, we might be able to recognize it if we got really close.

And have you?
I think so, but I don't know so.

How about the importance of food in the yoga practice?
Your food program is very important. *Abhyasa*, practice, and consistency with how we live our life, how and when we sleep, what we eat. The practice will teach us. When we are doing the practice, often habits that impede the practice will fall away of their own accord without someone telling you that you must stop smoking pot, you must stop eating meat, blah blah blah. People still say those things, but if we have the basic understanding of Ayurveda and our constitution and we have an understanding of the *gunas* and the elements, we will start to figure it out. And even if we don't have that understanding, through trial and error we will figure out what works and what doesn't work.

Why would it matter what you ate for asana *practice or other practices?*
Well, if you put it in the context of yoga practice, with a picture of yogic practice, the state of yoga will only be possible if the *sattvic* energy is predominant in our system. So if we are doing things contrary to that by

consuming *rajasic* and *tamasic* foods, participating in *rajasic* and *tamasic* activities, and so forth, obviously that state is going to be hard to attain. So the commonsense thing is to do what is helpful and don't do what is not helpful. Food, sleep, how we use substances, all of that is part of our daily life.

You obviously see ashtanga *yoga as a spiritual practice, but can you say something about the subtler aspects? What makes it spiritual?*
The magic of the *ashtanga* practice is the spanning and integration of all the different levels of our being, from the grossest level of our flesh and bones and musculature and structure to the most subtle level of the *nadis* and how the energy is flowing in our system. When we practice with *ujjayi* breathing and *drishti* and some awareness of the *bandhas*, this integration naturally starts to happen. So if we are really doing the practice, it can't help but happen even if that is not what we are looking for in the beginning.

And why would you call that spiritual?
I would define spirituality as anything that brings us closer to God. The more still our mind is, the less *vrittis* there are, the closer we are going to get. It's a natural outcome.

And you say the stillness of the mind results from asana *practice?*
The practice with all of its *bandhas* and ingredients.

How important is the philosophy of Shankaracharya, Guruji's family guru? Do you have any sense of how Guruji integrates the Advaita philosophy into his teaching?
I would not question how. It is integrated, period. It's integrated in Guruji's life, it's not a separate action or thought like, say, "Oh, I think I'll throw this into my teaching"—that's not how real teaching works. It's integrated. It's all there, it's a package deal, you can't separate it out.

It's all the same. I've been asked questions about Buddhism and different paths, dualistic, non-dualistic—well it's all the same. It's how you look at it. Anything that brings you closer to God is going to result in the same still mind. You might think of it in different ways or have on different-color glasses, but I believe it's all the same.

How do you incorporate Guruji's spiritual philosophy in the way that you teach?
Any way that I can. Any way that I am capable of. Any way that is appropriate for the students whom I am teaching.

As a teacher, my intention is threefold. To maintain the purity of the lineage and teach to the best of my capacity the pure tradition. Secondly, to exemplify the yoga lifestyle in all of its limbs and all of its aspects. Thirdly, to allow anybody—any practitioner—to experience the process of practice and to get a glimpse of the fruits of practice. For me, it's a package like that. I don't go through the thought process of "What should I do with these students today? What should I teach Jane and what should I teach John? What should I say?" There is not a thought process in that way. The practice is quite liberating for those of us who are teaching because it is a system. And having experienced the practice, if it is integrated we will find a way to communicate it to our students. There isn't a script, there isn't a teacher-training program and a test that we take to teach this yoga. The test is our life.

Do you think Westerners have an unrealistic view of the path of yoga?
Mostly I think there is a lot of confusion about what is yoga. You ask ten different people on the street in the West, there will be ten different answers.

What do you think Westerners are looking for through practice?
Some are looking for a healthy body, some are looking for someone to fix them, some are looking for a new dress size, some are looking for God. Again, there's a lot of confusion and there are a lot of differences.

You said earlier that your understanding is that yoga is about finding God. But I think for many Westerners that is fairly remote, and perhaps for you it also was not your immediate experience. How does one move from doing this physical asana *practice to something so subtle as that?*
It's a natural progression if you are really practicing. Students sign up for the fast train to God. Who wants to be healthy, feel good, and find something that works, that gives us some peace of mind? And that's probably the point at which the practitioner realizes that, wow, something is happening with my mind! There is some contentment there. There is some

peace there, this is a good thing, more is happening than on the physical level. We are not going to experience *samadhi*, experience God or the divine, with many *vrittis* in our mind. So the calmer one becomes, the closer we get. It's integration, it's a natural progression.

Still, the jump from body . . . yes, we can see the mind is a big obstacle, but getting to God is an enormous step.
I don't think it's always a huge leap. I think it sneaks in there.

Can you say something about that?
The practice works. It works all the levels. It's a package deal. So as different as we are as individuals, we can have different levels of acceptance or denial or acknowledgments, but it will creep in there one way or another.

I guess the question is, what is the relationship between God, the mind, and the body?
That would be yoga. Body and mind linked with the breath, how the breath works in the human system. Because of our system of *nadis*, we have the capacity to cultivate a predominance of *sattvic* energy in the system. So through all of our practices—in what we eat and how we sleep and how we practice and how we use our breath and all the different facets—if the *sattvic* energy is being cultivated, the *nadis* are putting it out. It will become integrated. The link is there. We have the capacity within our system to make the connection. The vehicle for that is the breath, which would mean that the state of yoga would be accessible to any human being that is alive and breathing.

How do the vrittis *reduce? What's the procedure by which God reveals himself?*
Most of us need to practice. Fortunately we have a practice, we have a system, we have a lineage, we have a package that is pretty clearly spelled out for us. What a gift! So we practice. This is not an era where we came in just ready to be enlightened, we weren't born into that state. We were born into *Kali Yuga*. Some of us were born into the Western culture. It's who we are and it's when we are, and we are in an era that requires effort, requires practice for most of us. It's a time of technology.

Technology also implies technique. We need techniques, we need some help, and we have them, so why not use them?

What do you think are the most foremost considerations for a lifelong healthy yoga practice? And as we get on in life, with sustaining it?
The practice inevitably will change form as we grow, as we age, as we come into different *ashrams* [stages] of life. The essence remains the same.

What do you have to consider? What do you have to think about? Or do you think it will just naturally change and evolve without you?
It's a lot of common sense and appropriateness.

Some people don't have common sense. Can you perhaps—
Slowly, slowly. As we practice, if we look at the actual practice itself, I think we should let our breath guide us when we are not in the presence of our guru or teacher. First off, we have a guru. Some of us have Western teachers as well. Even when we are practicing by ourselves, which I do most of the year, the breath will teach us. The breath has an intelligence, and if we listen to it, we'll know, it will become obvious. If your breath is spastic and strained, you are obviously pushing too hard. I think that would be our biggest guide or barometer.

Some students will never be able to achieve the more advanced postures. Do you think they have less hope of a spiritual evolution?
The essence of the practice and what happens energetically in our system, in our mind, is accessible to anyone who has the capacity to believe.

Then what would be the function of the advanced asanas?
To provide a challenge to those individuals where it would be appropriate, those with strong bodies and enthusiasm and energy. The advanced practice is not appropriate for everyone. It's not appropriate for most, but it does certainly exemplify the strength and grace that we have as human beings.

Would you like to share some final thoughts?
I have extreme gratitude for Guruji, for his family, the lineage, and on a

broader scale gratitude to have a system, a program to practice, to follow, when so many people are floundering without a method. Having a method and a system I believe automatically reduces the *vrittis* in our minds. We don't have to think about, well what should I do today? Or which one of these yoga classes should I go to? Or what should I do with my students today? It's spelled out for us, and I'm grateful for that, to have a system, a guru, even to have faith or trust in something or someone, where most of my life I didn't have that. I have my parents, who I always love and respect.

One time when I was working in the corporate world, taking some sort of a leadership-management seminar, and one of the questions as we were brainstorming and writing down on the easels with all the little markers and everything was: Who are your heroes? You couldn't say your parents and it needed to be someone who is alive today. This was before I met Guruji. And I was in this corporate workshop drawing an absolute blank, one of those moments I won't forget. I didn't have a hero. I didn't have some figure outside of my parents I could really look to and totally trust and respect as a guide. And there was a feeling of really being lost at sea at that point. But fortunately that didn't last forever. Again, it goes back to gratitude for having a system, having a guru, having teachers in my life who inspired me and have allowed me to make some decisions and be very clear about my intentions and my role in life.

Mysore, 2009

Sharmila Mahesh

Sharmila Mahesh had the rare privilege of being born in a family of yogis. She began her yoga practice at the age of twelve with her brother, Sharath. In 1991 she married and moved to Bangalore, eventually opened her own yoga school, and now teaches many local and foreign students in several locations in that busy metropolis.

How old were you when you started practicing?
I was eight years old when I started. We used to see all the other students, so we also started doing the yoga practice.

You just imitated?
Yes, initially. Later, when I was maybe twelve, I started seriously doing yoga.

Were you living in the same house with Guruji?
My father was away for work in Dubai, so we had to stay in my grandparents' house. He has been a great grandfather. I was brought up by him and my grandmother. When I was in school he would bring lunch for me in the afternoons. He used to wash my clothes and he took a lot of care of me and my brother. He made sure we ate good food. He did all the arrangements for my wedding. He was the backbone for me in my life.

Do you remember seeing your grandfather practicing yoga?
It was amazing. He used to finish all the housework and the yoga teaching and then he would practice.

How was it different watching Guruji practice from watching his students practice?
The style was the same, but the postures that he did were amazing. He was so flexible. He was sixty years old by then and [still] very strong.

Did ladies and men practice in separate rooms?
No, all of them were together, but in the morning class they had one or two sessions of ladies upstairs. Some classes were mixed and some classes were only for ladies.

Do you remember seeing Guruji with Krishnamacharya?
I recollect seeing Krishnamacharya once. He was ninety-one when some of the foreign students wanted to see him, so our whole family went to Madras to his house. I was very small.

Does Guruji talk about his guru?
Yes, he talks a lot about how Krishnamacharya used to teach him and how disciplined he was during his practice.

Do you remember Guruji touching his feet?
As soon as he saw the guru he touched his feet and took blessing from him.

Guruji is a great Sanskrit scholar. Does he bring his knowledge of Sanskrit into the house?
All the *pujas* are done in Sanskrit, all the mantras are in Sanskrit. But we don't talk in Sanskrit.

And you do puja *every day.*
We get up in the morning, have a bath, and do *puja*. We burn a ghee lamp and offer flowers with mantras, that's the basic thing that we do for daily *puja*. That's what all the ladies in India do.

Do you have any special stories about Guruji that you like to tell?
When he was young, he wanted to study Sanskrit, but they didn't have any outlets in his village, so after they did his thread ceremony, he took whatever money he received and ran away to Mysore. Back in the village the only opportunity he had was to look after the farm or the cows, so he

ran away to Mysore where he stayed at a free hostel. There he went to this free school and started studying Sanskrit. He met Krishnamacharya and started learning yoga along with his Sanskrit studies. Then one day the king had a competition in his court and Guruji had to represent yoga. He did a demonstration. The king was very happy with him and gave him a place to live and food to eat, which allowed him to spend more time studying Sanskrit. So that's how he started his life.

When Amma died you all moved back in together again.
My grandfather was very attached to my grandmother. He used to cry looking at her photo. The bond for sixty years, you can't just get over it in one or two days. We thought it was a good idea staying together, so he also can have freedom and we can give him sufficient care, just as Amma used to do for him. So we all moved into the same house.

What would you say is the most important thing he has taught you?
First of all, he has taught us how to follow every step of *ashtanga* yoga. You have to be honest, don't steal, you have to be humble. On each and every step he guided us on how to lead our lives. This helped us in our careers as teachers. He used to tell us, "You have to be disciplined, you have to concentrate, focus in your life." That has helped us a lot. The most important thing you have to do is to be disciplined and to focus on whatever you do.

Guruji built a temple in Kowshika dedicated to Shankaracharya. What kind of role does Shankaracharya play in the family worship?
Shankaracharya is our guru. The temple is mostly dedicated to my grandmother and my uncle Ramesh, who was also very much into Shankaracharya. It is a memory for them.

Did your two uncles, Ramesh and Manju, influence your childhood and your yoga practice?
Yoga practice was done only with my grandfather. Sharath has helped me lately. Manju went to America when I was eight or nine, and didn't come back for nearly ten years. Ramesh stayed with us. He was a very good uncle. He did wonderful yoga practice, amazing, he did all the *asanas* well and he was dedicated to God. He used to do all his daily *pujas* really well and he was very humble.

Did you have any idea how much Guruji would become involved in the West?

Definitely. He was totally dedicated to yoga. All he focused on was yoga. I remember an incident which illustrates how dedicated he was. One day he was on the scooter and he had an accident. There was a big cut on his forehead, a really big cut. My friend and I took him to the doctor for stitches. He was bleeding and had bruises over his face. We told him, "You better rest tomorrow." It was around seven o'clock in the evening. I told him, "Don't go to the yoga *shala* tomorrow." Early morning, I get up and he's already awake at 3 a.m. teaching. Many times, helping students into *shirshasana* [headstand], people have kicked him in the face. He lost three teeth, but he didn't care. He was in class the next day. So you can see how much dedication he's got. I knew he was going to spread yoga all over the world. I was very sure because of his dedication.

He has a lot of willpower.

He used to cycle before there were scooters in Mysore. He used to drop me at school sometimes on the cycle. But then he wanted to learn to drive a scooter. He was seventy years old and he wanted to drive a scooter, so one of the students taught him how to drive at the age of seventy! Now he's ready to drive a car, too, but they probably won't give him a license.

Guruji and Amma were very poor in the beginning.

Guruji was not poor. He was a rich man in his village. They were all agriculturists, and my great-grandfather used to be a priest. But Guruji got out. He wanted his own life. That's why he left the village. He wanted to build his own empire. That was his main goal in life. They had to struggle to build this empire. Sometimes they didn't even have food. My granny never let out to others that they didn't have food that day. She used to keep a vessel at the washing place and pretend she had food. He was not poor, but he struggled a lot in the beginning.

What do you think is special about Guruji as a teacher?

He is very strict and disciplined. He treats all the students the same way, he does not discriminate. When he is teaching, it's to perfect the *asanas* and for the student to know more about yoga. He's the same in his life: simplicity, no enmity, treating everyone equal. I like that. He was the same person before he was famous. And he says to us, "You should never be proud and say, 'I have everything,' or God will take everything away." He teaches us to be the same person all the time. You should feel you are getting only twenty rupees a month, as we used to get in the olden days. You have to have contentment. That is the great thinking of my grandfather.

He used to give instructions about how to live your life in the privacy of home. Can you say something about other lessons or suggestions he would give?
He expected us to be simple and never allowed us to feel our family was famous. He treats everybody the same way he has always done, all his relatives and friends.

Do you think it has to do with the Advaita philosophy—being one, everything is God, everything is the same?
Yeah, I think after you practice yoga for a long time you become very simple and all the eight limbs will be working. That's what I feel with my teaching. A lot of people have become simple; most of them have become vegetarians. The yoga helps you control the mind, body, everything. It balances your sleep, it balances your food. It's a purification of the body. We don't realize it, but it happens. He ate pure, *sattvic* food cooked by Amma, and I think that is the light. You can see the enlightenment in Guruji. After a while, when you practice *ashtanga* yoga, everything is like this. I've seen it with my students, too. Lots of people have given up smoking, they can't drink alcohol—after the practice, the body can't take it. It's a sign of purification.

How important is family?
Guruji's family is very important to him. Only two things he thinks of in his life. First is the students. He is totally into the students, involved, with yoga and philosophy. And he is so devoted to the family, his grandchildren, his great-grandchildren, his daughter, his son. He gets very emotional. It's very important to him. He gives 100 percent to the family and to yoga.

Does he think about students outside the classroom?
Yes. He talks about the students all the time. This person has done this,

he is like that. He or she has to improve on that posture. And he tells many things about Krishnamacharya and his teachings, and how he taught with Krishnamacharya.

They were teaching together?
He went with Krishnamacharya to north India. They wanted to spread yoga, so they formed a team and went to teach people in the north.

What else did he tell you about his studies with Krishnamacharya?
Krishnamacharya was very strict. One day, a student was asking lots of questions: "Why do you have to do *bandha*? Why do you have to do this?" And Krishnamacharya got mad. "Why do you eat with your mouth? Why don't you eat from another outlet of your body?" So he was a very strong teacher. He was with Krishnamacharya for twenty-six years. He's got energy from him.

I seem to remember Krishnamacharya also thought Guruji was very strong. Isn't there a story about Amma, and how Krishnamacharya says to Amma, "Be careful, he's a very strong man, he'll bring you Chamundi Hill"?
When Amma wanted to marry Guruji, the horoscope didn't match, so Amma's father said, "I don't think you'll be very happy." She had another offer from a wealthy person. Amma said, "I'm not going to marry that wealthy man, I'm going to marry Pattabhi. I'll never starve because he has so much strength. He might work hard as a coolie to keep me happy." She said that and got married to my grandfather when she was fourteen years old. And it was on her birthday they got married.

When did they start living together as husband and wife?
Two or three years after the marriage.

How do you see Guruji getting older? Is he affected by that?
Mentally, he is very strong. Because of the yoga, his bones, everything is so strong. He has not lost hope; he keeps going on. He goes out and buys vegetables and brings them to the house, and does his banking, sits in the car. He has not been in hospital since 1993. It is only the last year [2008] that he had a problem.

How did Guruji become established as a teacher?
In olden days when Guruji was teaching yoga, he used to call the local people and ask them to do yoga, but very few people used to come. One day he demonstrated in the court of the maharaja, and Guruji was doing *asanas* so well the maharaja gave him five rupees. Five rupees was like five lakhs now. He kept the five rupees for a long time. The maharaja was impressed and gave him free housing, free food, and he said, "You can stay in the kingdom and learn Sanskrit." He gave him a *shala* at the Sanskrit College so he could teach yoga. He taught there for years. He used to work very hard, day and night. Not so many local people came to learn. That's why he had to go to Western countries to teach, because Western people were more interested in yoga. He made his own *shala* in the back of his house. One of his students gave him a loan. He started teaching local people, but very few would come. Slowly Westerners started to come and they were more interested. It made him want to go to Western countries because he saw the devotion in them. He saw them changing their lives, so he went to Western countries to teach. Now it is spread all over the world.

He really likes Western students because he sees the devotion in them, devotion toward the guru and devotion toward the yoga.

Now students are coming from all over the world. Only in America was it popular. Slowly you can see it in the UK. Now it's also popular in Japan, in European countries, Finland, Copenhagen—everywhere they are doing *ashtanga* yoga. *Ashtanga* has become globalized.

How do you imagine it will continue in the future?
You should have quality students. People should be aware of certified teachers. People should find out who is a good teacher. *Ashtanga* yoga is just not commercial. You have to follow the traditional way of learning. Only then will you get satisfaction within you. You shouldn't learn yoga to make money. You should feel it's for yourself. Then you get the contentment and it changes your life.

Try the classes for a month and see how it changes your body. It shouldn't be done like aerobics, it should be done traditionally in the Mysore style.

Guruji always says he received this teaching from Krishnamacharya and continued to teach exactly the way he was taught. Yet nobody else teaches

*like Guruji. Krishnamacharya started teaching differently, then Desikachar
started teaching one way, Iyengar started teaching another way.*
He said he didn't want Guruji to change anything. The only changes Guruji made was he invented *surya namaskara* A and B, where you pray to the sun God. The rest was designed before, and he adopted the breathing and the *vinyasa* systems. Everything he was taught he has adopted. But he has done research while teaching, too.

He wanted to do everything the traditional way. Students have to come, do the yoga, learn with the guru. Only if the guru agrees, can you go and teach. Nowadays yoga has become so commercial everybody wants a certificate in one or two months. That doesn't happen in *ashtanga*. They have to study and deepen their understanding over many years, and then start teaching.

*People are in a big hurry to start to teach. It takes away some of your energy
for your own practice if you start teaching too soon, and you are just going
to hurt your students. The longer you can wait, the better.*
At least seven years they have to practice.

Anything else you would like to add?
Yoga is very good for pregnant ladies. Many students practice *ashtanga* yoga when they are pregnant. Under the guidance of a guru, they can do yoga. I feel that they should do it. Pregnant women should do yoga.

Bangalore, 2009

A Global Community

•

Joseph Dunham

Joseph Dunham was an unlikely candidate to settle in Mysore. His life was transformed through his assocation with Guruji and Amma, having spent eleven years traveling the world with them on teaching tours. He continues to live in Mysore, where he opens his comfortable home to a new generation of yoga students.

Why don't you start by telling me how you met Guruji.
I came to study with Guruji for one month in May—no, December of 1992.

What were the circumstances that led you to Mysore?
I was traveling around the world, which I had never done before, and I had stopped off in Crete to go to an *ashtanga* yoga intensive, which I didn't know anything about, and the first day I hated the practice, having studied other kinds of yoga. The second day, I was too tired to think. And the third day, I fell in love with it. I ended up staying an extra week. It was a two-week program and I stayed for three weeks. Derek Ireland gave me Guruji's address. I was on my way to Nepal trekking, and I came down here and knocked on Guruji's door and asked him if I could study with him.

Why did Derek give you his address?
Because I was going to be in the area and I was thinking of going to India.

Okay, so you knocked on Guruji's door . . .
And asked him if I could study with him for what I considered an in-

credible amount of time: four weeks. I didn't think I could endure living in Mysore for four whole weeks, but I asked him if I could study, and he said, "How long?" and I said I could stay for a month and he said, "That's not enough time." Somebody in the room said, "Two months?" And Guruji said, "You need three months," and somebody said I would stay for three months and he said, "Very good, you come tomorrow."

And that somebody was you?
There was nobody else in the room. But it didn't feel like me. I couldn't believe I said it, but as I walked out the door and I said to my friend Annie—she was walking in the door to see Guruji—"I can't believe it," I said, "I just told that man I was going to say in this two-bit burg for three frigging months." She said, "It's going to go by in a snap of a finger." At the end of three months, I said, "Guruji I have good news and bad news. The good news is I made it through three months and the bad news is I want to stay." He said, "Very good, very good." So I stayed for five months, and after that I ended up escorting him and his wife around the world for six months and it evolved into a position of escorting and organizing all of Guruji's tours and living with the family when they were on tour for the next eleven years.

Before we get into tours, why don't you tell me a little bit about your impressions of Guruji and of Amma. Let's start with Guruji, when you first met him, when you first started working with him. You were used to other kinds of yoga, you weren't used to Indian teachers, or practicing in India for that matter.
For some reason, I don't know why, he and I just had a very quick bonding. I felt very close to him, very comfortable around him and his wife. Very respectful people and most honorable and pleasant. It took me many months to call him Guruji. I just called him sir for many months. But he and I just felt comfortable around each other.

And how was the practice working on you? You made it through those three months very quickly and you wanted to stay.
I was overwhelmed with the practice. I had never experienced anything like this before. I had never done a practice more than a few weeks at a time. I would go to an intensive and study for a couple of weeks and not

have a practice after that, so I was very taken with it, with the structure and the intensity of it. When I first signed up for *ashtanga* yoga in Crete, it was described to me as a hard practice, but if you work very hard you will progress, and I love to work, which is why I got into it and it was exactly that: I was making progress. Well, my first day, I did *surya namaskara* A and *surya namaskara* B and Guruji said, "That's enough now, you take *padmasana*," and I said, "Okay, what's that?" And they put me, Sharath and Guruji put me in *padmasana* the first class. I started at forty-four years old, so I never thought I was going to get into *padmasana*. A couple of weeks later I was muscling myself into it. And I was very drawn to the people who were here and felt very comfortable and very alive and life just felt very full.

You stayed five months and then Guruji was going to go on tour. How did escorting him evolve?

I was spending some time with the woman who was the liaison for all of the teachers who were hosting him, and she came into my home one day and said, "He is not going," in shock. And I said, "Why not?" On this trip, it's six months' traveling. She said, "I don't know, he doesn't want to go." So many phone calls were made, many people were crying, begging. About a week later he said he was going to go again, and a week after that he said he wasn't going to go. I'd been told the last time they set up one of these tours, the day of the departure he just said no, and didn't go. And I asked, "Is anybody actually traveling with him?" and they said no, but of course people will take him to the airport and people will pick him up at the other end. And having traveled a considerable amount myself, I knew it was a huge job just going through customs, finding flights, connecting flights, being on the plane, not taking food. He's a very important person to us, but to everyone else he's a little guy in a sheet who doesn't speak English very well. So I could see how he'd have problems, and I had the time because I had taken a year to make this trip. My first stop was Crete, my second stop was Nepal, my next stop was here, and I had the time. So I went and knocked on his door and asked if he'd like me to go with him, to travel with him. And he was very excited. In retrospect, that's what he was waiting for. In this culture, it's too direct to ask for something, it's always done indirectly, it has to be figured out. Culturally, it wasn't acceptable to say that he wanted somebody to come with him.

He was just waiting for somebody to figure it out, and I just happened to be there, with the time. And so we traveled for six months: Guruji, his wife, and I. And after that, when asked to go somewhere, he said, "Joseph is not coming, I am not going." So it pretty much evolved into this position.

You traveled with him and Amma for several years, and that kind of work is particularly stressful, so spending that kind of time with him is also particularly precious. What was it like to travel with him, to arrange things, how he was on the airplanes, how he was preparing to travel, how he was when it was time for his classes to start? Obviously he made an impression or you wouldn't have kept on going.

That's the paramount point: you don't do something like this, take an eleven-year chunk out of your life, plop it on the table, without some consideration, of course. But he was, they were both so appreciative, and I could see, it was very obvious, that this position needed to be filled for him to be able to get out to see people. He couldn't and wouldn't do it on his own, and when I was observing the interaction with all the students, he would tell people to come to India and they would. I'd heard so many things about Pattabhi Jois, but until you meet him . . . He is very much like the *ashtanga* practice itself: you can hear all day long about it; until you do it, you don't have a clue what they're talking about. It's all experiential, and so is Pattabhi Jois. He's very experiential. You can hear all kinds of things, but when you meet him, it's a completely different story, it's never what you've heard. It's like describing what it would be like to jump out of an airplane with a parachute on. You can talk about it all day but until you experience it, you won't know what it's about. When I saw the reaction of people who met him on tour who couldn't make it to India, and the way he would encourage them to come to India, they would come to India, and it was just very obvious to me that he needed to get out, in my opinion, to meet people. When I was here the first time, there were a dozen or fourteen students, fifteen students maximum, and as friends have told me, ten years before there were the same amount of students, so it hadn't changed in ten years. But when we got out and met people, there was a tidal wave. When he was able to make contact with people, everything started. All the pieces were in place with the teaching that was going on, and at the same time he was coming in, so it started, and now quite often there's hundreds of students in Mysore at one time.

But he had been going in the 1980s and the '70s, traveling also. What do you think changed in the 1990s?
I think that the teachers that were established at that time [the '90s] were bringing up a whole new group, and he was meeting a larger group of people. There were very sporadic little groups of students when he was traveling before, from what I understand. That's what I mean by a perfect storm: the teaching that was going on and creating this foundation, and then he was actually going there and meeting them, and I think that all came together just at the right time. From what I understand, he made a few trips. I don't think he made too many.

He went in '79, '80, '82, '85, '87, and '89.
Well, he was building up. We were traveling just about every year when I started traveling with him, if not twice a year. Sometimes we'd go to Australia and then to America. It was a lot of trips and a different format. When he started, we were going one month at each place, and then it got down to two weeks, and then one trip we did thirteen cities in fifteen weeks. But of course, that was the last tour. They were all last tours, as far as I was told—from the first one.

Can you recall a few anecdotes about Guruji on your travels? Did they travel heavy, did they travel light, did they eat out in restaurants?
No, they didn't eat out in restaurants. We did have to bring quite a bit of food for Amma to prepare. As a Brahmin, he can only have food that is prepared by a Brahmin. We went to two restaurants that I can remember, one in London and one in Singapore. Both of them were Brahmin restaurants. And he was not very impressed with the food. He liked home-cooked food.

And how did they fare on the airplane?
On the airplane, he would always make a big drama about the fast he would have to go through, but I always brought a big bag of fruit and chocolate, and apparently it's just an assumed fact that all of the Swiss chocolatiers are Brahmin because that chocolate all disappeared, so did the fruit. [*Laughter*]

Amma ate chocolate also?
Amma ate chocolate also.

Very nice.

It was awkward for the stewardesses to be told they weren't going to eat, which I always explained to them. But they were comfortable. I always wore a suit and a tie when I traveled with them. It helped expedite things. No problems in the eleven years I traveled with Guruji. Thank God everything went well.

How did he prepare himself? Did he pack at the last minute?
No, no, he was always prepared to travel. If we were in India, and it was a travel day, he would teach a class. Even though the flight was leaving at night and it was five o'clock in the morning, the class was very fast-paced. And he always wanted to be at the airport very, very early.

The first time I flew with him to Geneva to New York, I had actually gone back to America and I met them in Paris. Some students had brought them to France, and I met them and we went to a yoga conference in Zinal, in Switzerland. A woman from Denmark had come down to be with me for the week and had to leave the day before we were traveling. So I explained to Guruji I had to take her to the airport in Geneva about three hours away, put her on the plane, and the next day we would go. Our flight to New York was leaving at one o'clock, I gave him the name of the hotel I'd be staying at, and the phone number, and I said, "I'll just meet you at the airport at eleven o'clock." I could tell he wasn't really happy. This was on a Thursday. The flight was on a Saturday. Friday he came and asked me again what was going to happen on Saturday. I told him the story again. And he apparently went up to the woman I was taking to the airport, was watching her very closely all day, and finally came up to her, took her hand, and said, "Tomorrow Joseph is coming with me, maybe later he is coming to Denmark, maybe later you are coming to India, but tomorrow Joseph is coming with me." It was very sweet, I thought. So I finally got everything together and drove her to the airport and went to the hotel. The next morning, I woke up at six o'clock, ordered some coffee, went to shave, and the phone rang right away after I'd hung it up. I thought they must have been confused about what coffee I wanted or something and I picked up the phone and it was Lino [Miele]. "Good morning, Joseph." Lino was driving Guruji in from Zinal.

"Joseph, we are at the airport."

I said, "Lino, it's six o'clock in the morning. What are you doing at the airport?"

"Well," he said, "two o'clock in the morning there was a knock on my door and Guruji said, 'Get up.'"

"But," I said, "the plane isn't leaving until one." And he said, "I know, but Guruji wants you to come out to the airport now."

"I just woke up," I told him. "I'll be there at ten. I have my practice to do and I'm not going to come out there. It's a lovely airport, I was just there last night. Tell them to enjoy it and I will be there."

It was very cute. I came out and met them at ten o'clock and we went to New York and all was well. He wasn't sure I was going to be there at all. He thought maybe I had gone to Denmark.

I remember one story you told me, how after practice you were going some-where to meet some people—I don't remember the situation. You hadn't had time to change your clothes and you were in your sweaty clothes and going down the elevator with him. He turned and looked you up and down, and he said, "You're going like that?"

That was in London. We were staying in a beautiful mansion and we were going to Buckingham Palace. Everybody was in a hurry to go, and I came down, and because I was running around doing a lot of stuff I didn't have a chance to change my clothes, and he looked at me and said, "Like that?" And I was, "Yes, sir, no problem." I know when I am being told to change my clothes at fifty-something years old. And Sharath was, "No, no, he's not saying that—"

"Yes, he's saying that," I said, and I ran up and changed my clothes and came back down with my sports coat on, and he said, "Better, much better."

And I said, "Better?"

He said, "Much better."

He's a fastidious person, that Guruji.

Yes, and I was not presentable. We might run into the queen. You never know.

What happened when your tenure basically came to an end?

Eleven years is a long time. It's a big chunk of anyone's life. It was a pleasure and an honor to have been in that position and I was grateful for the opportunity and the life it presented, and they had accepted me and, you know, things move on. It was time for that transition to happen.

Some of the things were really awkward, but it was appropriate, so I just bowed out and Sharath was certainly in a position to take care of his family. He didn't need me holding his hand.

What are you doing now?
Now I'm living very happily in this little two-bit town that I didn't think I could make it through a month in. I teach some yoga when traveling, and my real work is investing in the stock market online.

How is your life in Mysore?
My life in Mysore is full and sweet but simple, which is a good thing for me. It keeps me focused. It's a lovely and an unusual circumstance that so many of these very alive *ashtanga* yoga people are coming from all over the world to be here. And friends that I have made over the years . . . everybody comes here and I'm always meeting friends and forming rich friendships with people that are very familiar from the first time I meet them. I don't know it like Guruji knows it, but he has told me that a lot of people who come to him are yogis from a past life. I don't know that like he does, but I am very comfortable around them when I first meet them. And it's a unique living environment. It's like living in New York or Maui, somewhere that everyone wants to go to for one reason for another. You get a mass gathering of this tribe here, which is a very rich experience for me. It's quite fascinating. Everything's been a positive experience.

What have been your impressions of Guruji over the past year and couple months he's been sick. You were here when he first went into the hospital, and you saw him in the hospital, you saw him get out of the hospital and go back to the hospital and go back again.
You know, we should all be so lucky to live our dream. At ninety-two, my impressions are that he's secure, he's comfortable, and he's very, very fragile. But his sense of humor is keen, and that's something I've always focused on, and the brightness is in his eyes but his body is finally just acting like ninety-two years and he's just very, very fragile. Each night, sitting in his bedroom watching television and chatting and having to work at breathing, labored breathing, and in the most comfortable circumstance he could be in. He's just fragile. He's certainly acting his age. His family is taking excellent care of him.

What is his spirit?
His spirit is good.

Here's a man who has a tremendous amount of knowledge and a tremendous amount of practical experience with yoga. Do you see that he has moved into this stage of life with that supporting him, that there is some yogic sensibility in how he's feeling in his decay?
In his decay? I think, with his age. My experience with Guruji, my life with him, has very much, as you say with the practice, been 99 percent practice and 1 percent talking, and our communication has been 1 percent talking other than on a very pleasant level and 99 percent experiential. We look at each other. It's a lot of eye communication, not specifically verbal other than that he loves to laugh. I can remember one story. When we were at the old *shala*, he came in with a letter from some student he didn't know, and this person was coming, so he was going around the room, "Do you know this person?" Nobody knew this person, and finally somebody said, "Yes, I know this person."

Now you think he'd want to know if he was a yoga teacher, what sort of practice he had. The only thing he asked about this letter from this person was, "Happy student?" And the person who knew him said, "Yes." And he said, "Ah, good." That's all he wanted to know, didn't want to know anything else, that's all that mattered.

When I'm with him, he knows that I'm trying to keep things light and joke with him, and I gauge how his mental facilities are doing and how he responds to that. We have a light communication on that level, but I can tell he cherishes it. And the look I get whenever I walk in the room: he always smiles. Maybe he's just thinking about my practice. [*Laughter*] He could be.

Mysore, 2009

John Scott

John Scott trained as an industrial designer in New Zealand and discovered *ashtanga* yoga through Derek Ireland, a devoted and enthusiastic student of Guruji's who passed away in 1998. Two of the most widely distributed charts of the primary and intermediate series were drawn by John. His book on *ashtanga* yoga was a bestseller in England.

What first attracted you to ashtanga *yoga?*
I was working at a holistic health and fitness center. At that time I was an avid windsurfer, and one of the options at the center, apart from windsurfing, tai chi, and a number of alternative options, was yoga. The yoga wasn't of interest until I saw or met Derek Ireland. Initially I thought Derek was an American football player, but it turned out that he was an English soccer player. And anyway, before he arrived at the center, his fame was widely talked about, and the image of him was of quite an amazing man.

I was awestruck by his physical presence as well as his personality. And when I saw him practice, I was amazed by what a man with his physique could actually do. In those days I never believed that strong bulky muscles could actually do splits. So when I saw Derek doing his personal practice I was turned on by it. The feeling was, "Wow! That *is* possible! I would like to do that myself, and I would like to look like that." It was quite a vanity thing initially, an exercise system that would give you that fitness.

When I started doing the practice, because I got into the breath and the movement of that breath, I was hooked by the feeling. And because of that hook I continued practicing. Derek was an inspirational man. He was my first teacher. Because he was very grateful to Pattabhi Jois, his advice was, "John, as soon as you get the opportunity, go to Mysore and study with Pattabhi Jois."

Eighteen months later, I went to Pattabhi Jois, having had really only three months with Derek. Derek's advice was to go to Pattabhi Jois and say you're a complete beginner. So I said to Pattabhi Jois, "Derek is my teacher, but he said to start with you from the beginning," which I did. And on the very first day I remember being so nervous, excitedly nervous, but also afraid. The atmosphere in the room itself was very, very powerful, and the senior students there at the time were very impressive.

Guruji was not explaining very much as you practiced, but he prompted me where I needed prompting right from the beginning. And because he was on me in terms of his energy and his eyes and his hands, my adrenals must have been pumping, and halfway through the standing postures, I was shaking like a leaf. He said, "Now you sit down and take rest," which I was very glad of.

I felt very privileged to have started that way with Pattabhi Jois, because now he's very busy, so busy that when you go there, especially if you've had another teacher introducing you to the practice, you can be overlooked on the first few days. But being a complete beginner when the numbers were low, his eyes were on you, his hands were on you, and it was very intense. So for me it was very fortunate to start in the earlier days and I can say Pattabhi Jois has taken me posture by posture through my entire practice in the traditional method of teaching: first you take *surya namaskara* and then you add, one by one. I've actually experienced that from the master himself.

Can you describe the yoga shala *and the impression it made on you when you first went in there?*
Pattabhi Jois's yoga *shala* is in his own family home and it's in a little suburb of Mysore. Going to it, you wouldn't know you are going to a yoga center. Everybody knows where it is, all the rickshaw drivers know how to get there. You're walking down what would be described as a back street, there's cows wandering free. As you approach Pattabhi Jois's place, first of all you notice a lot of bikes and various other modes of transport parked outside. And as you enter into his foyer and there are stacks of shoes, already you begin to feel there are a lot of things happening. By this stage, you've heard the noise, the typical *ujjayi* sound, and some people will say the walls are breathing. And when you look into the space,

you are hit with the heat and just the energy of the people in there, and there is no noise apart from the breath and Pattabhi Jois giving a few sharp instructions.

Do you feel that Guruji's way of teaching has changed over the years?
In essence, Pattabhi Jois's teaching has remained the same for the whole time I've been with him, for about ten years. He's had to modify slightly the time, just the economics of time, because of the number of students, but essentially his teaching has remained very traditional, very classic for all that time.

Can you expand a little on how he teaches?
In Pattabhi Jois's method of teaching, he will take a beginner and will talk a beginner through [practice], counting [the *vinyasas*] in Sanskrit, and his method of teaching is that what he tells you, he expects you to remember the next day, which means he doesn't always have to repeat his information. He expects you to remember it. If you don't, he gets quite cross. By putting that pressure on his students, a student's personal discipline is tested and improved and you're made responsible, so all he has to do is look at you and the discipline is there. You have an energetic connection with his *shakti*, his energy.

If he then sees you incorrectly doing something, he will give you verbal instruction, a verbal adjustment—"Straight," "Move your arm" or hand—or a place to look [*drishti*]. If you still don't get that correct, he may have to come and physically adjust you, which is the term "being adjusted," where the teacher puts you in the posture. And when Pattabhi Jois in Mysore puts you in the *asana*, when you get home, you remember.

So his method is, while you are hot and sweaty and under a state of increased adrenaline because you're pumping there, he puts you into the posture and you just have to submit. On many occasions, I had tried to resist his adjustment and just felt his adjustment intensify, and over the years I've learned you have to look him in the eye, which isn't the correct *drishti*, look him in the eye and submit and have the faith that he isn't going to put you into something further than you can go. In the submitting or even just the yielding to his pressure, my body has changed over the years. In fact, now when he adjusts me I feel so secure.

Would you say there is a spiritual essence to the way Guruji teaches?
Guruji teaches a very traditional method of yoga and he doesn't preach anything to you. I call that teaching with the right of inquiry. If you ask Guruji something, he will answer. He won't give you information unless you need it. On the aspect of spirituality, he sets an example. It's by the example that you learn more of the other aspects of the eight limbs of yoga. And when you watch Guruji in the morning, when he comes into the room chanting, and he's lighting incense, and he's paying homage to his own father and teacher and children, and he goes about his own ritualistic routine every day. And by observing, you begin to learn a little about how people need a ritualistic pattern to begin the day.

How he enters the room, how he works in the room, and how he leaves—and I think a lot of his spiritual teaching is by example. But it's only by the years looked on retrospectively, how he's related to you over the years, you'll see it's not only the *asana*, you'll see that there is much more than the *asana*. When you have issues come up, how he'll handle those issues, and how you witness the issues come up with the other students and how he handles their issues. And how sometimes it feels contrived, but then if you look at him again with a lot of hindsight, you'll see he's just being natural and identifying with who you are and working on you as an individual. So you may be in a group of twelve people but you still are very much an individual and there is no general instruction on how he passes information. He is a very spiritual man and, without having to force it on you, I think you share it with him.

One criticism of ashtanga *yoga is that it's perceived as a standardized form of yoga, and what you're saying is really it's a very individual teaching.*
Ashtanga yoga practice is a very universal, very standardized sequence. We all have the same sequence to work with at varying levels of ability. What is different is each individual's mind, each individual's interpretation of that sequence. A number of other schools will criticize the system in terms of you are all doing the same thing, or if you do it this way, all you do is burn the body up—I've heard several times that it overheats the body and the fire just burns the body up.

The way I look at and respond to that is that there is nothing wrong with any kind of system, it's the attitude that one practices with. What's magic about the system is the fact that it's a set format, you have got something that is constant, that doesn't vary. You can then refer back to it as the mind fluctuates. Over the years of teaching, if you compare all the students you have taken through the system, the same system, from that constant benchmark or guideline you can see how the mind of each individual changes and how each personality is different. It's important to have a consistent practice because as soon as you vary a system, then you run into another variant. So I admire Pattabhi Jois for taking on what Krishnamacharya gave him as a set format, or they worked out together as a set format, and continuing it over the years. I would imagine if you questioned Pattabhi Jois, through that consistent sequence he has been able to understand the individual.

How does the ashtanga *practice affect people? How would you say transformation happens through it?*
The effect that *ashtanga* yoga has on the practitioner is a very personal thing. When people start working the system of breath/movement synchronicity, and when they actually start to develop the breath/*bandha* control, everybody then has an inner awakening where the breath is always the releasing. Pattabhi Jois will say, getting back to the spiritual matter, that the inhalation or inspiration is the inspiration of God—taking God in—and the exhalation or expiration is giving to God. Because everybody is working with that nature of inhalation and exhalation, when challenged through the sequencing of the *asanas*, eventually they yield to this constant synchronizing, and many times barriers or blocks will be presented to each practitioner, so each practitioner then has a learning opportunity. And this is how the system works: we are all faced with our individual growth. So anyone who takes on *ashtanga* will grow and will grow quite quickly if they continue with a daily practice.

Initially, when I was introduced to it, it was a vanity thing. Once I got into the breath, that changed. I then realized I was on a journey which was more important than the external world. And now that I've actually matured another ten years, what my practice looks like, what my body looks like, is not important anymore. What is important now is the appreciation of the breath and the rhythm of the breath when I practice and where that breath takes me. I remember when I first visited David Williams, he said, "All I teach now is *ujjayi pranayama* and *mula bandha*," and back then I sort of laughed, but now I appreciate that nearly all the senior practitioners and teachers, what they try and acquire after all is the breath and the *bandhas*. So you start working with the true essence of the practice and the true essence is your personal growth which is accessed by the breath.

How do you incorporate Guruji's teaching in the way that you teach?
I started teaching before I had the grace of Pattabhi Jois to teach. He likes, or wants his students to share this practice. So in other words, people can actually start teaching before they are so-called "qualified." When I first started teaching, I modeled myself on my first teacher, Derek Ireland. He had such an effect on me. He had quite a different style of presentation than Pattabhi Jois, called "led" or "talked-through" primary. In the beginning, I was very enthusiastic but naïve, and I feel as if I served my teaching apprenticeship through the experience of ten years of teaching in that style, and it's taken seven years to change from doing a talked-through-style class to Pattabhi Jois's self-practice class. I wish I had taught self-practice many years ago because if you teach only led classes, it can be very dangerous in the sense that you are presenting it the same way to each individual, and it doesn't work that way. You have the same thing but then you want to see the way that each individual relates to it. When you teach self-practice then you can have that direct relationship—individual student to individual practice—using the same method. So I now teach self-practice, but initially I was a consumer yoga teacher, meaning you needed an income to survive. I am now in a fortunate position and can model myself on Pattabhi Jois instead of a studio, reduce my numbers to ten, and then really honor and respect the system for that one-to-one instruction where you are taking an individual through their practice.

Now Guruji teaches the so-called led style when he is abroad. Do you understand how that fits into his teaching method?
When Pattabhi Jois teaches abroad, which I haven't had the opportunity or privilege to experience, he does a led class. But the people he has in the led class have already been practicing for many years and have been taken through a standard, so they can then go to one of those led classes. I believe the energy is very high, the count is exact, and it's very demanding. I'd love to do one of them. He is not actually instructing, he is leading people through it and all it is, is inhalation, exhalation, and a correct count of the *vinyasa*. When he went to New Zealand, the level

wasn't there for him to do in that manner, so he did a half-primary for the beginners. He didn't take the beginners right through, but if you work on a numbers and commercial basis and you have more than three or four people beginning at the same time, then you have to lead them through. The question is, how far do you lead them? You can talk through a practice in that manner, if you can really be strict on how far you take them, then it's okay. But if you take a fresh bunch of people all the way through, that's irresponsible. Pattabhi Jois has a certain level of practitioner that he takes through that led class.

What would you say is the difference between practice and teaching? What is the relationship between your practice and your teaching?
As a practitioner, the biggest sacrifice you can make is to teach. Teaching takes so much out of your own practice, especially if you teach in the morning, Mysore style, because the morning is the best time for your own individual practice. So I feel I make the greatest sacrifice to give up my practice time to teach. Then the actual adjusting is a very physical workout, and without already having practiced, it's quite taxing on the body. But if you work it as a yoga practice and choreograph yourself to the class, it can be another practice. I feel very privileged to be a teacher of this method because I think of the teaching as another practice. And I have learned so much from teaching that I have a circle of yoga practice and yoga teaching. When I am doing my own practice, I digest and I process and I feed into a class. And I take from the class what I observe on ten students, fifteen students, in a workshop twenty, thirty students, observe how they all relate to the information that has been given them. What I see in class, I take and reprocess in my own practice, so in fact the dialogue that goes on in my own practice is my own class. Some days it's intense in terms of a dialogue. I have to try to separate that out to be able to do my own individual-focused practice, to get to that inner breath, to get to that inner meditative quality that's there. So sometimes I have to confront an inner turmoil: my own practice is very much a scientific project. My mind is also a class, so I have a double bind there. I'm practicing and teaching. It's all in one, and some days I manage to get in a just-John practice. But that circle of energy that goes around has been very important to me in terms of my evolution. I've learned a lot from my classes. I've created a lot of monsters in terms of how I've presented things over the years, but I've been able to correct those and I've been

able to correct them in my own practice. But I think there is a conflict between teaching and practicing.

Have you injured yourself, and what do you see as the role of pain, injury, or opening?
On the subject of injury, I always think of Graeme Northfield, and when I was going through a very intense knee phase, Graeme said to me, "John, it's just an acute awareness." So from that day onward I've related to the word "injury" not as injury. In conversations, I sometimes use the word "injury" to know what we are talking about, but in a yoga practice there shouldn't be such a thing as injury. If one has injured oneself during yoga, then they have broken the first and the second principles of *ashtanga*, the *yamas* and the *niyamas*. One is being violent to oneself, and one is being greedy or materialistic. So when we reappraise the word "injury" and call it "acute awareness," then we learn that a blockage, or the energy stopping that has occurred, is a teaching. And everybody needs to be able to work through to understand what it is that has caused the so-called injury. So when you call it an acute awareness, by being acutely aware of what's happening, you learn what caused it, why it happened, and what you can do about healing it or growing past it. The term "work through," it is a terrible term. You've got to understand it and then treat it with respect and through that understanding to work with, and breathe through it, and grow.

Yes, I have injured myself, and most of the time it's been related to my ego. If we are too materialistic about our practice, what it looks like and how advanced it is, then you're going to get injured. But that injury will teach you something. It'll teach you humility for a start, and indeed, it's a good one, for most of us will go through injuries because our ego is so out there that we aren't humble enough to be on bended knee. Before I actually touched Guruji's feet [in respect] it was a period that I had knee problems, and subsequently I now understand that the knee is about going forward or change of direction and also the ego, and I've had some ego conflicts. And I finally asked Pattabhi Jois, I said, "Guruji, you know I don't touch your feet?" He said, "Yes." I said, "Should I touch your feet?" He said, "Yes." I said, "Guruji why should I touch your feet?" He said, "For three reasons. One, I'm older than you," so respect. "Two, because I'm your teacher, I'm your guru," again a sign of respect. And, "Thirdly, if you touch your guru's feet, all bad is going, only good is coming." And at that particular time, when finally I asked him something and he gave me the answers, I felt the respect just came out to touch his feet. I could only go down on one knee because the other knee was so swollen.

And I had an ego clash with my very first teacher, Derek, and once all these issues were resolved, I was able to go down on both knees. So it teaches you humility, and again that all ties in with acute awareness. What were you doing that would cause the knee to be injured? Eventually it comes back to, as Guruji says, "Stiff body, stiff mind!"—broken knee, broken mind! The body is expressing what's happening in your mind. So when you solve this stuff up here [in the mind], it's all anatomical. You start to go back: Where's the source of movement coming from? The source of movement is coming from the hip, so you become more acutely aware of how you go into lotus rather than being all egotistical about it and just ramming it [the foot] in there. So the word "injury" is just a word we use to communicate with the people on the outside. But working with it inside, it's an acute awareness.

Do you think ashtanga *yoga attracts a particular kind of person?*
It definitely attracts people who have a very obsessive nature or an addictive nature. I think the practice itself can be very addictive, which is clever. So anyone who's had a drug habit, for example, is perfect because you can swap one addiction for the yoga practice addiction. Now when you start working with the addiction of yoga, the not doing the yoga is a yoga in itself. For five years I could say categorically I didn't miss one day of practice. I was that addicted, and I was that scared to not do it for fear of letting it go. So within the practice there are carrots hanging out in front of you to go further and further and further, but it's always there, too, the system is always testing you. So I think these are some of the reasons why Pattabhi Jois puts in the full and dark moon to give us the opportunity to not practice. So the people with obsessive natures are also challenged within the practice to let go of the practice. Well, we have to release from *padmasana*. [Laughter—John has been sitting in lotus position for the interview.]

How has your relationship with Guruji changed over the years?
I have a very special relationship with Guruji. I think most of the earlier students will have very special relationships with Guruji. For me, he's a

bit like a granddad, he's also like a father, and sometimes he's very much like a guru. Many times I've contemplated looking for a guru, like a spiritual guru or someone that has *siddhis* [magical powers]. Westerners like to see people manifest things [magically] and stuff like that. It's quite silly, because many of the times I looked at that question and then I look at Guruji and I say, "He is the one!" Guruji is my guru, I feel it with a tremendous amount of love and respect. I see the relationship he has with all of his students. He loves every one of his students and he cares about every one of his students and he has a great memory for all the students that have gone before. My personal relationship with him hasn't really changed. I've always had respect and admiration for him. I couldn't touch his feet in the beginning because that wasn't my culture, it wasn't my custom, but the way I related to him was, rather than shaking his hand, which is just a Western thing and didn't feel right, I went to hug him. So when I hugged Guruji, he hugged me back. Now it wasn't like just a blank hug or a stiff-board hug. He actually hugged me like a father hug or a friend hug. And I feel with him, the relationship that I've had with Guruji, he never expected anything of me, but he has a way of getting me to work my best. He's been strict with me, but at the same time he's also given me lots of encouragement and praise in his own way. He has pressed many buttons, but when he's pressed my buttons there's been no sort of aggression or bad judgment or unkindness. And one particular time, he pressed my ego button. All he did was mirror me, and that's when I really realized that he was being a true mirror and he mirrored who I was. And I think after that period that I went through I had a greater respect for him. I can now call him up on the phone and he will know who I am and he will have a conversation with me. It's very special to have that connection with him. He will ask me how my family is, how my children are. He doesn't just think of you as an *asana*, he thinks of you as a person, and a person who has a life and a family, and that family is really very much included in his family. All I can say is that he's a warm, loving man.

Do you have any anecdotes, stories of your time with Guruji?
I think the funniest one was when Guruji was priming me for the third series. I'd come back to Mysore, and he said, "You come back, start third series." It was before Sharmila's wedding. And Shammie's wedding was becoming very expensive and it was time-consuming for Guruji and

he was getting very tired. Prior to the wedding, he said, "Oh, no new *asanas*"—he was saying this to all the students—"Wedding, very busy, very busy. After wedding, new *asana* after wedding." Personally, he said to me, "John Scott, after wedding, starting third series." So during the wedding, here I am having the wedding breakfast and he said, "John Scott, you eat sweets, you eat more sweets, sweets good, make you strong for third series." So, anyway, I ate all the sweets and after the wedding, on the first week after the wedding, I was wise enough not to ask him straightaway for the beginning of the third series. Up to this stage, I had never asked Guruji for a new posture. Anyway, come about the second or third day I thought it must be about time, Guruji is going to start me. But he didn't start me. So I finally took the bait, and I said to Guruji, "When starting third series?" He said, "Oh, not ready yet, not ready yet." And my ego went boom, down to my boots. And I thought, "He said to me before, 'After wedding, starting third series,' during the wedding he said, 'Eat more sweets, make you strong.'" So instantly I got in a mood and I didn't smile at Guruji, I didn't say hi to Guruji, I didn't say goodbye to Guruji, I just did my practice and went out. And he mirrored that completely. So finally I said to Sharath, "Sharath, why is Guruji not starting me on third series?" And Sharath said, "Guruji doesn't think you are good enough." And the ego was really low because Guruji had primed me for it with all this encouragement. And it wasn't until I went to one of the Saturday-afternoon theory sessions which he used to do—and I loved the theory sessions because he'd always tell stories and the introduction to yoga was always, "*Ashtanga* yoga: *yama, niyama, asana, pranayama, pratyahara, dharana, dhyana, samadhi* . . ." And then he would tell the story about the little boy who had some *siddhis* and how he went off to Benares [a city in north India] and he's meditating. And at first I thought he went off to the market to get some bananas just because of his accent. And over the years I had heard the story several times, so I could see the confusion in other people, thinking that when he said Benares he was saying "bananas." Anyway, after the theory class I had eye contact with him and he managed to get a smile out of me. At the end of the class he said to me, "John Scott, how are you?" It was like I hadn't seen him for weeks and I just looked at him and said, "Fine, Guruji." And he gave me this big smile so I just had to smile back at him. And the very next week I started third series. That's quite strange. He finally got me to ask for the postures because I never asked for postures. And I think that was his subtle way of getting my ego to finally express itself because he knew I had one but hadn't displayed it up to then, and he managed to get it to the surface. I always think fondly of that time.

Penzance, 1999

Lino Miele

Lino Miele is well known for publishing the book *Ashtanga Yoga*, a collection of the *vinyasas* of the primary and intermediate series, which he cataloged under Guruji's guidance. He has established many schools in Finland and Norway, and also maintains a school in Rome, Italy, where he lives with his wife and son.

How did you find Guruji?
Actually, you know who discovered Guruji? My wife, Tina. She was—how do you say in English?—stubborn in her search for a guru. She was looking for a guru, we were looking everywhere, and eventually found Guruji's address in the book by André van Lysebeth.

And so we went to Mysore. At a Krishna temple they told us that he was a very well-known master and, "You should go over there." And so we met Guruji.

We pulled back the curtain across the door to the *shala*, looked inside, and I remember Tina said, "What's happening over here?" And we saw at least six to eight sweating bodies, breathing very strong breath, and Guruji was helping one and helping the other one—bing bang boom! And she got a little scared, you know, and said, "He's not going to push me!"—because she was doing the mild yoga, you know, so seeing Guruji helping everybody in very difficult poses was a little shocking.

But after, you know, speaking with him, we released our fear. But I will say it took me a few years to understand the system. I was speaking to myself, I was repeating what others were doing, I thought I was understanding the system, but it took me, oh, four years I believe, four or five—until we met in Lille in 1993.

I still did not have enough respect for him. I had already started the advanced [series in Mysore], and, he look at me and said, "Tomorrow, you start primary." I looked at him and said, "No, Guruji, tomorrow I start intermediate." He look at me and said, "You start primary!" "Guruji, I know what I'm doing, trust me. I start intermediate." He started to yell. He was mad! And there was Amma next to him and she tried speaking in Kannada to him to calm down. I don't know what she told him, he was woowoowoowoowoowoowoowoo. And I said, "Guruji, give me a chance, I come to intermediate," because there were three classes in the morning, 5 a.m. intermediate, 6:30 a.m. and 8 a.m. primary. So I told him, "I come at five," and he was mad. I said, "No, Guruji, I'm here for only a few days." Then the next day I went at eight o'clock, sat down, and he walk in the room wearing a *lungi*. He didn't say anything, he look at me, then he start the class, finish the class, and he come in front of me. I was sitting down and he say, "What time you start?"

I look at him, I didn't answer. He said, "Five a.m." Of course, he was a little upset with me. He looked at me, and I believe I start to understand better my guru, and I hoped he was content, pleased with my practice, but he didn't say anything. After one week, we went to give a demonstration in Zinal, Switzerland, so it was good. Then I start my relationship with Guruji.

There was this Frenchman, he asked me, "But Lino, do you understand Guruji?" I say, "Of course I do." I thought I did. "But you know that he's repeating, '*Ekam, dve, trini, chatvari*'—what's that?" "Numbers, and he repeats all the time the same numbers," I said. He said, "No! I have a piece of paper and there are different numbers, what is this?" "I don't know."

Everybody was asking Guruji about a [teaching] certificate. Amma, she answered, "Oh, a certificate! You take a test, exam. Like me and Guruji." I say, "Which test?" She say, "Yeah, we took a test with Krishnamacharya. So you want a certificate, you take a test." "What kind of test?" "Exam," she says, "each *asana* has its own *vinyasa*. When we trained with him, he was calling a name of the *asana*, let's say *pasasana*, and after that he would say, '*Ashto*,' the eighth *vinyasa* of *pasasana*, so we were to jump into the eighth *vinyasa*. Was it inhaling or exhaling? Was it the posture itself, or a movement, what is this? And that was the test for all the six series." She told me that Guruji used to wake up during the night and give numbers. [*Laughter*] Guruji was calling out a name, "*Krounchasana*, six-teen!" like this, he was just dreaming. Guruji was just laughing as she told us.

So I spoke with the Frenchman, and I told him the story that Amma told me. "This is interesting," he said. "We should do research." And then we start to do the research. So we did the first series, the second series, the third series with Guruji, and after one year we finished the fourth se-ries. And I was very pleased, of course, you know, that he explained this system to me.

But the *vinyasa* system is not only the inhale-exhale, there is also the *vinyasa* of each pose, how many *vinyasa*, and so on. So the book came out, but it was not a book, it was research, it was my research with Gu-ruji. And then we decided together to make a book, and he even told me, I remember, "You make ten thousand copies," and I said, "Yes, Guruji, how much we should sell each copy?" "One hundred dollars." "Guruji, one hundred dollars, one copy?" "Yes. This book, one hundred dollars." I think it's too much, but at that time I didn't understand Guruji very well. When he says one hundred dollars, it's not that we sell for one hundred dollars, it was the value of the book, that was the one hundred dollars. You cannot sell a book for one hundred dollars. Do you remember the first one? It was only the *vinyasa*. The benefits [of the postures] were not there.

What about third and fourth series?
That is another story.

The book is coming?
No, no, the book is there, it's ready. Did you see the new edition?

Yes.
John Scott did the drawing of the third series, now he is supposed to do the drawing of the fourth, so we included the advanced A into the first and second series book. I made the photocopy of the book from the com-puter, I sent it to Guruji, as usual—he gives the approval over everything. After two weeks, I call. "Guruji, did you receive the book?" "Yes." "Guruji, what do you think about the book?" "Good, well done, but take the last part out." "Which part, Guruji?" "Advanced A—we don't want." I say, "Guruji, you mean that you don't want advanced A?" And he say, "We

don't want." "Okay, Guruji, we take it out, bye-bye." We hang up the phone. After two days I call back. "I want to speak with Sharath," and he says, "No, Sharath is not here." "Guruji, last time you told me that you don't want advanced A, I have to take out advanced A from the book." He say, "We don't want." "Okay, Guruji," and I hang up. After one week, I call back again. I say, "Guruji, you sure that we don't want advanced A?" He say, "We don't want. Finished!" "Okay, Guruji. I take it out for you," and I hang up the phone.

I took out advanced A. John sent an e-mail to Eddie Stern, who was in Mysore, to ask Guruji why he don't want advanced A. It was an extra check, you know, sometimes we don't understand, and he said, "People will look [at the book] and people will repeat [imitate], and that is no good." And he was right, that was a good answer. You see, people look at the book, look at advanced A, they want to do it, the ego is very high, and they break themselves. For what reason? There is no reason to do this. So he said, "We don't want. In the future, maybe in the future, when people are more ready to understand *ashtanga* better." So I have the book, but it's in the drawer.

That time you went to do the demonstration in Switzerland, there was a yoga conference and Guruji saw what was happening and said, okay, we'll show them what real yoga is.
Yes. Guruji was invited for one week teaching over there, I believe. Guruji didn't understand very well what was happening. So we told Guruji, "Guruji, we will come with you."

We went with him and he start to teach. But the room they gave us, actually they didn't give us a good room, they gave us the bar, where you drink. The bar was a big bar, with all the liquors, everything on the bar, and we had this bar to use and Guruji was teaching yoga there.

I tell you this because, you know, the man, the human being of Guruji. "I'm teaching, I don't care, you give me this, I take this, no problem." It's not that he presents himself, "I am the best." He just says, "Give me the bar, okay." We were a little upset because we feel uncomfortable. "What do you mean, my guru comes and you give the bar to teach?" He didn't say anything.

Two days later I was looking at a *big* guru, another guru, he had not spoken for twenty-five years, so he was just writing words. And he asks, "What do you want to do?," to the audience, and we were maybe fifty people. "What do you want to do? What do you want to start with? To start with *pranayama*, meditation? Just tell."

Nobody was speaking. No answer. I say okay, I get up and say, "Start them with *asana*, we warm up, can you show us something?" So he took off his shirt and I look at him and what's happening? I saw his belly button to one side and down. I don't remember if it was on the right or the left, it was not in the center. I look. And a friend of mine, another teacher, says, "What's wrong with this man? Look at his belly button. Look at this energy!" I'm looking at the belly button, I get up, I leave. This was around two in the afternoon, and around four the same man run after me, he say, "Come, come! Guruji wants to speak to you." So I went.

This was the first time that Guruji called me out, so I went in his room. Guruji say, "What did you do today?" I did my practice, I did help, because we were helping him teach in the morning, and he say, "No, no, no. After. In the afternoon, what did you do?" I went to work, I went to do third series. "No, no, no, you went to the conference!" Ah yes, I went. "Then what happen?" "I look at the man, I didn't like, I get up, I left." "Why did you leave?" "Guruji, why I left? His belly button was one side and down. What kind of energy has this man, you know? I left, I know the belly button has to be center." There is a technique, if you know how to channel the energy, actually the belly button could move. A few years back, a great teacher in the north show me how to place the belly button in the same position. It looked strange.

So Guruji said, "The belly button is down, tomorrow come!"

We went. Guruji walk inside. He didn't want to sit on the floor, he ask for a chair and he sit right in front of him, on the chair, looking at him. Ammaji sat on the floor, look at him. And he start, the man start. Guruji was very serious-looking. Happens that one of these teachers was the translator for Guruji, so wherever Guruji went, he was next to him. He said, "Lino I have to go to the toilet."

He get up. Amma saw him go outside. I saw Amma leaving, I went after her. Outside, Amma start to laugh and after one minute everyone walk outside, all the *ashtanga* group. Guruji walk outside, laughing.

"Everybody in my room." We went to his room. He told the translator, "You go downstairs to the office and speak to the other teacher and we give a demonstration in two days. We will show them what yoga is." And then the demonstration came out. There is a video of this demonstration,

I don't know if you ever saw this video, I never saw it myself, but they sell it in the States.

They say that it is a very good video because Guruji starts to give the best of himself in this conference, because there were six of us giving demonstration and maybe more than one hundred teachers looking at us and Guruji explaining in Sanskrit and in English.

I believe it was the first demonstration that Pattabhi Jois give in France or Switzerland. And from that we start to understand, I start to understand that I didn't know, I still don't know. There is too much to ask, too much to write with Pattabhi Jois. So this is how my relationship started with him.

Did Ammaji understand everything, do you think?
I know she did *ashtanga* yoga, so she knew. Every time I was finished with practice in Mysore, I was passing by and all the time she knew that I was not drinking coffee, but every day she was offering me coffee, and asking, "How are you?" and was like this and like that, she was really good. You know, it was a big loss not only for the students, not only for the family, but for everybody. She was the—how do you say in English?—the link between us and Guruji.

We felt it, because in Guruji's yoga *shala*, it is like *this* and it is like this *no question*. But outside, Guruji's a human being—he's laughing, and they are cooking together. She was a big loss.

When she died, we went over there. Guruji, he was crying and saying, "What I'm going to do with my life?"

I have a feeling that Guruji gives more of himself to the students now. He's there every day, talking, very open, very loving. Something has really changed. What he was giving to Amma, he's giving more to the students.
I know there are many, many—how do you say?—silly questions are asked and that is natural, you know, but Guruji is the type of guru that they should have precise questions. To understand his knowledge and not, "Guruji, how are you?" or "Are you vegetarian?" or "What do you eat, or should I eat?" or something like that. Because when we were working with the *ashtanga* yoga book and *Yoga Mala*, when Guruji starts, he gives from his heart and he comes out with a lot of speaking, speaking, speaking. Many things come from him, many.

So what is the essence of this teaching, do you think?
It's very clear for me: the *vinyasa* system. *Vinyasa* for me is the essence of his teaching. Forget about the system, but the *vinyasa* itself, synchronized breath and movement, yeah that might be the gross part. *Vinyasa* has another meaning. *Vinyasa* is spirituality, the way you move, the way you feel inside, and that is *vinyasa*, too, and that is the breath. He's so precise that he calls it the scientific method. Think about this: Who are you to call it scientific? Can you prove? Yes, he can prove. It is a scientific method. He's so precise, and that many people don't understand. When you are watching the video, first and second series, he's very precise. Hear him leading the class, he's very precise. When, how to inhale, how to exhale, how to move, and so on.

What do you think is the connection between this precise instruction and the spiritual aspect of what he is teaching?
If you know the system, how to breathe, how to move, it goes very deep, deep, deep inside. Touching the essence, touching the soul, like that is the link. I read once that somebody ask Krishnamacharya, "What is yoga?" And the answer is: "Breath and movement."

What's the relationship between this system and the eight limbs, in your view?
It's very like what Guruji is teaching all the time. He's teaching that when we speak of the eight limbs, the first two are very difficult to achieve—*yama* and *niyama*. So there is *asana*. With the *asana*, with the purification [through *asana* practice], cleansing the system, you clean up your mind.

You start doing *yoga chikitsa* [primary series]. Why? To take away, to prevent all the illness. So he's teaching: you start with the *asana*. It's not like when reading a book you say, "Now I know everything." With this system, you clean yourself up and you change your attitude. This is my experience and my students' experience. So the teaching starts with *asana*. It can speak to you, it can tell us many things, but it's not the complete truth.

With the purification, with the system, with Guruji, how come after many years people around you say, "Hey, you look better, your eyes . . . you look different to me"? If you think, "I have to be good! I have to be good! I have to be good!" does it work? No. Do it and all is coming! Why?

He is right! And the power, if you want to call it the power, of Guruji, the strength of the system is this. There is no other, you see? Yoga is experience. You do it and you see what happens. Yoga is for everybody, but not everybody can do *ashtanga*, especially because it works deep, deep inside of us. Start from the *asana*, slowly, slowly. Guruji, when he used to tell us, I was beginning to understand. Now, after more than ten years, I start to understand better.

He speaks about the *vinyasa* system in *Yoga Mala*. He even speaks about meditation, *dhyana*, also he speaks about the *drishti*, the breath, the movement, the *asana* and *dhyana*, of course the *bandhas*, the technique to channel the energy. At this point, you're doing yoga, otherwise its just exercise. And he's right. You experience it within yourself, and that is the best way.

What type of changes have you personally experienced through this practice, and what do you see happening in your students?
In my practice, you know, I was very proud. [*Laughter*] Even my ego, I could not control it, I was *rrrr*, like this, like that, and the practice cut me down, even mentally, you know? It's quite demanding, the practice. If you survive, somebody wrote, do the practice and if you survive, for sure you change. Even my thinking is changing. What kind of book I'm looking at, reading is changing, but mostly you see it in the family, with your friends, with your students, in the way they look at you.

Many people—no smile on the face. It takes maybe two years and then they smile. It's good, that effect is wonderful, you know, but you don't need to do the advanced A, B, C, D [advanced postures] to reach this point. Absolutely not.

What is the use of the advanced asanas?
In my experience, the advanced makes my mind lucid, more lucid, I understand better. And when I do advanced, if I have any problems in my mind, it's like I resolve the problem and my mind is clear and I feel much much better.

But you know what Guruji was saying, how it works deeper. Inside is the fruit. Try [to go] deeper inside. Of course we should be prepared. Many people don't do it and they blame the *ashtanga*. "*Ashtanga* did this to me and it's . . ." No, no! You did this to yourself! Many people feel pain. "I feel this, why?" The breath is very important, the quality of the breath is very important, and the length of the breath is very important. To reach this state of mind, to calm down.

The length of the inhale and exhale being the same—
Yes, yes, inhale and exhale with the movement, for this reason they called it the psychic breath. Why? It works inside, it gives time for your ribs and your body to open up, you are aware of the movement, you are aware of the inhale, you are aware of the exhale, your mind calms down.

I never heard that expression before—the psychic breath. Is that your invention?
Absolutely not.

Where does it come from?
You can read in the *Hatha Yoga Pradipika*, there are two meanings of *ujjayi* breathing. One is victorious breath and one is psychic breath. I read in *Hatha Yoga Pradipika* translated by Satyananda.

Reading something like that gives more value to what Guruji is teaching, because according to my experience with Guruji, he is teaching a long breath. I did a practice of ten seconds each inhalation, ten seconds each exhalation, then it takes three hours, the primary series! It's very hard to maintain the same length. I think about how it works on your body and your mind, with all the *bandhas* and everything.

I've heard him say twenty seconds for each inhalation and exhalation.
Even twenty-five. I look at him, I say, "I think it's too much!" He say, "No." [*Laughter*] But of course, when we do the practice over there [back home], we speed up, because there is not too much time.

What do you see your role as a teacher to be?
My path first is to make people understand the breath, for me most important is the breath; then the movement, then comes the *asana*. What we call the perfect *asana* takes a long, long time. Some *asanas* take five, six, seven years. You spend many years to calm down the mind with the breath with the *vinyasa* system. I wrote a book with Pattabhi Jois, to make them understand how to work with the breath. Just like that, that is my part. Many other teachers do the same. For me, I emphasize more, in the beginning, the *vinyasa* system. The breath, the movement, where

to look, and how to work the *bandhas*. Each teacher is different, so we give according to our personality.

Are people still practicing in the same way as they were twenty years ago, do you think?
If they follow Guruji. The problem with us as human beings, in the long run, being a teacher, we like to change things around and we like to include this but not this. This we write in a book, "according to the way Pattabhi Jois teaches," which is not the truth! But who knows? Can we tell these people, "It's not the way Pattabhi Jois is teaching, why you write down? Why use his name?" What can I say? When we spoke about this with Pattabhi Jois, Pattabhi Jois said, "Lino, when people are ready. When there are two books, let's face it, they know which has value. In the long run, people start to understand."

Two books?
He meant if there is *Yoga Mala* and then another book speaking about *ashtanga*, in the long run we understand which is the book of value, if you are really into the practice. I hope in fifty years, when he won't be with us anymore, it won't be a mess, that everybody, every teacher say, "No it's this, no it's that, no it's that, no it's that." Now there is a line to follow according to Guruji. It's this one. That's right. But people say he's changing all the time.

Do you think he teaches people differently?
At the beginning, yes. Of course, as a teacher you don't change the system. If I cannot do that particular *asana*, if I cannot do that particular *drishti*, of course you change it. But that does not mean you are changing the system, you are adapting.

Does he change it when he teaches?
Does he adapt it, you mean? Sometimes he was telling me something and there was someone else who was not ready to accept this teaching [who heard his instructions to Lino] and they were repeating the same. But it was for me at that point [in practice] but maybe it was not a final pose, maybe it was not a final *drishti*, but they think, "Because he is doing it, so should I." That is why, when researching the book, I asked many, many times to make sure I had it right. And that is the final

[word]. But it causes some confusion because Guruji tells a student one thing because of where they are in their practice and they say to me, "Guruji told me to look at the foot, but in your book it says look at the nose." That's okay, look at the foot, when you are ready you will look at the nose. But there is always evolution and the book may not be final. But it is one thing changing the system which has been there for many, many years, and another changing the *drishti*.

What did you notice from the correct drishtis?
It has to do with directing the energy, moving the energy. I always felt that his teaching was subtle and he was always working on that focus of moving energy and directing your attention and focus to certain things. But only when necessary would he correct you.

He would get you to work on a certain thing for some time, and then when he felt it was necessary he would adjust something. He would never be in a hurry. He would change things gradually, he may give you only one or two instructions in a six-month period, and gradually he would adjust things. Not in one day. He would look for certain things, and when he felt the time was right, he would introduce something else.

Koralam, 2000

Peter Sanson

Peter Sanson grew up on a farm in New Zealand. He left for Mysore in 1989, having no experience in *ashtanga* yoga, and has spent years studying with Guruji. Peter is considered one of the old students, and always has a calm and collected view of his practice.

How is it that you first started doing yoga?
This Australian woman came to stay at my friend's house when I was at university, and my friend rang me up and said, "This woman has come to stay at my house, she eats bean sprouts and peanut butter on rice wafers and does yoga." I went to my friend's house about a week later, and my friend and I did a class with her in the garage. I did two classes with her. Since that moment, I've done yoga.

Was that ashtanga *yoga?*
No, she was a student of B. K. S. Iyengar. She had just come from Pune.

How old were you when you did yoga in the garage?
About twenty-one. I came here [to Mysore] when I was twenty-four. After university I was doing *hatha* yoga once per week, Wednesday nights at six. I went every week with a guy called Michael Jones. The teacher at the university recommended me to go to a school in Sydney, but I ended up in Queensland. I was in a health-food shop and saw a sign for Nicki Know and James Brian, so I studied with them. Nicki and James were doing Iyengar. They came to know of *ashtanga* through *Yoga Journal*. It had an article in 1987 by Jane McMullen.

Nicki and James decided to come to India in 1988—had written to Guruji and gotten permission to come—and asked me if I wanted to come with them. Then I wrote to Guruji, and it took some time to get a reply, and I had to get a visa, so I ended up coming in January 1989.

What happened when you got to India?
Man, it was wild. I got to Chennai and took the train from Chennai to Mysore. It was a bit of a shock. I met Guruji at the old *shala*.

What were your first impressions of Guruji and the shala?
At the *shala* I was met by Guruji wearing a dhoti with a thread over his shoulder. He asked me for my letter and told me, "Sit down." He said nothing for some time, and I became quite anxious and started thinking he might reject me as his student! Finally, he told me to return the next morning at 6 a.m.

But you did not really know any ashtanga *yoga?*
At that stage I did not know any. I didn't even know a sun salute.

How did Guruji teach you?
He started me at six in the morning in the upstairs room with an Indian lady, and the regular class was going on downstairs. They were mainly quite advanced practitioners at that time. I looked in the window and heard them breathing, and that freaked me out. It was a good thing that Guruji took me upstairs. I stayed for six months.

What was it like?
It was nerve-racking. He taught me the sun salute, and then he went downstairs and would come back after some time. I remember that I built up to doing twenty-four of the sun salutes. He started me on A, and in one week I was doing twelve of A and twelve of B and then sitting down and doing the breathing. That was my program. Then slowly he taught me the standing positions, the two *padangushtasanas*, then the two *trikonasanas*. Slowly like that.

Was the Indian lady learning at the same rate as you?
Similar. She was more advanced than me. She was flexible, I was stiff.

How long did he keep you upstairs?
Quite some time, for at least a month, because I can't recall going down-

stairs for quite a while. But then at some stage the class downstairs got quite small, by April or May the students were getting less when the heat came, it was only half, maybe a dozen students. And then he brought me downstairs.

After you had been doing all the other yoga, and then you started the ashtanga yoga, how did it strike you? What was the impression you had of the actual practice?
I loved it. It was much more active and I liked the way Guruji was teaching it, and it was a much shorter practice. At first I was practicing only half an hour. I was used to doing a lot more *asanas* before that. [Now] I was doing very few and a lot of repetition and I was really enjoying it from the first moment.

How about the idea of yoga being a physical or spiritual practice? Was that ever a question for you?
The question never came up because I didn't see it as one or the other. I was just doing the practice and enjoying it, and enjoying being with Guruji and feeling really good. It touched me on a deep level, and being with Guruji was like nothing else I had ever experienced before.

In the past you have characterized Guruji's teachings as being very subtle.
Very subtle. He is very much completely in the moment with people, so you connect with him in the moment on that level. He is very subtle in how he works with you in terms of your personality, emotions, any physical or mental blocks, and he knew how to move the energy and move through subtle layers with you.

I remember you talking about ardha baddha paschimattanasna, *that you had stiff knees.*
I couldn't bend at all at first. Even though I had done quite a bit of yoga, I couldn't make a lot of *asanas*. He was very hands-on, he would get hold of you and mold you into things. You had to surrender to his adjustments, and then you would be safe. If you tried to resist anything you were in serious trouble. Many times I could hear things tearing in my body—like the sound of sheets ripping—I thought I was going to be finished. But in the end I would just let go, and surrender up to him, and allow him to take me into the different *asanas*, and then I was safe.

He could just feel where he wanted you to be.
Yeah, exactly.

Were there times when you were all by yourself?
That first year I was here. By the end of May all the Western students had left, and then I joined the Indian class at 5 a.m. That was in the monsoon. I was having the time of my life.

Was the energy different between the Western and Indian class?
Very much so. The Indian students were much more relaxed about their approach, and would often stop and chat among themselves, especially when Guruji left the room for coffee.

Did their approach make an impact on the way you decided to practice?
They were not so into pushing or straining, they weren't so hung up on who was doing what *asana*; their practice was more like a gentle daily ritual. I really liked the way they were practicing. It left a lasting impression on me.

I remember that one guy who used to get up and fix his hair every few asanas.
[*Laughter*] Yeah, they would sometimes skip out on a few things here and there also.

How about Guruji? Was his teaching style or attitude different between the two classes?
He was still quite strict with them also. He was pretty much the same, as far as I can remember. But they were more relaxed and familiar with Guruji than we were.

Were they coming primarily for health issues, or were they just doing their practice?
Guruji had a few therapy cases at that time, even with the Westerners.

What kinds did you see?
People with spinal or heart problems. A lot of the Indians were older and had health issues.

Did you ever watch his therapy?
Yes, he taught them in the same class. He had them on simple, modified programs, adjusting them. According to their capacity, he would adjust and slowly work with them. Just simplified everything down, but still *ashtanga* yoga.

Who was the gentleman who was popping nitroglycerin tablets?
Alexander. He had severe gout and heart problems. He had a mild heart attack on the street to Nagarathna's and I remember thinking, thank God that Graeme Northfield was here because he was a registered nurse, and if Alexander had a heart attack in class, Graeme would know what to do!

Guruji put him on a diet and had him doing very gentle Sun salutations. Within one month he was off his tablets. His diet was restricted to what he could hold in his two hands. He really improved. He stayed here more than twelve or eighteen months studying.

What about Amma? Did she give you tips on your practice?
Yes, one or two. *Mula bandhasana.* She used to keep a check on the yoga students. She was quite involved in the school. Because we were so few, she would know all of us also, and would quite often call us in for a cup of coffee. From time to time we would have a meal at Guruji's house, which was nice. She was a lovely lady. She was the only person I ever heard tell off Guruji.

She always used to know who had back pain, who had knee pain.
Very much so. She kept a little bit of a check.

Eventually you started teaching yoga, but you did not start off wanting to be a yoga teacher.
When I came back one time, a lady named Judy Colbert, who was living in Gisborne, asked me to come and show her what I was doing, so I showed her a little of what I learned from Guruji. And I think there were two or three people who became interested at that time, so I showed them a few sun salutations and a few simple things. I was helping them on a Monday night, and that's how my class began. I had that Monday-night class for about ten years.

Did Guruji ever give you any tips on teaching?
Not really, because I was too scared to even mention to him that I was teaching that class. I didn't discuss it with him, but I did ask him one time about teaching yoga, and he told me first that I should complete fifth series and learn Sanskrit. So I put my head down and just focused on my practice.

What kind of changes have you seen in your life and in the lives of other practitioners?
Guruji and his teachings changed my life. I'd graduated from university in New Zealand and was set to start a career in property valuation. But after I started to practice with Guruji, my entire focus was on yoga. I would stay in Mysore till my money ran out, then return to New Zealand and work on the family farm—fencing, pruning trees, doing general work.

When people start practicing I notice their body shape change quite dramatically, sometimes their faces can even take on a different appearance. I guess it is a reflection of the changes happening on quite a deep level. Also I find it interesting how quickly new practitioners adjust their diets after starting the *ashtanga*.

Did you ever see Guruji as a healer?
I had total faith in Guruji from the start. He was a teacher, a healer, and a psychologist—all essential qualities for a yoga teacher. He connected immediately with people, understanding their experiences, and was very supportive of whatever anyone was going through. Often things would arise in the practice, and Guruji would help. Not always did things directly connect with the *asanas*, but more with life. I think all the students were learning a great deal about themselves, and it was helpful to have advice from someone so wise.

What about the other limbs? Tell me about your thoughts on everything that comes after yama, niyama, asana. *How is it integral or not to what Guruji is teaching?*
To me, Guruji embodied everything that comes after. It was all integrated from the start. My understanding was that it was an integrated practice, all of the limbs of yoga are integrated into the practice. That is my un-

derstanding to this day, and in fact the more I practice the more I understand how integrated it is with the breathing. He was working in a very focused way with the breathing from the first moment, and I realized that it was a very meditative experience, and automatically the other limbs, such as the behavioral limbs and diet, started coming into it from the start. I was so awed by him that it took me nearly a year before I summoned the courage to touch his feet.

Did you feel that he was a healer of sorts, or perhaps that he had psychological insights into the nature of the students he was teaching?
I think those are essential qualities for a yoga teacher anyway, and he was able very easily to connect with people directly in the moment and go with whatever their experience was, and that was a very special quality he had. To be very present and in the moment with the student, and very supportive of whatever anyone was going through.

Do you remember any particular situation?
I can't remember in particular, but many times stuff comes up with the practice, and Guruji could quite often help with what was arising. A lot of the things coming up weren't necessarily to do with the *asanas* but with lessons that I was learning about life. Coming to know my own nature a little bit.

And as for the practice itself?
He was a master at details. You wouldn't think it, but he paid a lot of attention to the details. The pointing of the toes, the position of the hands. Everything. Right from the first moment there were certain details that he was very strong on always. Certain things that he would emphasize: *drishtis*, breathing, many small things. Certain things he would emphasize and you would have to do them before he would move you along. He would look for a level of proficiency in each *asana*. He was much bigger on details than people would imagine.

What was the most important thing you have learned?
The most important thing I learned from Guruji is the need for patience. Guruji once kept me on the same *asana* for seven years, which broke down a lot of physical and mental barriers. He taught everyone individu-

ally, intuitively, and from the heart. When Guruji finally moved me to the next *asana*, I realized the specific *asana* didn't matter; it was more important to focus on the level of attention one brings to the practice.

Was he doing any conferences or lectures back then?
Yes, he would call a conference from time to time on the weekend, and we would come and he would discuss some certain something. Not too many, from time to time. A lot of it went over my head in the early days. On a more personal level, he would call you into his office and test you on the names of the *asanas*, you had to know the names of the *asanas*, and that was nerve-racking because I didn't know the names at first. And you had to know the *vinyasas*, also.

Would he make you do the asana?
In the early days, on one or two occasions. From time to time he would tell me that I should start studying Sanskrit. I tried a little, mainly to learn the Aditya Hridayam. I started slowly with a local scholar.

What do you know about his personal practices, or the Yoga Korunta, *or his practices with Krishnamacharya?*
Only from the stories he would tell. He would talk about Krishnamacharya from time to time. He had tremendous respect for him, the utmost respect for his teacher. He would also talk about the *Yoga Korunta* from time to time. He knew parts of it by heart and would quote from it as they related to what you might be working with, especially having to do with the *vinyasas*, that you must do them, with the breathing, the *drishtis*, and working with *mula* and *uddiyana bandha*. In conference, these were the things that he would talk about.

These are the things that you would say are the essence of his practice?
Definitely. He always emphasized correct breathing and *drishtis*, and working with the *bandhas*.

What do you see as the central importance of correct breathing? If a student comes and asks you, "What's up with this breathing thing, why do I have to breathe?"
It is the central thing to this whole practice. Without that, it is not a yoga practice. Everything is moving with the breath on so many levels.

How about mula *and* uddiyana bandha?
Also very important, on an energetic level. Without that, it is not the same practice. Once I started to work with the *bandhas* with Guruji, my body became light and the energy started to move smoothly. He would have us work on it right from the start with upward and downward dog, emphasizing in upward dog to tighten the anus and in downward dog to look at the navel and pull up from the groin and below the navel. Not all the time, but from time to time he would get us to work with it. He would always correct the *drishtis*.

What did you notice from the correct drishtis?
It has to do with directing the energy, moving the energy. I always felt that his teaching was subtle and he was always working on that focus of moving energy and directing your attention and focus to certain things. But only when necessary would he correct you. He would get you to work on a certain thing for some time, and then when he felt it was necessary he would adjust something. He would never be in a hurry. He would change things gradually, he may give you only one or two instructions in a six-month period, and gradually he would adjust things. Not in one day. He would look for certain things, and when he felt the time was right, he would introduce something else.

As Guruji began to get a little older, what changes did you see in how he was teaching?
In the early years he was incredibly strong. I recall him being incredibly strong until two years ago, actually, so I didn't notice too many changes in terms of his teaching. In the teaching, he didn't seem to age. There really weren't any changes. It was pretty much exactly the same because he just had, even though he was aging, boundless energy. I did notice a change after Amma died. That affected him a lot. But in his teaching, he was just as strict.

Even after he got sick two years ago, he didn't get the idea that it was anything more than a temporary lay up for him, that he needed to rest for a while but that he would be back teaching soon.
Even last year with the led classes he taught, he was still going strong, except that he started getting tired easily. That was the main physical change.

Can you say something about Guruji's character/personality?
There was no mucking about with Guruji. He was a very disciplined man, with a strong character, and deeply religious—this permeated his whole way of life—but he could be very playful and had a good sense of humor.

There is one thing Guruji said that has really stuck with me over the years. He pointed to his heart and said, "There is a small box sitting here. / In that box is sitting Atman. / Turn your attention here. That is yoga." I will never forget that. I always felt he was a very heart-centered man, loving toward his students and doing all he could to support us on our journey.

Mysore, 2009

Rolf Naujokat

Rolf Naujokat arrived in India in the 1970s, and immersed himself in the ancient ways of Indian spirituality, living with *sadhus* and traveling as a mendicant. Meeting Guruji proved transformational. Rolf resides in Goa, as he has for the past twenty years, where he teaches *ashtanga* yoga with love and enthusiasm.

Can you tell me the story of how you came to India?
It was in '73 or '74, and I came actually on that hippie road—Istanbul, Afghanistan, and then Pakistan, India—not knowing much about yoga but being more into that hippie trip. After India, I came to a place in Hyderabad, which changed my approach in life. I got in touch with what is called "yoga" and it went deeper and deeper. So there it was that I met my first guru; this *babaji* brought me on the path of yoga. And there everything started for me. And then in '75 I had established already a daily practice, not *ashtanga* but *hatha* yoga in a traditional way with *pranayama* and a lot of *kriya* and sitting practice. So I really had my little *sadhana*, with days of fasting and different kinds of things in the way of yoga and that stayed with me until now.

The style has changed over the years. And then I had a time when I was practicing Iyengar yoga for seven years, and then I changed into *ashtanga*. I met *ashtanga* in '80 to '83 when I lived with Danny Paradise and Cliff Barber, who were practicing *ashtanga* yoga and I was doing Iyengar then. And they turned me on to *ashtanga* and the four sequences. So I practiced . . . not regularly. And I was still doing Iyengar and teaching Iyengar. It was old-style Iyengar; there were less props, still a lot of jumpings. It was very pleasant.

But slowly *ashtanga* took over more and more, and I kept practicing and teaching the other way, which was fine because I see yoga as a one-ness and I don't see so many differences in different systems. It's more about the nature of people and how it fits to them. And then finally, in the beginning of the '90s, I came to Guruji. And then, when I met Guruji, it was very clear. There was no question. I just saw him and I was like, "Yeah, that's my teacher." There it carries on; there is guru *shakti*; *shakti* manifest in this man. Then I stayed, and came every year at least one time a year, mostly between three and six months. Sometimes I came two times a year, depending on how my financial situation was. It was easy because I lived in Goa and it was only fifteen hours' bus ride from Mysore.

That's why I was able to spend quite some time there, but it was mainly all in the small *shala* [in Lakshmipuram]. And in the beginning when I came, there were maybe eight people [practicing] in the *shala* [at a time]. Then the next year twelve, and then there were two shifts of twelve people, and that was for a long time like that. And after came more and more people. This time in the small *shala* was very important for me. The attention from Guruji was just full-on. He was always there with us. There was no moment when he wasn't with us. You knew he was adjusting always one of us. And Sharath started also to teach and so there were two of them. Often we were trying not to get adjusted, so they were always there with our practice. They knew our practice and it was a connection, which was not so much based in words and vocalization but more in feeling the body—how Guruji touches us one day and then the next day. You see that every opening he achieves in a different way, and he adjusts us to bring us to another level, depending on what the *asana* was and where we were in the practice. And Sharath just grew up in the grace of Guruji to become a teacher. And over the years he developed amazingly until he's now taking over the whole thing. But these times for me were the precious times. The big *shala* is amazing, but it's just differ-ent. But I feel I received most of the blessings there [in the old *shala*]. It was a bit of a family, with Guruji, and Amma making coffee, and every student knowing each other. In the afternoon we cooked together. It was a very, very graceful and special time. And Guruji just became a channel of guru *shakti* which manifested through him. And the more I was ready to receive, the more I was able to receive. That was my arrival and time in Mysore, in short words.

Can you say something about Guruji, his personality, how he teaches, what his energy is like, and how he treated you personally?

He treated me in a way that I felt I needed it. I had a little bit, or quite a bit of an ego when I came there. In some way, he broke it down. He was always shouting at me in the practice, always shouting, always correcting. But it was not in a mean way, in a way it was to eliminate something which was not necessary. And after he was very friendly, loving, and receptive. We would meet in the market and he was buying fruit or vegetables and he was very sweet. But during the teaching, he was very firm and straightforward, there was no bullshit. I feel his teaching in those days was very personal. When I saw how he adjusted or he taught a pose or some part of the sequence to some people, and how he taught it to other people, even if they were learning the same *asana* and the same sequence, it was taught so that the person could understand it the way they were able to learn it. So I felt it was very personal, the teaching in those days, even if it was eight or twelve people in the room. And you were just feeling that both Sharath and Guruji know your practice and know where to help, where to adjust and where not to adjust. What I really loved in the beginning, it was just eight of us and I had the first shift. Later, when there were more shifts, I was allowed to sit maybe the next two shifts and see how he and Sharath were adjusting. And this was a big, big learning process for me, and many of those things I received there I use now when I'm teaching or when I have students. Yeah, it was a big learning process.

Can you describe a little bit what it is that Guruji teaches?

The *asana* aspect you know: it is a system that is still practiced now more or less the same. But it matters how it is brought over individually to people. And it brought me to a point where I got confronted by my blockages, or discomfort in myself, or what you can call very simply "ego." And to a point where you can't let go anymore without anger or attachment until it just falls off; it's not a pulling off. Something, it just falls off. And it was how Guruji is and was teaching, and I think other students experience it very different.

I felt him very, very close to my process of call it "waking up" or something like that. And also, somehow, when I think back to that moment there on the mat, and especially when I stayed focused on my breath again and again, how it concentrated the mind. It was like bringing me into the here and now on that mat in that moment of sweating, in that moment of being in his arms adjusting and feeling a kind of love or whatever you call it coming over from him. It is very subtle, difficult to put into words, somehow making it less, toning it down.

Individually, he is something very special. And I often felt it was like a kind of *shakti* that comes through him using his body and mind. Sri Pattabhi Jois was a tool, which was so ripe and ready that it allowed his *shakti* to pass through him and give it to other people, bringing them to their own practice. I think what Guruji wants to do in his teaching is to bring us to our own practice, not to just depend on a certain school or teacher. This is my idea and how I received it. That's why I went there for three or six months of practice, and then I came back here to Goa, taught a bit and kept up my practice. When I was ready next year, I went back. So in this case, I feel he is giving that—bringing you into your own practice and that's what the whole thing is about.

And the yoga is about remembering that we are already one with the divinity and that we've never left it. Only the illusion of the mind makes us different, pulls us into this aspect of dualism. I feel all the teachers I had taught me that, and during the time when I came to Guruji it was just a continuation of this guru *shakti* manifesting through him in this way. I like to put it this way because I know no other words to use or explain it. And the thing is, in a certain moment when we are getting also older, you feel that it is much more subtle. It's not just about putting your legs behind the head or grabbing your ankles. What happens with the practice of the system is a bit beyond the *asana* aspect. The *asana* and the breathing system is a tool to bring you or us to that point of a nondualistic view of God, not just by reading about it in books but by experiencing it inside. Also, again and again, the aspect of letting go—because the older you get, you can't just throw yourself into *kapotasana*. You need a few breaths to go in and open, to be in that process of doing. Somewhere you realize the message that yoga is much more than *asana*, and I think that is what Guruji wants to teach us, and he's an example of it.

Guruji always talks about the starting point of ashtanga *yoga being the* asana *practice, the third limb of* ashtanga *yoga. Why do you think that is the case?*

By doing all the *asana* and sweating a lot, it's very simple: a lot of toxins and blockages are getting removed from the body and then this vehicle, this physical body/mind organism feels good, and *prana*, energy, can flow freely. Also, the waves of the mind become quiet, more quiet, more quiet, and at a certain moment there is that point of stillness in you, which is not like a state of static stillness but a moving stillness which is maybe what you feel sometimes makes you breathe. Maybe it goes in this direction and you experience what it actually is. So in one way, the *asanas* are the first step and I agree with it and it's good. For some people it takes longer and some people shorter, for some people very long, until they get a glimpse of what is beyond the *asana*.

How important is the householder lifestyle for Guruji?
Maybe just to show it's possible to lead a yogic life even as a householder. Maybe there is more meaning behind it, but just to see it is possible to do it, that it is not such a step into the extreme ascetic life.

You've spent a lot of time in north India with more of a sadhu *culture, and then being in south India with this more Brahminical and Advaita approach. Do you see much difference between the two as far as yoga practice goes?*
I think first, many of the *sadhus*, especially the Shivaite *sadhus*, have a totally Advaita non-dualistic approach. And many of them have been Brahmins or were born in a high caste and they just threw it away. They are born in the caste system and they leave it behind. And many of them do practice *asana* and *pranayama*, maybe not the *ashtanga* system, but *ashtanga* yoga in the way it was described by Patanjali. So I don't see so much difference. I think the lineage of Krishnamacharya and where he comes from are mostly householders, but that is just a part of it, you know. To again show that it is possible to lead a yogic life of self-realization as a householder or as an ascetic in the end it doesn't matter. When this point of realization has happened, then the question, whether it is a household system or a *baba* in the jungle, doesn't matter. The way the realization has happened, it just happened, then there is no matter of difference, there is no dualism anymore.

Do you think it's more challenging to be a householder?
Maybe it's according to your *samskaras*. For some people, it's just their way to be a householder. That's how it is. It's not worse than somebody

who sits by the river alone or lives in an ashram. These are only outer circumstances. When they are standing next to each other, for example, on
the mat, it doesn't matter if it is a householder from New York or a hippie from England; on the mat they sweat the same and go through the
same process, and that's what happens inside, the process. It may appear
different, but at the end to realize that, in the oneness of truth, there it is
the same. This is how I feel about it, it doesn't have to be necessarily
true. That's just my approach to it. So I don't like to see a difference and
say one is more difficult than the other. It's according to our *samskaras*,
what we are into here.

*How do you the see the relationship between what Guruji teaches and what
he calls* ashtanga *yoga and the Patanjali yoga of* The Yoga Sutras?
I think often in the system that Guruji teaches, people forget the other
parts and think only of the poses. They often forget that actually this aspect of *ahimsa* should be done in my own practice for me—to have a little respect, that I don't need to reach a pose today, just give my body the
time to grow into it and approach it with that aspect of *ahimsa*, with love,
with gentleness to myself. Often it is forgotten and then at this point,
often, people get injured or injure themselves and they say, "Oh it's *ashtanga* yoga." It's not, it's mostly them where they bring all their baggage
from their daily life onto the mat and want to do the things in the same
way that they do their daily life, in their jobs—to approach, to reach, to
be goal-oriented. I think what Guruji is teaching, *ashtanga*, is no different
than what Patanjali is teaching. I think there is no difference. It's just
what people make out of it, a big misunderstanding, and we can all see
that.

How do you think we came to make such a mistake?
Conditioning from our daily life in the past. And you see often after some
years people change and change their approach. Maybe they have to hurt
themselves in that process, that sometimes happens—often it happens!
But it's not necessary. Often Guruji tried to stop them or make it a bit
playful, take the serious aspect out of it. Playful means not stupid and
lazy, it means more like, with a bit of joy in it. He tries to bring that with
the laughter. And laughing, maybe people fall out of the pose and do not
take it so seriously. But on the other hand, when people get on the mat

they are already angry and if the neighbor accidentally puts their feet on their mat, you know . . .

People bring all their baggage. Guruji was very good at illuminating that especially when he knows the people. Again this point of personally working with people in a system of *ashtanga* where everybody does more or less the same primary, intermediate, or advanced series. So the whole practice system is a tool to wake up. It can be. The chance is there.

What is the other option, if you don't wake up?
That you drop it sooner or later.

How do you see Guruji bringing in the teaching of Shankaracharya and Advaita Vedanta? Generally speaking we think of Patanjali yoga as dualistic.
Is it really a dualistic approach? Or is it only seeing the dualistic illusion and letting it go? Making ourselves realize and see the dualism as an illusion to make us ready for seeing the non-dualistic aspect of God or divinity. Different people reach realization differently. Different people receive Guruji's teaching in different ways. I can eat only so much as I can digest. When I try to eat more, I will get sick. So if I can eat a little and I can digest, I receive more than when I try to get it all. The message is big and it takes some time and maybe that's why Guruji likes people to come for a long time, and more regularly. You can see people changing, and their approach to what yoga is changing.

Guruji always says 99 percent practice, 1 percent theory. What do you understand is the theory part?
I think that's it. I think 99 percent practice and 1 percent theory—that's perfect. It's also not only 99 percent [*asana*] practice; it's also in everything. There's so much theory going around in the world. There's so much theory on many aspects of life, and so much less practice. So a little practice is much better than all the theory. Somebody who sits every day maybe just half an hour in silence or does *japa kriya* for half an hour or half an hour on his mat lives during this half hour this way of life. It is better than reading hundreds of books and having all this theoretical knowledge in the head, but where nothing manifests. I know people who know a lot of the scriptures. They know the slogans and can speak them and think them, but in their daily approach to life they don't really man-

ifest. I don't judge them, I just see that. So I think 99 percent practice in many aspects of life is very useful. And a little theory to put it into words.

So you think it's a suggestion about how one should think about practicing rather than how we weigh the importance of one against the other.
One time Guruji said in a conference, "*Ujjayi* breathing, you keep it twenty-four hours." When you are aware of your breath, it brings you back to that point. It is the shortest way to that essence inside you that makes you breathe, that makes a plant grow, that makes meditation happen. I think the shortest way toward it, or one of the shortest ways, is through the breath. So when you say, "Oh you keep *ujjayi* breathing twenty-four hours a day," this means something like 99 percent practice, not only the two hours on the mat. You can be with your breath in your work, in your garden, even when you dance, when you sit on the bus or travel. It means practice not only for two hours but in our daily life, in our approach to situations and everything we experience. Maybe I misunderstand, but that's the way I understand it.

Why do you think breathing is so important in yoga?
It's the first and the last thing we do. You come out and if you don't breathe, you don't stay in this human body. And when you leave, it's the last thing you do.

How does it become part of a sadhana, *part of a practice? Why is it such a useful tool in the practice?*
It's the closest thing to death of the physical body. Without food, you can survive for one month. Without water maybe also quite a long time. But without breath, a very short time. I have met some yogis who can stay a long time also without breath. It's one of the closest ways to, let's call it, self-realization and to make meditation happen—through the breath. You feel it as a very simple, grounding aspect. When your breath is even, and you go through [the practice], there is this moving in stillness within you and a certain kind of bliss happens. You cannot deny it, it just happens. When there is not . . . "Wow, I have to bind in *marichyasana*!" No, you don't even think about that! You just go in with the breath and out. But it takes time. One time Guruji said, "You need to do one *asana* ten thousand times to be able to understand it." When he said that it touched me, and I felt it was true. And after some years of practice, doing the

same poses, something changes, but that is very individual and every-body should find out for themselves.

Guruji always talks about devotion, bhakti, *and praying to God. Why do you think it's so important?*
Yoga cannot happen without devotion; without *bhakti*, it's not possible. People say, "There are so many different kinds of yoga, whichever kind you feel, fits to you." If you have no devotion, no *bhakti*, it's not happen-ing, it's just not happening. Each musician hears it when he is in a certain state in his devotion and love for his music. This makes the music hap-pen, otherwise no music happens. And that is with everything, especially with the yoga. When there's no devotion in it, it's a lamp without oil.

And what do you think it is most important to be devoted to?
People in India devote themselves to a certain deity and worship that deity—for example, Krishna. They see it in the form [a physical repre-sentation], and in a certain moment that form melts away and it is just a devotion to the unmanifested aspect of divinity. And in the practice we can do that, too, in *ashtanga* yoga, the devotion in that can bring us to that same point.

What about guru bhakti?
Guru *bhakti* grows, it grows inside. Nobody can make it happen, it just grows. It is like when the seed germinates, it comes out like a little plant and grows into a tree, it's beyond words, beyond giving flowers, beyond giving money, beyond all that shit. It just grows in your heart toward your master. And it comes out as something greater than thankfulness. And I think the guru feels when it is growing. When Krishna's devotee instead of giving Krishna the fruit of the banana, gave him the peel? She was so into the study of love for Krishna, so she gave him the peel with-out noticing, and Krishna just ate the peel. And then other devotees shouted, "You just ate the peel!" "No," he said, "I just ate the *bhakti* of the devotee."

Do you think Guruji teaches a set system of yoga, or does he teach each per-son individually?
Within the frame of that system, he was teaching people individually. In the small *shala*, I saw how he adjusted different people in the same pose

in a different way, taught them how to handle it in different ways, and it was the same structured system. There lies a lot of individuality and personal approach.

What's the value of practicing every day for years and years? How does that change one's inner experience?
Regular practice is a sort of *tapas*, what they call in India *tapasya*. Some yogis stand for twelve years on one leg, and some for twelve years only eat *phalahari*. With the *asana* practice, some keep it going for a long time. I know some *babas* in their late eighties and nineties who still have a strong *asana* practice. So it is a *tapasya*, and the *tapasya* is purifying not only for this mind/body organism but also for developing guru *bhakti*, which is actually *bhakti* to divinity, to God, to whatever, which makes us at a certain moment become one and to burn away a lot of hang-ups. They say burn away, but I feel more that they fall away. And a daily practice helps, and a certain kind of discipline. Many people say, "Oh, this makes you framed and rigid," and in a certain way that's true, but it makes the ground fertile to be spontaneous. On this level, if you have a daily practice, always somehow the *nadis* remain quite clean and the body in its different *koshas* [sheaths] is also quite pure, and this gives fertile ground for the Atman to realize its union with the *paramatman*, your own union with God. After some years, that daily practice is not like "Oh, I have to go on the mat," it's "Yeah, I can go on my mat."

How important is it to have a teacher?
If you want to learn music and play sitar it's good to have a teacher, to know the scales and the idea of the instrument. Let's call it on that level, to learn *asana*, to put your body in a certain way, to make it happen easily. On that level a teacher is quite important. But the teacher, I think, should really always encourage the student to self-practice, you know, but still give guidance and maybe suggestions of how to work and approach it. When this teacher happens to become a guru, this is like the plant of the guru *bhakti*, it can grow. With *ashtanga*, there's Guruji and the older students who teach younger students. I feel like actually we are all the same, you know. I often have the feeling not that I am teaching, more that I transmit something that was given to me, and I try to communicate it in a way so that these people get it. I communicate something, but it's not my creation. I just transmit something.

You made the comparison with music a few times. Do you see a relationship between yoga and art?
Yoga is an art. There's no question about that for me.

What about the subtle aspects of the practice? Do you feel they're somehow integrated with asana *practice? Do you naturally evolve toward* pratyahara, dharana, dhyana, samadhi *through just doing* asana *practice? Or do you need something else?*
It grows out of that. Most people, after doing *asana* practice for some time, want to sit [meditate], you know, sooner or later, often later. Then the next step is doing *pranayama*. It's such a beautiful thing, such a final touch. When you are able to sit there without pain and guide your breath without even trying, the idea of not to control, just with love guide your breath in a certain way. It's an extension of the *asana* practice. It's not like one chapter, next chapter. The whole thing is one, and it merges with the next one: *pratyahara, dharana, dhyana,* and at the end maybe even *samadhi* happens. It's a process where you grow.

What do you think the ultimate goal is, according to Guruji? Where is this practice taking us?
Forget the idea of goal. As long as there is an idea of goal there is still too much ego effort involved. "Don't worry, just do your practice and all is coming." What is "all is coming"? "All is coming" is maybe that moment where I realize, I am already there, I don't have to go anywhere anymore, there never has been anywhere to go. It was always there, I am always in it, inheriting this divinity through this body/mind organism. Goal. I don't like that word so much. It can create misunderstanding.

If you are a teacher and you have a student, you want to do something. Maybe it's only to help them do what they want to do, but there has to be some goal, someplace you help them go to.
You can show them how to do the pose in a way that they can do it alone and guide them, but I don't have to put them onto the idea of a goal. They already have enough goals and aims. They come to you with *marichyasana* D and they think already of *kapotasana*—so why should I support that? Just bring them back to the moment and then let it grow into the next, which often is not that easy.

I wasn't suggesting you put it in the student's head. But in the teacher's head there has to be some agenda.
It didn't really work for me that way. It's individual from teacher to teacher, how they teach. When they know the practice of the student for some time, they know where to help or where to stop or better go this direction or that direction. Sometimes it can happen that the student shows you where the need is.

So it's the teacher following the student rather than the other way around. It's an interesting idea.
Or maybe walking together and you just hold the hand in difficult spots. I felt often that Guruji did just that, hold the hand as I pass over some difficult area. But again, it's according to each person's nature, and it works somehow because in the end it doesn't matter—whatever makes it work, wake up, that's fine.

How do you incorporate Guruji's philosophy in the way that you teach?
I think it means more or less living the same way of life, even if his was maybe a bit more involved. When you live it, then you can communicate it. When he was teaching, he gets up early, he does his practice, then he teaches. He has his *sadhana* before he teaches. It's a part of his daily life. And somehow the guidance or teaching of students is not separate anymore from your own practice, it spills over and becomes one. That's how it feels to me. I remember one time he took me to show me his room and his deerskin where he does his prayer and his *pranayama*. It was really nice. I saw the similarity with my little place in the morning.

What is the relationship between practice and teaching?
Without practice, not much teaching happens. Guruji practiced sixty, seventy years. Eventually there's just sitting practice, the *pranayama*. Practice is the basis of any teaching. If this is not happening, I would not believe in the teaching.

Guruji hasn't been practicing for quite a long time.
But before that there was fifty years of practice. I have done maybe thirty years and I feel already there is quite a little foundation, and quite a well where the groundwater has reached a certain level and flows. He showed me sometimes *shirshasana* and so on, but mainly he was doing *pranayama*

and sitting practice, and at a certain moment this becomes the essence. Many *asanas* just work toward being able to sit, you know, to be able to sit comfortably.

Cliff is seventy-five and he still has a practice going. Maybe he modifies it, but there is still a practice and that is something beautiful. But mainly he goes to the aspect of sitting. He is clean and pure so he can sit, he's allowed just to sit and it happens.

I like that analogy. You said that you find your source and then it overflows. That's beautiful.
Yeah, it's the groundwater you reach.

What is the importance of food in practice?
Big. Everybody who practices even a few weeks knows it is so, it's very clear. Like with your scooter or motorbike—what you put in, that's how it drives. If you put kerosene, you go nowhere. With food, it's the same. You put too much, even if it's good petrol, it flows over and it will not ride. With the body, it is the same. Balanced diet, not too much, not too little, in a good clean way. I think living as a vegetarian is a good idea. But it should not be forced on people. But they should get the information and a chance to try. What I experience in people who are eating a lot of animal products, when they start practicing, after one or two years the consumption of animal products reduces and at a certain moment it vanishes, just by a daily *asana* practice. Maybe it takes a long time, but it happens. And at a certain moment, these people, even without telling them, come to you and ask and then it's good, they are ready. And then you can give information about food. If you look at the Chinese Shaolin people, the traditional monks who practice this martial art were all vegetarian. People can get a lot of information nowadays. It's good to take as much as possible and look at how it fits for you, your body/mind organism, for your condition/constitution, if you eat maybe only raw or if you prefer more cooked food, or less at this time of the day. Everybody has a chance to find out individually. Even if you do not practice yoga, all humanity would be better off more vegetarian.

Can you say something about what the negative effect of inappropriate food on practice is?
Indigestion and bloating and a lot of disturbance in the mind. If the

stomach and the intestines are full and not clean and not eliminated, the mind is clouded and that makes everything a little more difficult.

What is most important to think about for a healthy lifelong practice?
Creating the circumstance around this. Find a nice place where you are. Have this little area where you put your mat and do your daily practice, so that it becomes something natural. Then it will take care of itself. When it has manifested in a certain way, it will take care of itself. Then even when you travel it will always happen, the chance to do your practice. You make it happen there and be thankful that it happens. Maybe you have to shift sometimes from here to there. That, too, is part of the practice.

Would you change the practice as you become older?
I'm going to be fifty-five in two months. My practice has changed. I need to be a bit more warm to do certain poses. There are still some poses that I can still go in and out of like that, but for backbends I like to be warm and really give myself a few more breaths to take the pose. That's part of getting older and it also should be approached with thankfulness, in a nice way: thankful for this way of growing old. You realize you are not twenty-five anymore and it's fine. And if you have a daily practice, this practice is somehow taking care of the change that happens, a certain awareness arises that makes it work. And then you don't have to change too much. Maybe you are a bit more slow, but it is still there and you remain very thankful for it. And in the end whatever you can keep, whatever will remain, is just perfect as it is.

Do you think Indians and Westerners need to practice differently?
I think individuals anyhow practice different. And even if you do the same, it is different than mine and that's how it is. I notice Indians have a more light-and-easy approach to the practice. Some foreigners also, men who have dropped a lot of baggage and do not take it too seriously, you know, just a bit playful. In the end I think it's very individual.

So you see that as a positive thing. They don't actually need to do it in such a heavy way; they are freer somehow.
Like I say, the practice takes care of it anyhow. If you don't reach it today, maybe next week it happens, that's fine. But you did today what you had

to do, what you're able to do, and that's amazing. Even just put your mat down and do a few *surya namaskaras* and you are there, the few *surya namaskaras* with peace and joy—beautiful. And after some time a few *surya namaskaras* become advanced A or B. It's the same attitude inside. We say, in the beginning is *ahimsa*—be gentle and loving with yourself. Also with your neighbor.

Most students won't be able to do the advanced asanas. *Do you think they have less opportunity for spiritual growth?*
No way. It doesn't matter.

Can you say something about advancement in the asanas *and the meaning of that?*
Guruji said one time, "People practice primary and intermediate, it keeps you going very well and gives you the basis to be able to sit." Advanced series are beautiful to do and I love it and I'm still thankful for what I can do. But sometimes you see people, especially young people and some older people, they just do half primary, they are so aware and in the moment with it and it's so beautiful, going in and out with the breath, and some are hurrying through advanced series and look like a horse with a carrot. Realization can happen with *asana* or without *asana* because it's already there. The woman who works the whole time in the kitchen, the moment she does that with all her devotion and all her love can find realization there. Or the man who works in the garden. Other people choose the way of yoga. The moment there is devotion toward God, the first step takes you there directly. Yoga is a useful tool and you should do it with love and keep it clean and nice. It's a tool that removes the veil of dust off our inner being, and is one way. In one of the old scriptures, Shiva says to Parvati, "There are as many ways as there are creatures on this earth."

Can you say something about Amma's role in Guruji's life and how her death affected him?
Amma, she was like the mother, not only for Guruji but also for all the students when we were in the small *shala*. She was like a joyful reflection of what happened in the *shala*. Her presence gave a lot of stability to everything that was going on there, and especially to Guruji. And when she died, when she left her body, it was a very sad moment and I never

saw Guruji like that, never, even when we saw him sometimes sick. That moment when she left, he was ready to leave also, not because he was physically sick. It felt like he was ready to leave. When he recovered he became healthy again, but that moment was very sad.

What do you think helped him to recover?
Teaching and the sharing of love with a lot of his students and devotees, and maybe the feeling that Amma wanted him to carry on.

What are you most thankful for?
It is the whole package. It's the meeting with Guruji, the receiving of the teaching, the time I was allowed to spend in his presence. One of the biggest things I feel thankful for, which I even feel keeps the practice going, is that it manifests in my life in such a way that I'm allowed to share it. I think that is a big thing. Thankfulness also because I'm allowed to make my living with something I love to do myself and that is actually, you should not forget, something also very special. You don't do something you hate to do to make your bread. You do something that you love and you receive your daily needs. And that is the way of Guruji's teaching, and the practice is taken care of also.

Goa, 2009

Nick Evans

While healing himself from a rare form of cancer, Nick Evans began learning yoga. He eventually made his way to Mysore, where he spent several years studying with Guruji. He has immersed himself in many aspects of yoga practice during his journey toward health and self-discovery.

How and when did you become interested in yoga?
I suppose, initially, I grew up with a very spiritually oriented mom. When I was a young boy, about seven, my mother was doing Transcendental Meditation and so I was taken off to learn Transcendental Meditation— a children's version of it—so it was in the environment at home. And I did that for about seven years, until I was about thirteen or fourteen, at which point I discovered punk-rock music and being naughty, and forgot all about it.

Then at the age of twenty-eight, after about ten years in the music industry in London, having lived a life as far away from meditation and spirituality and practice as you could possibly get, I fell very ill with a rare and aggressive cancer and went through chemotherapy, radiotherapy, and several reconstructive operations. And it was clear I needed to change the way I was living dramatically, because I had a terrible sense of fear and sadness. And I had some experiences during the illness that started to acclimatize me to a different way to approaching life.

After the treatment was ended, I did maybe six months of going to a gym and doing a bit of tai chi, and sometime in 1999 I went to the Greek Islands. [My tai chi teacher] told me about this place in Crete called Yoga Plus and this fellow who taught a particular style of yoga, a moving style of yoga. And because tai chi was a moving practice, that got me interested. So I went to Yoga Plus in Crete, and Radha and Pierre showed me the basic standing sequence and I think somewhere in the second week I began having a tangible sense of hope, having come out of this really horrific experience with the treatment of the cancer, and I got the feeling, a kind of glimpse of a new world of possibilities that comes maybe once or twice in a lifetime, if you are lucky.

It was very clear that this breathing, moving, gazing, squeezing [*mula bandha*] thing that they teach you in *ashtanga* was profound. It got me as a kind of paradigm for living your life, as they say. I was scared that I would get cancer again. During the cancer experience there was a time when the fear and anxiety were so great that it became physically difficult to manage basic functions. I was terrified. With that fear came a physical holding which made it very difficult to pass the chemotherapy drugs from my body into the toilet—terrible pain trying to poo. And I made a discovery, that when I let go of the effort, not only going to the toilet but even to get well . . . I had some sort of epiphany, where I said, "Look! I'm not beating my heart, I'm not assimilating the oxygen in my bloodstream, I'm not digesting my food, I'm not making my ears hear and my legs walk. I didn't design this vehicle I'm sitting in, I *find* myself in it, I *find* myself in this situation. I have to give the decision about it getting well or dying back to the one that designed this thing we find ourselves in, not just the body but the entire thing." And somehow that sense of abdication of personal responsibility made me relax. There are moments when you taste that: "Oh, I do feel better with that way of thinking, that approach seems to let my body release, and therefore allows me to go to the toilet." And really, all I was concerned about was going to the toilet without this searing pain.

So I went to Crete, and later on there was guilt, because prior to the illness my behavior had become compulsive and addictive and, I suppose, *tamasic*—to use yoga terminology. There was guilt, there was pain, there was a sense that I had taken a wrong turn in life. I'd had an introduction to spirituality early on and I had an overwhelming sense that I turned in the wrong direction. My therapist, Gestalt therapist, who I went to see to deal with the compulsive behavior, introduced some ideas, and one of them, I remember her saying to me, was that when I talk, I used to gesticulate quite a lot, I would be quite animated, like I was doing tai chi with my arms. She was very clever. She brought a picture of

Derek Ireland [of Yoga Plus in Crete] doing *prasarita padottanasana*. And I looked at him, and he was very muscular with lots of hair and had a physical language I could relate to, and when I got through the treatment, when I was looking for a place to unwind and go for a holiday with my then-partner, who is half Indian and had a family history with yoga and some of these things, she responded to the idea. They did tai chi at Yoga Plus as well, so it was almost as if the story was written.

It was a suggestion to you, and you just followed that.
I just followed that, I mean this idea of abdicating, surrendering, and taking advice. I had always been a kind of controlling person and quite big for my boots, quite full of myself. This sense of letting go had caught on because there had been practical results in very important ways, you know.

Then you connected the idea of doing yoga or tai chi with being more capable of letting go, with relaxation and also a new modality of living.
Correct. Tai chi is about flow and *ashtanga* was about flow but much more, in a way, refined. Tai chi sort of inferred it, that feeling of breathing and moving was there but it wasn't delineated, it wasn't "Look at the tip of your nose, squeeze." These are very precise directions for getting back to basics. And again, this idea of surrendering to instructions, this idea of somebody saying, "This is what you are going to be doing, this is how you are going to be doing it. It's simple, don't complicate it." And it was again: "I remember this! This is how I got through the toilet thing with the cancer." Just sort of letting go and letting someone else tell you what to do, this letting it happen, which immediately resonated with me because of that aspect of my character that was less developed. And I think generally when we come into contact with a part of ourselves that is less developed or less familiar, there's a sense of wonder that's kind of spiritual. Halfway through the second week of practicing every day, I felt like a little kid.

Then I went to Glastonbury rock festival at the end of the holiday and saw all these people rocking and rolling and having partied for days on end and they looked terrible. And instead of having this feeling of, "It's exotic and exciting, rock and roll," I just thought how dull and ugly this all looks. I then realized my interest lay elsewhere, because I discovered a new technology that was better than sex, drugs, and rock and roll for getting that sense of communion. Whereas previously I had got by by being greedy and a bit desperate.

Interesting that you saw a picture of Derek Ireland, who happened to die of cancer. Was he still alive at the time?
No, he'd gone.

That's interesting, he sort of inspired you but you probably didn't know that.
I didn't know, I didn't know. What a guy, like a lion.

How did you become interested in studying with Guruji, and when did you first meet him?
At Yoga Plus, I heard people talking about him. I heard Radha talking about him. I heard, "All is God." I heard, "Do your practice, all is coming." I heard all sorts of funny tales, that he liked gold and he kissed the girls. Because I had my mother's version of spirituality, it wasn't what I considered to be the conventional view of what a spiritual master was supposed to be like, but that seemed intriguing—so there was a conundrum there.

So just to clarify, it was because he seemed unusual and radical in the spiritual tradition that it appealed to you specifically.
Yes, and also the practice itself.

Did you connect with the practice immediately?
Yes, and if you connect with it, it's like you've got to go to the source. That is like my entire involvement with music, you've got to get to the heart of the thing. Getting to the real thing and everything else was gravy, really. That was my understanding.

You were looking for reality, truth.
Yeah.

Some experience of reality.
Definitely.

Before you even knew that it was a spiritual quest.
Yeah, and also, as I said before, it was clear to me that there was something about the sequence of movements and the way the sequence of movements was conveyed that required you to surrender to someone else, to an external system, to a method, to a thing you didn't understand and know about yourself so you had to surrender.

Why was that important to you?
Because it was so contrary to my nature, which had been about control and effort and dominance.

And this way you felt you could . . .
Get well.

Change your modality and become a different person.
Yes, exactly. I went first to a fellow who taught in London, in between my work in Wandsworth and my home in West London. It was a bit outside the traditional *ashtanga* thing, but he taught a led class and he played a bit of music—he was a bit of a rocker, too. I went to him two or three times a week for maybe six months and then I saw this video of Lino and found out that Lino did a thing in Kovalam [south India], and I heard the breathing on Lino's video and the Sanskrit counting . . . and so he was my next bus stop and I went to see Lino. And Lino said some interesting things and had a certain flavor about him that was very attractive and very interesting. And then I heard the way that Lino was talking. I went back and closed down my company and my relationship disintegrated and five weeks later I went to Mysore, very early on in my practice.

What year was this?
I went to Lino in 2000 and I went to Mysore in January 2001.

Can you describe your arrival in Mysore and your first meeting with Guruji? What was your first impression?
I had fallen in love with a girl and she was sort of my chaperone, she was deeper into the practice than I was. She was reading *The Yoga Sutras*, she was involved already, and she sort of held my hand and was in a way my first guru, you know, because I trusted her. She guided me and she was the one who said, "I'm going to Mysore next. You can come and meet me

there." And I thought, "Okay, okay." So she met me at the train and I went to see [Guruji]. I was still feeling quite cynical and skeptical about just handing someone my unfettered devotion. I remember looking at him and seeing Sharath and being quite guarded with it all and not being instantly taken and not really understanding. He was a sort of rotund fellow. I was used to yogis being skinny people in all the pictures I had seen, so I was sort of a bit taken aback. He had Calvin Klein underwear on and I thought, "This is peculiar." Some of the discrepancies I heard about in Yoga Plus were in evidence to a degree.

He wasn't trying to be nice to anyone, he was quite gruff in a way, and he counted my money. So initially, there was no feeling that I was obliged or interested in surrendering to him or acknowledging his authority. I thought he was going to teach me this set of movements, these sequences, and I didn't really have a sense of a methodology that extended beyond the immediately physical. But then later on in that first three-month trip both he and Sharath said interesting things to me that were very insightful about my character. Guruji said, "Ah, you danger man!" And that was sharp, very sharp, because I had had this surgery, I had a weakness, I had a reconstructed stomach-wall muscle, so there was a weakness. I was quite crooked in my backbends. I remember saying to Sharath, "I'm very weak here," and pointing to one side of my stomach and Sharath saying, "No, you are very weak here," and pointing to my head, my mind, you know, yeah! And being quite shocked, first of all Guruji saying, "You danger man," and thinking, "Oh my God I've been rumbled, that's outrageous. How did he get that? Is it that obvious?" There didn't seem to be any nonsense or any kind of airs or graces. It was very direct and quite, I wouldn't say brutal, but very, very cutting. They weren't being polite. And being from Britain, where politeness is held in high regard, it was a shock. So that was the first occasion where my skepticism was softened. Then, on the second trip, I had some considerable shifts and changes and incidents.

How was your experience practicing in the shala? *How was that for you on the first trip? And how was it different on subsequent trips? What kind of initial impressions did you have, and how did that change when you went back on the second trip?*
Right from the beginning there was a very, very clear sense that what was

happening on the surface was not what was really happening. It was in the small *shala*, so there were big queues on the stairs. There seemed to be a lot of tension on the stairs, which I thought was weird, considering we were all there being yogis.

People were queuing to go into the room to practice?
Yes, to practice. The room held twelve people. Guruji sat on a plastic stool in the corner, sometimes working quite physically but then for other periods of time not doing anything and sleeping—he seemed to be sleeping to me. So that was what was going on, he's not doing anything! And that was very weird. But I noticed he was still watching. Watching very closely, and I felt his watching had almost a physical effect. There was heat in his gaze, almost like you were in the spotlight even when he wasn't actually physically looking at you. A little bit of interest coming, like, "Oh you, who are you? What are you about? Who are you?"

Interest on his part?
Yeah, a little bit. It built over the months. I was there two and a half, maybe three months, and I felt that the interest started to grow. And I also felt there were people in the queue, maybe Hamish [Hendry] from London or some different people that I spoke to, who said interesting things, and it became clear that perfecting this physical sequence of movements and making it look nice and doing it all properly was not what was going on, or was not what was interesting about this. But it wasn't just Guruji and Sharath in the room but the people in the room and the intensity of that focused practice, it was the comments that the other people were making as well.

What was it they were suggesting that this was about?
A depth of presence, focus, and becoming less and less distracted bit by bit by bit—that was the thing that would grow. I also started hearing people talk about the "witness," this idea of the witness. That clicked. And I remembered some of the moments when I had been in a lot of pain and frightened, and that peace that I found, that letting go—when that happened—I was aligned or identified with the watching itself. So that definitely clicked. This idea that the purpose of this was to be watching.

So the other students were important for you.
Because Guruji and Sharath didn't say very much, and I could read that
these were very real people and also pretty nice to me.

Why do you think they didn't say very much?
Well, now I know. I think then I didn't. Because there's a lot of wisdom in
silence and in the sound of breathing. And a teacher that creates a space
that allows you to drop into the sound of the breathing and the focus on
the *tristhana*, the three points of attention, and doesn't distract you from
that being the primary component of the practice, is giving you something
very, very, very precious even if you don't know that it's very, very, very precious. And it is golden, as a lot of us now know, priceless. We all know. I
think that people who engage and connect with the practice in an atmosphere of silence and devotion and acknowledgment of where it's come
from can experience very, very deep states of meditation quite quickly.

*I want to go back to you saying that something really shifted in your second
trip.*
First of all, the first trip I was still involved with a sort of romance with
the practice. It was the practice I was falling in love with and Guruji was
a side issue. The second trip, that sort of changed. There was an incident. After the second month, my partner left—well, we separated—and
I was very, very sad, a bit shaky, and anxious. At the same time the
motorbike-rental people came around and changed the motorbike I was
familiar with riding, with another motorbike that I wasn't familiar with.
The following morning I was also due to pay for my second month. So I
took my wad of rupees, got on this funny motorbike, and I had just had a
feeling that the whole world was different, partially because my girlfriend
had left and I was doing it on my own. I was in Lakshmipuram and I was
feeling a little bit vulnerable and unsteady generally and I was doing a little bit of intermediate on the second trip—maybe that had something to
do with it. First thing Guruji asked me for was the money. So I paid him
and he counted the money very slowly, then I sat on the staircase, it was
very early in the morning, waiting to practice, with some very old students in front of me who people respected a great deal, and who I understood I should respect also.

Then Guruji came out of the room and started shouting at someone.
I didn't know who it was because I had headphones on and I was listen-

ing to some chanting and was in my own world. I didn't think he could possibly be interested in me. Somebody prodded me and said, "He's talking to you!" And I pulled the headphones off and Guruji was saying, "You, you miss your spot." I thought, "I don't have a spot"—other students have spots but I didn't have a spot, I didn't know anything about all that and I was doing my best to be seen and not heard, you know, and just keep my head down. "You! You! You come, you come, you miss your spot." He was furious. "You! Why not listen? You come, you come."

And the space he was talking about was the space in front of his plastic stool. So, "Oh, okay, okay"—I sort of staggered down the stairs and tried to compose myself and got in there and started practicing at his feet, really. And again this thing of being gazed at, stared at, had a whole different degree of intensity in my mind and I could never say that this was really anything other than in my mind. I don't know, but my experience was that I was almost being lifted by him, or scrutinized by him, to such an extent that it wasn't the physical movements or the postures or the shapes that I was making, or even the breathing that was being monitored. But it was my behavior, my spirit, my essence that was being observed. I felt very observed and looked at deeply, and quite shocked and a bit frightened. And he looked very different to me, his face looked different and big—he's quite a little guy, he'd gotten older. By the time I got there he was probably eighty-something.

Was this experience sustained for you throughout that second trip or was it just that one moment?
In my *ashtanga* mythology, it's become quite a story. If I had been interested in having my astrology looked at at that point maybe it would have been a pivotal alignment in my chart. Because not only was it the day I paid, the day the motorbike was changed, and the day after my girlfriend had left, but later on in the day I drove on this little borrowed bike to Srirangapatna, where I had some friends living out at the river. And halfway there I was knocked off my bike by a bus and had my foot badly injured and I had surgery in a hospital in Nazarbad and the ends of my toes were basically sewn back on. It was raining, it was a very bleak experience, and I was shaky.

Was it the same day?
Yes, the same day as this thing with Guruji. So I went under a bus. The

bike was flattened. Somehow ten Indian guys picked me up and took me across the road and into the one hospital with an orthopedic doctor, the one guy in Karnataka who could set bones. And I was asking, "Do I get to keep my toes?" You know, it was heavy. Anyway, some friends came and picked me up, finally.

I went back to the *shala* because I paid that morning. In my mind I was, "Oh, I've given all that money, what shall I do? What shall I do?" And I went back, and he had my money, which was very peculiar, and he seemed . . . he didn't say, "I thought this was going to happen to you," but there was something that he was expecting. Then again, maybe I'm reading more into it. But all in all, in my personal mythology, in my reading of the whole thing, I had a deep sense of déjà vu, that this was a set piece and he was prepared for it somehow or connected with it somehow. So it's quite a grand tale, you know, but at the time . . .

You said he had your money ready for you.
He took the money for one class and said, "One class I'm giving." Then he gave me the rest and he said, "You resting, one month resting."

By that time, the whole thing was different. My idea that India really did have a powerful effect on one, and that this teacher was not just someone showing you sequences of movements and pushing you, was a lot more established. Logic didn't seem to be applying here. This is just really, bloody weird. And whatever is going on in that little room with this guy and all these people is really strange and I didn't really have a solution or an answer.

When you say "strange," do you mean that you felt that they had some kind of insight into what was going on with you?
I felt that there was energy being worked with, that there was power, it was all a bit magical. When I was little, and I was doing the TM, you repeated this syllable you were given over and over and over in your head. It was as if the vibration of the syllable almost massaged your whole being at a deep level and you'd go into quite a strange state of meditation, maybe a light sound, a whine in your ear, a feeling like vibrating somehow—and I started to get a sense of that there.

And what was happening on the surface. There were a lot of people crying in the finishing room, and that was regular, you know, if you go into a very open intimate feeling with friends, it's palpable, you can tell, you can feel it. It's not something that the logical mind can quantify or necessarily explain with words. But there was a feeling of tenderness, of openness, that maybe some of them were touching something that they had not had contact with since they were children. And that is certainly how I felt, that I was reconnecting with a silence, a solitude, a place inside that was very, very touching.

It won't let you down, for example, and you feel touched. It's a very important thing, but as a simple mechanical practice, as an intellectual understanding, you'll never be able to convey that. Somebody gives you a gift on your birthday and you really get a sense that they thought about it and they've given it to you because they know you and understand you and they care about you a great deal and it touches you—that was what I was feeling, there in his house, presided over by him, unexplained and unspoken.

Can you say something about Guruji as a teacher?
He's like the whole orchestra. He doesn't just have one way, he can find a way for everyone. So he sees you and your spirit and the aspects of your character that are competent and good and that may be lacking and not so rounded, and he seems to be able to do that with everyone. He doesn't overcomplicate it, he keeps it really simple. There are three really powerful techniques: the breathing method, coordinating the movement with the breath; the *drishti*; and the squeezing, the *bandhas*. He doesn't get extremely technical, he doesn't talk about anatomy, he doesn't talk about complicated energetic concepts. He keeps it incredibly simple. It takes a brave person not to appeal to a person's, particularly a Westerner's, need for information. You know, that kind of information, it's incredibly simple: "Breathe!" "You breathe!" "You do!" "No, no, no, don't think, you do!" And it's so effective.

Why is it effective?
Because we Westerners don't like being told what to do, don't like surrendering, because, "No, I want to have a think about it, ruminate with it, wrestle with it, and put my point across." And there is no way for you to go but, "Okay, he means business." There is no denying he means business, but with the people who are vulnerable and have a difficult time, he is the gentlest creature, the gentlest father figure. So he goes from having this terrible, intense authority to commanding your attention

and your respect with very few words, just with presence, to being very, very supportive and kind, and he encompasses the whole lot in between. That's a balanced range of abilities, and he's correct, so with the people he approaches, he gets it right. He gets it right over and over and over again with a huge range of personalities and bodies. His tone and his approach seem to be appropriate every time. I can't really say that with absolute certainty because I don't know, but from what I've seen.

There is something about the way he restricts the information, if that is the correct way to put it, that is intentional.
Yes, I agree with you. It's a huge cliché, but less is more. He knows. When people [at a] conference would say, "Guruji, can you tell me about the *kleshas* or the *granthis* or the *vayus*" or get into some esoteric line of questioning: "I am telling, you are not understanding." He'll tell, he'll quote from scriptures, he'll chant his textural evidence, memorized and understood and experienced himself, he can go straight to four or five texts with his own opinion, with a body of knowledge that has been around eight thousand years, depending on where you look for your evidence. So he will talk to you about that stuff and he will respond to people, depending on who is asking the question. But generally, he is saying to people, "Do it, don't talk about it. Do it, don't think about it: *Yogas chitta vritti nirodhah*"—the cessations of the mental fluctuations. When the mind quiets down, you will start to taste something of yoga, and asking lots and lots of esoteric questions is not going to give you the insight you are looking for. By asking these questions, therefore, "You are asking, I am telling, [but] you are not understanding."

I asked a few questions on one of the trips. I had a hernia and I asked him about that and he gave me a prescription, a yoga *asana* prescription to do. He said surgery is not necessary. He said, "You do. I am telling. You are doing, it is going." And, you know, pretty much he's right. It's not completely cured, but I've gotten very little problem with the hernia over the years.

I was going every year. I went for longer and longer stints and my trust for him, my love for him, got bigger and bigger and bigger. I really do like him ever so much now, and I love to kneel down and touch his feet and say thank you. I feel like he held my hand and led me out of a dark place. And any insights I had, or impetus or any initial galvanizing encouragement I had for changing my life from the cancer issue, his method, his being there, the contact I had with him, which usually just involved touching his feet, maybe occasionally having a little more, not very much, I felt like I had a guide, some more comfortable person who accepted himself—and that stuff is priceless. Quite difficult for me now, with hindsight, to go back and see what technique he used, because it was almost beyond words and technique, it was love, really. But a sort of fatherly, strict sort of love. But I really do have the feeling that he believed in me more than I believed in myself.

The year before last, we were in Lakshmipuram and my partner found a copy of the *Mysore Star* blowing around on the floor and it was a yoga issue which had all of the yoga teachers in Mysore and a big picture of Pattabhi Jois with a famous basketball player on the cover. It was the Pattabhi Jois issue of the *Mysore Star*, essentially, with interviews with Sharath and all the other people in Mysore, with four pages of photographs. And in the interview with Pattabhi Jois, they were asking him, "What makes you think this yoga can cure diabetes? What makes you think you can cure?" And he told this story about Krishnamacharya giving him a [sick] man to heal [through yoga]. And he said, "Many people who are ill come to Mysore to see me. I have one student, Nick, who comes every year." I couldn't believe it.

Sometimes I would go to touch his feet and he would ignore me or wouldn't have any interest in even acknowledging me that day. But the next day, after seeing this paper that I took home with me and was all sort of excited about and telling people about and quietly proud of, I went to touch his feet and he sort of gazed at me and started laughing his head off. And I didn't get into it with him, and maybe I'm assigning too much importance to it, but I really had the sense that he's sensitive. I'm not saying that he saw me in his mind's eye pick up the paper—

Maybe he saw your pride and thought it was funny.
Yes, more likely.

Do you see Guruji as a healer?
Yes.

What qualities does he embody that lead you to say that?
When I look at his face and when I'm in his presence, I think he knows that there is one eternal infinite power living in us all and making all this

happen and grow and move. It's making the sun go up and making all the galaxies not fall into themselves. In his tradition, they call it Ishvara. Not only Guruji and his guru but his family have spent generations and generations and generations acknowledging and working with this power and understanding that this power is what's real, and what we perceive to be reality is a covering, or the clothes that this power wears. When your primary contact is with this power, with this source of being, and that's something that you've inherited in the work that your parents have done and the work that their parents have done and their parents have done and the work that the entire culture has done—regarding that as the way life works. Not that we are all separate people striving for our own. And I think that light shines through you, and I think that light shines through him. I think he knows. He says, "All is God."

He makes no bones about it. In *Yoga Mala*, he says, "Nothing is achieved . . ." I can't remember the exact quote, I don't want to misquote him. I think the quote is something along the lines, "Nothing in the universe is done by individual will alone, that is definite . . . All is God. Practice, practice and all is coming." And I think there is less between him and that understanding than other people and that understanding.

How does that play into his healing powers?
Because when he puts his hands on you, when he smiles at you, when he is with you, that's what's with you. That understanding, that firm belief, established understanding, knowledge, is what pours out of him. And of course it's everywhere all the time, but because we are so enmeshed in our bodies and our histories and resistance and fear, we don't contact it. We don't make a connection with it. But when he touches us, it is like light flowing from him into us. Healing love, knowledge, power, forgiveness, kindness . . . you are already perfect. He knows it, we don't know it. He knows it, he touches us, and with absolute certainly he knows that to be the case. We don't. We go, "Oh yes," but arrogance and personal self-preservation get in the way.

How does he penetrate through that?
Well, in a way he doesn't. It does. And he allows it to by not taking any credit and not staking personal ownership. He doesn't say, "I'm a guru, I'm enlightened." He's just pretty funny, simple, sweet. I don't want to underestimate, downplay his gravitas as a scholar and as an academic

and as a serious teacher—but that his way is very charming and light and playful and sweet. He's like a big kid. You look into his eyes and it's like looking into the face of a child. He thinks it's funny. "How are you? What news? What news?" "Oh, no news, Guruji. Oh, no news." He thinks it's pretty funny. And that lightness transfers itself to you.

But then there've been times when it just appears to be the opposite, when I felt irritated, lost with all this. I'm back feeling tight and all that resistance and then he seems to respond in another way, he takes on a much more gruff demeanor and would maybe say something quite cutting, unkind, or nothing at all. And for months on end you are ignored, and you have no sense from him that you even exist, and you have to deal with that, because of course it's nice when your teacher pays you a bit of attention. So the whole range is there, and I've thought quite a lot about these moments that have been meaningful to me, and feel as though I was somehow singled out as being of interest or special, but the reality [is that] for much, much, much of the time that I spent in Mysore, years on end, I was just completely ignored. I felt I was completely ignored.

Not getting as much attention as you felt you deserved is not the same thing as being ignored.
Correct, correct, thank you. And that taught me.

During the last period when Guruji was teaching in the shala, *he would tend to pick one or two students to work intensively with, and your girl-friend Eva was one of his favorites during a period where he was ignoring you.*
He really liked Eva, he liked her a lot. She was a bright light. But why is he giving my girlfriend so much attention and being increasingly more gruff with me and cold with me? And she was getting a lot of warmth and love, and it was like I was being toughened up. And yeah, he gave Eva an enormous amount of attention, really seemed to take a big shine to her and seemed to despise me. [*Laughter*] I was, "Oh my God, he loves her and he hates me!" And it went on for months and months and months.

After that trip, where he gave Eva a lot of attention and a lot of postures and I didn't get much, but I got shouted at a lot, and any opportunity to make me look stupid in the led classes he took—"You! Skinny man, incorrect!"—there was a lot of it coming my way and I was really feeling like, "Oh my God, I'm an idiot."

That time I really didn't get a chance to say goodbye to Guruji, but I saw Sharath, and I left knowing that my father was very ill with some sort of tumor, some illness. And Sharath sat me down—well, we went upstairs for coffee—and he said, "Nick, you can trust this practice completely. You don't have to worry, the practice will take care of everything." He stared at me to reaffirm [what he had said]. And that was one of the moments when Sharath's presence in my life and in my practice increased, because that was a very clear establishing, a very clear, almost a promise or reassurance that connected [with me].

My father had a fatal cancer and after some months passed away. I spent those last months with him and I taught with my partner in Brighton and in Barcelona, and I had a terrible amount of pain in my body, aches and pains that might have been some sort of psychosomatic response, I don't know, I felt the sadness and the loss of my father . . . the knots and lumps and searing pain under my shoulder blades and all these things and also I was teaching quite actively, so my body was in pain for months. And I knew some of the pains very well. They didn't move and they had been there for a long time and I was compensating and there were things there that I thought had been there forever, in my lower back and sacrum and a bunch of stuff.

So when we finished the teaching in Barcelona, we went to Mysore early. They had been on a world tour and I hadn't seen them for maybe seven or eight months. Prior to that, I had been doing these long trips and staying there for a year. So this was the longest I hadn't seen them for a long time. And I was really desperate to see them. So we went early before we thought anyone else would be there. We had a little house in Gokulam that we kept and let out when we weren't there. They had come from France or something, and invited us upstairs for coffee. I told Sharath my father had died in some strained circumstances and I was interested in doing a *puja* to let go of him. I had brought his ashes with me, and Sharath organized a *puja* for me with their family priests out at the Kaveri [River]. I had an idea to maybe go to the Ganges and maybe put his ashes in the Ganges, but Sharath said, "No, no, you put the ashes where our family puts our ashes," and talked to Guruji in Kannada, "*Appa* [grandfather]!" I had never had a conversation apart from the hernia conversation, one or two little bits, really, with him before in that way.

Guruji sat opposite from me and talked to me about milk in France and milk in the other countries. He had been to Finland, I think, and [was talking about] fruit and milk. And I started looking at him and noticing how well he looked and what started off as a feeling—"He looks incredibly well"—then I thought, "Oh my God, he's sort of shining." And I felt very, very blissed out and trippy and quite high, and I remember saying to him, "Guruji, you look very, very well, in fact you look beautiful, in fact you look incredibly beautiful." And he started laughing at me and I was really radiating again with this sort of beautiful, I don't know what, love, for want of a better word. But this mean, grumpy granddad who was shouting at me all the time had been replaced with a shiny person.

Well, anyway, the whole thing lasted about eight minutes, maximum and I got up to go. I touched his feet and there wasn't a pain in my body. From head to toe I was completely pain free and I was pain free for the next two or three weeks. Some of them have surfaced again, but generally no. And that was a very weird, practical, tangible, physical encounter with something I don't have access to. I couldn't do that for someone else. I don't know how he did it, I don't know if he did it, I don't know how it was done, I don't know if I created it, I don't know, but I promise it happened.

What is it about the practice and Guruji that you felt was helpful in the healing process? Why do you think it's an effective method?
I don't know if it is for other people, but it was effective for me. It's what I understood he wanted of me and I had an instinctual feeling to trust him. But people should follow their hearts. And people should practice with the teachers whom they feel they can trust. In my case, at least, it served me well. Other people have different ways of approaching life, different ways of seeing, and that path of absolute surrender may not be the path for them. There is also discernment [as an alternative path], and different characters have different journeys to make and have come into these bodies to learn different lessons, and this will not work for everyone else. But at the same time, it is what I know and I'm not sure I would be truthful to try and convey a different approach. I saw a DVD released a couple years ago, a documentary, a guru documentary that Dominic and Rob made. There is a little extra on the DVD, which is an interview with Pattabhi Jois. I think Sharath is conducting the interview or translating the interview, and the question is, "What is the single most important quality in a good student?" and Guruji just says, "Obedience," and that's that. So he made it quite clear then, and he wasn't talking to

one individual student, he was talking to all the people who were going to watch and buy that DVD. That is quite clear, what he wants of us as students. And for me it was easy to give to him and maybe for some people it's not, and that's okay, too.

Does Guruji approach different students in different ways, or is it that each student has a different perception of their relationship?
I'm reluctant to speak about this in any kind of authoritative way because I've only known him for maybe eight years now.

But you must have seen hundreds of students?
Yeah, but I wasn't around much at the old *shala*, you know. There were a lot of people whose relationship with him was quite personal. What I've seen is how he deals with large numbers who are going to Mysore to meet the guru, to be with the guru, who have got a lot of preconceptions, maybe expectations, ideas about him. And what I've seen is this generic lesson that everyone seems to be invited to understand, which is sort of, "Calm down, get over yourself. Shhh! Shut up!" You know?

So it seems there are too many people around.
To get personal, individual relationships.

Would you say that Guruji teaches a standard form of practice, or would you say it's individually tailored for the practitioner?
I think it's a standard form that is individually tailored. It's like a piece of music by Mozart—a different conductor will emphasize different aspects of the same piece of music. So there will be a different rate at which the postures are given, different aspects of the practice are emphasized. Again, my feeling is that different people have got different energies, different vibrations, as it were, and he sees that and their rate of progress will be managed carefully. And the tone with which he approaches each person, in terms of their body and the way that they are practicing, the way that they are breathing. Some people he will try and calm down, and other people he will try and [snaps fingers], "You! Move back, move back, you!," sharpen up, get with it sort of thing. There is a range of approaches in that sense.

The sequence is like a formula or a medicine, a certain prescription. We all have the same organs, the same blood flowing through our bodies, the same limbs; generally speaking, all of us have the same physical composition basically, but with huge variations on the classical theme. So the *yoga chikitsa* is a classical theme, a classical prescription. Each thinning of the blood, cleaning, clearing the organs as a sort of generic human prescription is then applied at different rates for different—

Is it just the rates, or is there more to it? For instance, some people he seems to never adjust, and some people he is all over, with some people he's very intense.
Yeah, that seems to be true. There were some people he left alone and some he got more involved with physically. But my sense was that there was a general prescription worked with or moderated or intensified according to the rate at which the postures were given. And also the amount of attention and the way that attention was given. So maybe he would shout or encourage people to intensify the way they were practicing or to relax the way they were practicing. He would open some people or push some people or not push others, as you've said.

Have you had experiences with Guruji taking you to the limit of your physical and mental endurance and beyond?
I remember doing *karandavasana*. Again, I have a weakness in my stomach muscles, I remember him coming over and sort of . . . it's difficult to tell if he dropped me or pushed me over, but I looked up in horror, because I basically had been pushed onto Eva, who was practicing next to me in *supta kurmasana*. I had gone hurtling over and landed on top of her and it was a disaster, really, a little yoga Mysore disaster . . . at least it felt like a disaster at the time. And I looked up expecting him to say, sorry I pushed you, but he had a look of revulsion and disgust on his face. "You! Why? You bad man!" And it was a shock. I was expecting him to say, sorry. Instead of that he was like, "You disgust me." I was, "Okay, okay, you're the boss, end of story." And that was a shock.

And the backbending was strong for me. There were times when I had a lot of pain and Saraswathi was trying to get me to take my ankles. And a lot of times when I had pain, "Take a rest," Sharath said to me. When they moved into the big *shala* and there were more people, he was adjusting less and that kind of thing was happening less. And I felt he was doing things particularly for me less and less.

You have described instances where you were mentally quite disturbed, chal-lenged by his behavior, especially toward your partner. Did you feel like, "There is no way I can do this asana, I'm going to die!"—like you are totally exhausted, or you can't imagine yourself going to the next step, and he's helped you to transcend that?

I wouldn't say that he's singled me out and worked with me on a particu-lar *asana* and taken me that much further. Sharath, yes. By the time I was doing more advanced *asanas*, Guruji's involvement physically was significantly less than it had been. But I do feel that he has made com-ments about me as a person that have had an impact. For example, I would do a little halfhearted *nakrasana*, and, "You! Why not jumping? Why not?" So there were a lot of "Bad man!" comments directed to me at certain moments. In *karandavasana* it was difficult for me to come down and hold it and maintain it and come back up. And directing this gaze, this attention toward me in order to—"You! Skinny man, why not eating? You not eating! You eat!"—put more effort into it, I suppose, try harder here.

I'm trying to think of the *asanas* I was given and the adjustments I re-ceived. At the time when it's all happening you are in such an open place that, with the exception of those big events, like being knocked over or yelled at, it's all a blur, you know, just this sort of eight years of blur with the occasional shout, more a case of him walking past me, standing at my mat, and not doing anything physically, in a posture and noticing, "I'm much lighter," or remembering a posture I was having pain in, and without him saying or doing very much with me, but being in very close proximity, I noticed a lot more. Specific him-and-Nick, him-and-me things? Not that much, really. Just all these bits and bobs and anecdotes and things.

But it seems quite appropriate, considering your interest in the non-dual ap-proach, that he would be not so specific in the way he communicated with you, but that you could just absorb the general philosophy that he expresses.
Yes. Light, love, oneness. Yeah, really.

I've often heard Guruji say that he teaches real ashtanga yoga. What is your experience of Guruji as a teacher of true yoga?
He is not taking personal credit. He is not full of "me" and "mine." He is constantly referring to scriptural evidence, almost as though he is simply

a vessel for the teaching that he received from his guru and his family guru. He's very clear that he is simply passing on methods and techniques that were passed on to him unchanged. And the way that life came to meet him, with all these Westerners showing up at his door—instead of, "No, no, no, I teach Indians only, Brahmin only," it's "Okay, this is what life is presenting me. This is the way that the yoga wants to move. This is the way that these teachings seem to be taking naturally"—and rising to meet the occasion without a sense of personal involvement. You hear very, very little in the way of his personal opinion. All the emphasis seems to be on channeling, for want of a better word, giving voice to methods of teaching which have been preserved for generations and generations without coloring them, being really, really in service of the teachings not the other way around.

Why does Guruji emphasize the third limb of ashtanga *yoga as the starting point?*
If you have got a closed, rigid, stagnant, disease-ridden body, you will never know God or the purpose of yoga, which is to know reality as it truly is. Because you are worrying, you are uncomfortable. Because you are in pain, your physical body is a source of anxiety for you. Oxygen, energy-enriched oxygen, stretching and filling your body full of life force and vital energy, the energetic, living component of oxygen that you are filtering using a particular style of breathing. And then moving, building this heat, cleaning the organs, cleaning the blood, opening the joints, allowing the energy, the blood to move around the body unobstructed by the old physical patterns in your being. Allowing all the old physical patterns in your being to realign themselves, to let go, to release. So you stand a far greater chance of being comfortable in a body that God gave you.

If you are comfortable in the body, you stand a chance of being able to relax mentally because you have more fluidity physically. You are not as restricted physically, there is less likelihood of stagnation in your organs or in your blood, and if stagnation is less likely to take hold in your physical being, it's less likely to take hold in your mental being. So this cleaning, this washing out of habits, physical and mental habits, seems to allow a more peaceful state of mind to be a more consistent experience in your life. And when that's a more consistent experience in your life, you are a more relaxed person who can start to engage in the ideas of the *yamas* and *niyamas* with less resistance and you are more comfortable generally, and being more comfortable, you are more open to letting these difficulties emerge in your day-to-day living.

What we have is a body. We know that. Here it is. Nobody is going to deny that. The mind we can speculate about, difficult to be clear about the mind. But I don't think you'd find a human being without some identification with the body. So to enter the mental work, the quieting of the mind through the body is a very tangible physical approach that I think leaves very little room to argue with. We all want a healthy body. End of story. I mean, it's a pretty genius place to start. And the *ashtanga* practice seems to give you a vibrant, healthy body. In the end, that's the tendency. I don't say you don't go through enormous amounts of pain and difficulty along the way, but the general tendency is that the body becomes more open, stronger, more flexible, and steadier. And in turn the mind reflects that. And also you know if you've done something good for yourself every morning, you spend the rest of the day feeling all that much better about yourself.

How do you think this plays into more advanced practices?
The explanation I heard that resonated most with me was: each of these bodies that we inhabit is sort of like an electrical wire, and the cleaner the organism and nervous system, the more able the body is to channel or receive or live with greater amounts of life force or *prana* or electrical energy or chi. Since I took the *pranayama* that Pattabhi Jois taught us together, I feel that there is a lot more energy in my body, and I am able to manage that energy more effectively. I don't get ill so often, I am able to teach bigger groups of people without getting tired. It's like you are making the body available for increasing levels of energy, and *asanas* are preparatory. If too much energy is put through a copper wire that's too thin, the wire burns out. The reason the *asanas* are taught first is if you gain access to this energy with a body that hasn't done any preparatory work, it can cause enormous energetic problems, behavioral problems, physical problems. So I think there is a sequential approach to preparing the body for a greater level of life force.

What do you consider to be the essence of Guruji's teaching?
Ishvarapranidhana, surrender to God, acknowledging your body/mind's place in the grand scheme of things. You are the product of your environ-

ment, you do not exist separate from your environment, you are completely reliant on your environment for everything: oxygen, food, love. We are at one with our present moment and environment. If we believe ourselves to be separate from it, and separated from it, we will suffer. Yoga is an integration back to the totality. That is our yogic responsibility: to yoke, to join the sense of separation with the sense of the universal, and to have a tangible direct sense that we do not stop existing at the surface of our skin, that we extend upward and outward and in every direction. And that is what he is saying constantly.

Guruji emphasizes prayer and devotion to God. Why do you think he considers this to be so important?
I heard that Krishnamacharya, his guru, was asked, "What is the single most important aspect of yoga practice?" I might be simplifying this, and it's hearsay really, but he said of Patanjali, the yoga that we study, "*Ishvarapranidhana* [surrender to God] is the single most important aspect." I come back to this sense that there are techniques and approaches in this religious culture that allow you to surrender in a sequential way. So rather than some great catastrophe befalling you that forces you to surrender to the infinite power of life, that you have no control over, if you take Ishvara *deva*, a deity, a personification of infinity, then you can approach it in a physical emblem or representative, and talk to it and sing to it and offer it things and start to develop a relationship with it. It's a cliché, but God is love. It's impossible to know that until you start to love whatever idea you have of God that is comfortable, whether it's Jesus or Krishna.

For some people it's Shiva, Vishnu . . . and of course in India, they are colorful, they have personalities, they are easy to identify with, they have beautiful qualities and it is very, very easy to start to feel affection for them. Just in the same way that kids in America or Europe feel affection for Batman or Spider-Man, these characters have incredible qualities. When you start to familiarize yourself with the qualities, you look at the picture, you start to meditate on the qualities and familiarize yourself with the qualities of one particular deity—one that you already have a predisposition for—or maybe you can learn to love the Buddha and his teachings. The gods all become one.

Through daily offerings and daily practice you begin to share your life with this imagined personification of the unimaginable, and you approach it with humility every day, and you say, "I'm sorry, I need some help," or "I trust you to deliver me, I trust your decisions for me, I trust your infinite wisdom, I trust you because the universe functions and the fact that the universe functions is proof enough for me of your existence." The image you choose or that is chosen for you takes away a lot of the fear, because the gap is so big between little Nick and little Guy, who are trying to approach these big ancient huge concepts in an ancient language. They are like a vehicle to acclimatize you, to introduce you to something bigger than yourself and your own opinions and your own sense of preference. My experience is that it works. It facilitates the yogic process. It gives concepts that are intangible a way for the mind to chew them and meditate on them and become accustomed and familiar with them. I think Guruji grew up with that. Shankaracharya had nominated five deities for worship and Guruji inherited that practice and that approach to life. That was the *artha*, karma, and dharma: livelihood, the sensual life in the world, and dharma, upholding the tradition. I think that is the essence of the Indian tradition: responsibility. He's an orthodox Brahmin Hindu and so he took on board his responsibilities, his cultural, religious responsibilities, because they worked for his people, the Smarta Brahmins, for many generations. It's his job to preserve them and convey their effectiveness.

It's his duty within society to preserve that.
Yes.

He always says, "Pray, you should pray."
I really agree. It helped me a lot.

Guruji also says yoga is 99 percent practice, 1 percent theory. What's your understanding of the theory part?
Guruji says this is Patanjali yoga. It takes into account every facet of being human. And it's a teaching that allows you to have a sense of purpose. For me an interest in *The Yoga Sutras* came more quickly than the *Bhagavad Gita* or the *Upanishads*. I just generally allowed Indian spiritual prose and wisdom to soothe my spirit. Study became less of an academic pursuit and more of a kind of soothing my soul, for want of a better word. The practice somehow puts you in contact with a depth of silence that— maybe when you were busy rushing around not taking the time to

experience your breath, your body, your thoughts, the sensations in the moment—gives you a taste of depth, the depth of life. A natural interest in hearing about, and listening to, and reading bodies of wisdom that have gone before you that can somehow put words to this very existential, wordless experience that you have had in the practice. A natural hunger for spiritual study developed and I started to like meditating and having conversations with people about understanding God and meditation and what yoga was, and to have a certain sense of communion through the text that we can all look at and use as mirrors for our own experiences.

Boil it down, the theory part. In simple terms, what do you think that would be?
I'd go with Guruji's "All is God." He says, "You looking at wall. Not wall seeing, God seeing." Taking that leap of faith and seeing that the life around us is alive, and it's the livingness that is the lord, or the divinity. It's alive, it lives.

Do you see ashtanga *yoga as a spiritual practice?*
Yes.

It seems like you came into it looking for—
Health benefits.

But you acknowledge that some of the health benefits were mental. You made a jump from the mental to the spiritual.
I suppose that there were no health benefits without making the jump from the physical to the spiritual. But there are no guarantees, you are not in the position to make any guarantees, you can have the healthiest body imaginable and step out and a bus can run you over. If you get right with God, if you clean yourself up, if you behave as you wish others would treat you, you stand a greater chance of life treating you with kindness because you treat life with kindness, and this is very spiritual. Yoga teaches this practice, teaches you a depth of humility that I fail to see another practice teaching people.

Maybe I'm wrong, I didn't do *vipassana*, I didn't live in a cave for thirty months, but in the modern world, the way that people are going to their jobs and living their lives and going to buy their things, this practice seems to slot into a modern life and invite you to humble yourself. Humble people do not try to force life to behave in the way that they think it should. They accept life as it comes, they accept people as people come, and they accept the moment as the moment comes, and that makes for a special kind of quality of human being.

What would you say are the nonphysical aspects of the practice?
The sum of focusing on squeezing your *mula bandha*, gazing at the *drishti* and listening to the sound. Those three separate parts that seem to be separate elements becoming one element, one state. And that one state allows you to penetrate the moment with deeper awareness to almost the point when you feel like everything has slowed down into this timelessness. There are moments where you commence your practice with a very clear sense that it's you or me or your individual Self standing at the edge of your mat with your aches and pains, worries and preoccupations, but after fifteen, twenty minutes you are sweating and you are beginning, for periods of time, to lose yourself in it and there really is no one doing it. And there are moments when it really is as though you are observing the body performing the practice. You are not connected to it but the body's still doing it. I'm not saying that it's every time that I have that degree of distance from my body performing these sequences of movements and breath. But talk about witness culture, consciousness, there's a distance, a sense of observation that in the past I only experienced using drugs. [*Laughter*]

How important is the philosophy of Shankaracharya, Guruji's family guru?
For me that was big. I liked that a lot, it really resonated because it was so poetic. He sang, he was a poet. When I read what I read, when I understood what I understood, it felt to me that this sense "All is God" stems very specifically from the Smarta Brahmin Advaita view, and many of the texts say, ultimately, all the philosophies resolve themselves in Advaita.

I've read commentaries on *The Yoga Sutras* that say, effectively, the final step is when observer and observed are one and not separate, so Shiva and Shakti being Ardhanarishvara, contained within the one. They are the same organism, the same being, the same single being. So Shankaracharya was not, from my understanding, opposed to yogic practices, but emphasized that the purpose of yoga was to realize reality to be non-dual. I read one passage where he said the *nasagra*, the *drishti* at the tip of the nose, is everywhere you look. The one taste, the formless eternal brahman, is wherever you look. Yoga is constant meditation, is a permanent state of awareness that there is only one Lord, living this moment and every moment for everyone, one at a time. And the Lord is one, without a second—dissolve into that! This may give you a very different kind of life. And again I'm not a scholar, I'm just a baby [on the path of yoga].

How does Guruji integrate that into this system of philosophy which he is teaching?
Well, I think it's where he's leading everyone. I think he knows that there are sequences or prescriptions of practices or methods that can make the soil fertile for an appreciation of Shankaracharya's teaching, his non-dual teaching. And that a mind and a body that are disturbed are very unlikely to be enabled to engage in that in a meaningful way.

On one occasion, at the opening of an orphanage in Mysore, Guruji was the guest of honor and Swami Dayananda Saraswati, one of Shankaracharya's swamis—who I know Guruji's family loves and respects very much—translated Guruji's speech from Kannada into English. He said that the essence of Vedanta without yoga is useless, yoga without Vedanta is useless, they are mutually interrelated. So the knowledge that comes from yoga is non-dual awareness, and without non-dual awareness there is no yoga. Without yoga there can be no non-dual awareness. And Dayananda said we practice yoga for our lives, as separate bodies, as separate people, because we want to have good lives, lives that do good in the world: healthy lives, loving lives, caring lives—we do this while everything is one. The world is a beautiful place and deserves to be loved and respected. There is a big difference between a world that is at war and a world where people love and respect one another. We do yoga to understand the idea of duality, because if we don't understand the value of duality, we'll never understand the value of unity or oneness. And that was big. The two of them sat there beaming: this philosopher-teacher honoring Guruji's perspective and view, Guruji completely honoring and loving Dayananda's view, and the two being completely at one with one another with no contradiction whatsoever. It was wonderful, and I videoed it with my little camera and put it on my MySpace site, so it's there.

Patanjali seems to be presenting a dualist model of a human being by dividing our experiences into the material [prakriti] and the spiritual [purusa], but Guruji's favorite philosophy is Advaita Vedanta [non-dualist]. How do you see the relationship between these two systems of thought?

I think they are the same system of thought expressed in two different ways. Some people will be attracted to one of them and other people will be attracted to the other. I don't think there's any contradiction. It's like separating food from the flavor of the food when you taste it. The food is one. It has different qualities, it can be hot and sweet, it can be cold and bitter, there are different qualities within that food. Reality can be seen as that which changes *and* that which observes the change. The *purusha* is still, it never changes from when you were a baby, it's timeless, infinite, and ultimately formless and eternal. It watches through all of us, and everything that is perceived relies on the perceiving to exist. That which is perceived [nature] has no independent existence from the perceiver [soul]. Therefore, according to Advaita, that which is perceived and that which is perceiving are one because they cannot exist without one another.

At the point of kaivalya [liberation], the connection between the two is severed. Purusha continues to exist but prakriti no longer exists for purusha. They say the connection is beginningless but not endless.

How do you see this spiritual philosophy that Guruji is expounding fitting in modern Indian society? Do you think it's something that will survive and continue to be relevant?

He really has the Midas touch from the evidence that we have, if you observe the growth and the spread of *ashtanga* yoga, the way it's been managed, the way that he's brought it to people, or the way that it's grown of its own volition. Maybe it's not him, maybe it's the power of the practice itself that he inherited from Krishnamacharya and that Sharath has inherited from him. It's growing roots in Europe, Asia, and certainly seems to be growing deep roots especially in China and in Japan, and now there seem to be some teachers appearing in India, too. Because so many Indian professionals are living busy, stressful lives they will certainly benefit from the experience of this practice, just like the ambitious Westerners did. And in some ways, the Indians might embody it in another way because they are so much closer to the culture that spawned it. So they won't have to go through so many cultural filters or layers in order to re-connect with their own ancient wisdoms. It's going to be exciting; it's going to be interesting to see.

It's interesting, because you are suggesting, perhaps, exactly because of the cultural changes it becomes that much more important.
I am.

Because yoga was in decline for many years.
There are a lot more Indian students going to Mysore now.

Is there a special quality to Mysore and south India that makes it a support-ive context for studying yoga at K. Pattabhi Jois Ashtanga Yoga Institute?
I would say primarily it's a devotional context. This idea of acknowledg-ing and giving form to the idea of a higher power or the idea of an infi-nite, living, all-knowing being that does this [creates this reality]—they have this idea that the creator and creation are one. There is a living God here doing this and who needs to be worshipped and acknowledged and loved in the forms of these deities, so there are temples on every corner. They're all vegetarian, they are kind, they smile, they are not mean-spirited people. They are very welcoming. It's a sweet, sweet environ-ment that you arrive in, and if you've got impurities [in your system], they are purged out of you by the simple fact that the people in your environ-ment are used to behaving in such loving ways as part of their cultural, normal, daily duties. They respect their elders, they respect the children, the old people are wise ancestors, animals are sacred, the earth is the mother. Those aren't weird hippie ideas, those are the normal ideas. Those are the ideas that have functioned as the prevalent social concept for thousands of years. And there are also areas of the society that are changing. They are also interested in money and all sorts of modern things. But underlying all that there is an intimacy with paying your dues, acknowledging your maker, and there's a temple on every corner, and they are cool places, they are better than a pub, having a pint of beer. They are full of love and it's brilliant if you thought that religion was stuffy nonsense or brainwashing. Go to a festival, feel the feeling, and then come back and tell me it's for simpletons. Because these people are geniuses—they understand the purpose of human existence, which is to

love God, and they taught me that, Guruji taught me that, this practice taught me that. *Surya namaskara*, it's a physical prayer, whether you like it or not.

What is the ultimate aim of yoga according to Guruji?
According to Guruji, union. On many different levels there are many different purposes of yoga. I think you have to go to the highest one, which is to know God, because that encompasses all the others. Actually, I come back to the lecture that Dayananda and Guruji gave, where Dayananda was translating Guruji. Dayananda [translating Guruji] said, "We don't know who we are and we must understand; this is why we are here. It's not an option, we have to know."

Do you think it's obtainable?
When Guruji was asked in conference, "Sixth series—enlightenment possible?" "Yes, yes, enlightenment possible." "Guruji, fifth series—enlightenment possible?" "Yes, yes, enlightenment possible." "Fourth series, third series, second series, primary—enlightenment possible?" "Primary series, possible." And I think in *Yoga Mala* it says that knowledge is given by the grace of Brahma, is given by the grace of God. So whether an individual can do anything to achieve a personal result or not is a great yogic debate. I wouldn't dream of trying to answer that. What I do know is that yoga makes the situation sufficiently healthy and open for that knowledge to come if it's destined to. But whether you can control it? I don't think so. But that doesn't make practicing any less valuable.

Do you think our cultural conditioning creates a particularly large obstacle to obtaining that, and is there something we need to give up in order to achieve it?
Giving up the fruit of your actions. Understanding that it's the one that acts through all of us. The less you claim personal authorship for your actions, the more your actions seem to be loving and good. But all of us have a sense of personal authorship, and even when we think we don't, we probably do in a residual sense. I think it allows life to become more peaceful, and therefore knowledge of higher ideas and how to live a good life come more naturally than when you are trying to force yourself into it, because you have an idea of what a nice person should be doing. Also, the moment has a lot of wisdom, and I think if you tune in to the mo-

ment, and *ashtanga* yoga practice helps you do that, it will start happening more and more effortlessly, without a sense that you have to push your way into it, or be a good person. You can just let it happen rather than make it happen.

What I want to say, I suppose, is that I'm incredibly grateful to Guruji, Sharath, and Saraswathi for sharing this with people, with me, because I probably could have quite ended my life [without it]. Some of their senior teachers, the people I've studied with—Eddie [Stern] and Hamish [Hendry] come to mind—they are the ones who showed me how to maintain and sustain a practice with a certain attitude and shared some pearls of wisdom at specific moments that continue to flower in my mind. That it is ultimately about being a kinder, nicer, loving person, and that should be the focus in this practice. It's not about being better than anybody else. And if you've forgotten that, please remind yourself of it. Without that, this practice has no heart, so it needs to be performed with great gratitude, great devotion, and great love and respect for the people around you, the best that you can. We are all frail, we are all human, we are all limited, and we make mistakes. But every time you fall off the horse, get back on with humility and love. Really, keep doing that and you can't go far wrong, I think.

Penarth, 2008

Acknowledgments

The journey that has resulted in this book has been circuitous. What began as a documentary became a book instead, and making the book spurred back to life the documentary project, which had come to a standstill due to the twists and turns life sometimes brings.

To arrive where we are now has required the help of many people. First and foremost, thanks must be given to Guruji, his children Manju and Saraswathi, his grandchildren Shammie and Sharath, and his son-in-law, Mahesh. They arranged interviews, advised on whom to include, and gave their blessings and encouragement.

This project would not have come about without Lori Brungard, who was instrumental in most aspects of the earlier interviews, including shaping the questions, the recording, the financing, and the logistics.

Financial support came from Donald and Kathleen Brungard, who gave a generous donation to fund the early interviews, and from Daniel Loeb, an early champion of this project. Alan and Patricia Abramson generously gave a donation that helped secure our last interviews.

During the filming, our director of photography was Jefferson Spady, the sound recordists were Irin Strauss and Paul Zehrer, our gaffer was Paul Breen, and cameras were operated by Pilar Settlemeir and Zini Lardieri.

The material that we needed to transcribe was voluminous. For this, we had an intrepid team: Sylvia Chivaratanond, Anthony Enriquez, Pony Gentile, Deborah Harada, Nathalie Leiseing, Matana Roberts, and Jamie Waugh. Thanks are also due to Luc Georges for translating Brigitte Deroses; Dr. Anil Kumar, for N. V. Anantha Ramaiah; and Sunaad Raghuraam, for T. S. Krishnamurthi.

Heidi Lender assisted in the early stages of editing, and Stephanie

Gilgoff and Adina Konits helped to obtain the interviews with Heather Troud and Brad Ramsey. Malcolm Neo performed all the image scanning of archival photos of Guruji, including the cover photo—which was then turned into a work of art by Charlotte Strick.

Special thanks to Jeff Seroy of Farrar, Straus and Giroux, whose loving care brought it all together, and to Jocelyne and Lili Stern and Ruby and Josh Donahaye for their endless support, encouragement, and patience.

Lastly, we thank with immense gratitude the contributors of these interviews who opened their lives and hearts to us in order to recount their memories of the brilliant and loving man whom we all knew as Guruji: N. V. Anantha Ramaiah, T. S. Krishnamurthi, S. L. Bhyrappa, Norman Allen, Nancy Gilgoff, David Williams, Brad Ramsey, David Swenson, Tim Miller, Chuck Miller, Ricky Heiman, Mark and Joanne Darby, Annie Pace, Heather Troud, Richard Freeman, Tomas Zorzo, Graeme Northfield, Brigitte Deroses, Peter Sanson, Rolf Naujokat, Dena Kingsberg, Peter Greve, John Scott, Lino Miele, Joseph Dunham, and Nick Evans.